NeUroGastroenterology

With compliments

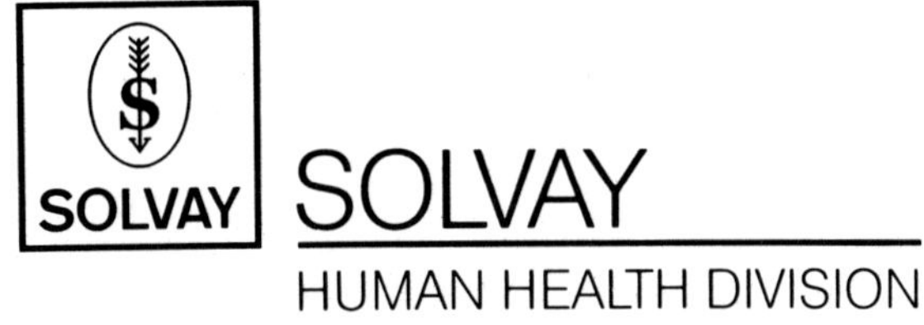

NeUroGastroenterology

Edited by
E. Corazziari

Walter de Gruyter
Berlin · New York 1996

Editor

Dr. E. Corazziari

Cattedra di Gastroenterologia I
Clinica Medica II
Universita „La Sapienza"
Policlinico Umberto I
V.le del Policlinico
00161 Roma
Italy

Die Deutsche Bibliothek — CIP-Einheitsaufnahme

NeUroGastroenterology / ed. by E. Corazziari. — Berlin ; New
York : de Gruyter, 1996
ISBN 3-11-015343-2
NE: Corazziari, Enrico [Hrsg.]

To my father

First-mentioned authors

Dr. E. Alcini
Università Cattolica de Sacro Cuore
Facoltà di Medicina e Chirurgia
„Agostino Gemelli"
Cattedra di Urologia
Largo Agostino Gemelli 8
I-00168 Roma

Dr. D. F. Altomare
Istituto di Clinica Chirurgicà
Università degli Studi di Bari
Piazza Giulio Cesare 11
I-70124 Bari

Dr. W. Artibani
Cattedra di Urologia
Università di Modena
Dipartimento di Chirurgia
Via de Pozzo 71
I-41100 Modena

Dr. F. Azpiroz
Digestive System Research Unit
Hospital General Vall d'Hebron
E-08035 Barcelona

Dr. D. Badiali
Cattedra di Gastroenterologia 1
Clinica Medica II
Policlinico Umberto I
Viale de Policlinico
I-00161 Roma

Dr. L. Buéno
Department of Pharmacology, INRA
180 Chemin de Tournefeuille
B. P. 3
F-31931 Toulouse Cedex

Dr. M. Camilleri
Mayo Clinic/Mayo Medical School
Gastroenterology Research Unit
200 First Street S. W.
Rochester MN 55905
USA

Dr. R. Caprilli
Cattedra di Gastroenterologia
Dipartimento di Medicina Interna
e Sanità Pubblica
Università de L'Aquila
Via S. Sisto 22 E
I-67100 L'Aquila

Dr. A. Carbone
Via B. Bardanzellu 44
I-00155 Roma

Dr. R. E. Clouse
Division of Gastroenterology
Department of Internal Medicine/
School of Medicine
Washington University in St. Louis
Children's Annex, Suite 417
One Barnes Hospital Plaza
St. Louis MO 63110
USA

Dr. D. De Grandis
Azienda Ospedaliera − Arcispedale S. Anna
Divisione Neurologica
C.so Giovecca 203
I-44100 Ferrara

Dr. M. Delvaux
Gastroenterology Unit
CHU Rangueil
F-31054 Toulouse

Dr. C. Di Lorenzo
Department of Pediatric Gastroenterology
Children's Hospital of Pittsburgh
3705 Fifth Avenue
Pittsburgh PA 15213
USA

Dr. D. A. Drossman
Digestive Diseases and Nutrition
Schol of Medicine/Department of Medicine
CB# 7080
Room 420 Burnett Womack Building
The University of North Carolina at Chapel
Hill
Chapel Hill NC 27599−7080
USA

Dr. G. A. Fava
Dipartimento di Psicologia
Università di Bologna
Viale Berti Pichat
I-40127 Bologna

Dr. C. J. Fowler
The National Hospital for Neurology and
Neurosurgery
Department of Uro-Neurology
Queen Square
GB-London WC1N 3BG

Dr. E. Gussoni
Kunkel Laboratory
Genetics Division
300 Longwood Avenue
Boston MA 02115
USA

Dr. R. Jian
Service de Gastroentérologie
Hôpital Saint-Louis
1, Avenue Claude Vellefaux
F-75010 Paris

Dr. S. Lyonnet
Laboratoire de Génétique et Unité de Re-
cherches sur les Handicaps Génétiques de l'En-
fant
Inserm − Hôpital des Enfants Malades
Tour Technique Lavoisier (2ième étage)
149 Rue de Sèvres
F-75743 Paris

Dr. C. D. Marsden
University Department of Clinical Neurology
Institute of Neurology
Queen Square
GB-London WC1N 3BG

Dr. C. J. Mathias
The National Hospital for Neurology and
Neurosurgery
Queen Square
GB-LondonWC1N 3BG

Dr. E. A. Mayer
Building 115, Room 116
Cure/Gastroenteric Biology Center
West Los Angeles
VA Medical Center
Los Angeles CA 90073
USA

Dr. P. J. Milla
Institute of Child Health
University of London
Hospital for Sick Children
30, Guildford Street
GB-London WC1N 1EH

Dr. H. Mönnikes
Medizinisches Zentrum für Innere Medizin
Philipps Universität
Baldinger Straße
D-35033 Marburg

Dr. R. J. Opsomer
Cliniques Saint-Luc
Division of Urology
Avenue Hippocrate 10
B-1200 Bruxelles

Dr. F. Pesce
Via Livorno 85
I-00162 Roma

Dr. R. F. Pfeiffer
Department of Neurology
University of Tennessee
411 Monroe Avenue
415 Link Building
Memphis TN 38163−4901
USA

Dr. E. M. M. Quigley
Department of Internal Medicine
Section of Gastroenterology and Hepatology
University of Nebraska Medical Center
600 South 42nd Street
Omaha NE 68198−2000
USA

Dr. R. Shaker
GI Division
Medical College of Wisconsin
Zablocki VA Medical Center
5000 West National Avenue
Milwaukee WI 53295
USA

Dr. A. Staiano
Dipartimento di Pediatria
Università „Federico II“
Via S. Pansini 5
I-80131 Napoli

Dr. F. Stocchi
Dipartimento di Scienze Neurologiche
Università „La Sapienza“
Viale dell'Università 30
I-00185 Roma

Dr. Ph. F. V. Van Kerrebroeck
University Hospital Nijmegen
Department of Urology
Geert Grooteplein 16
P. O. Box 9101
NL-6500 HB Nijmegen

Dr. J. Weber
Centre Hospitalier Universitaire de Rouen
Physiologie Digestive et Urinaire
Hopital Charles Nicolie
Pavillon Deroque 1er étage
1, Rue de Germont
F-76031 Rouen Cedex

Dr. W. E. Whitehead
Division of Digestive Diseases
CB# 7080, Room 326
Burnett Womack Building
The University of North Carolina
at Chapel Hill
Chapel Hill NC 27599−7080
USA

Contents

Preface

It is well-known that viscera are largely regulated by the Autonomic Nervous System (ANS) under the control of the Central Nervous System (CNS) which can profoundly affect their functions; the observations by Pavlov, where a trained dog can be conditioned to secrete gastric juice at the sound of a bell, or those by Oddi, Beamount and Almy, where anger, an embarrassing and/or aggressive dialogue modify gastric and colonic blood flow and secretion, are the experimental evidence of the everyday clinical experience of how much environmental factors can affect visceral functions via the CNS. It is not surprising, therefore, that CNS structural alterations, and relevant environmental and/or psychological stimuli, can lead to visceral alterations. Nonetheless, although constipation and other bowel dysfunctions are inevitable, and often severely invalidating, sequelae of spinal cord lesions, in their practice neurologists will direct their therapeutical efforts toward the CNS/somatic interactions, often overlooking the visceral disability. Similarly, gastrointestinal disturbances are frequently associated with psychological and/or environmental conditions and yet many psychiatrists will give little attention to the bowel dysfunction, directing their therapy towards the mind and mind/environmental interactions; gastroenterologists, and general practitioners, on the other hand, will focus their therapy on GI dysfunctions and give little attention to the psychological/environmental interactions. This situation is a consequence of the progressive segregation of medical disciplines, and the need continuously to improve knowledge, diagnosis and therapy of different organs inevitably leads to the use of technologies which, needing highly specialized personnel, further contribute to the segregation of patients in separate diagnostic-therapeutic areas.

This lack of interdisciplinary interaction becomes even more evident when considering those patients who, due to their age, need pediatric or geriatric counseling, or need the expertise of other specialists such as surgeons, gynecologists or oncologists for intercurrent disease. However, irrespective of the different specialistic approaches, visceral disturbances related to nervous structural alterations and/or psychosocial factors are far from being satisfactorily managed and, with their prevalence increasing, there is a growing need for physicians and other health staff to be able properly to diagnose and treat visceral disturbances in patients with neurological abnormalities and functional disorders. This demand cannot at present be met due to (a) the limited knowledge of the interactions between the nervous system and the visceral functions; (b) the lack of epidemiological data on the prevalence, severity and impact on quality of life of visceral disturbances in the various alterations of the nervous system;

(c) inadequate integration among specialists from the various disciplines dealing with these patients.

In the attempt to at least start a process of integration among some of the disciplines which share a common area of interest, the "Associazione per la NeUroGastroenterologia e la Motilità Gastrointestinale (ANEMGI)" has promoted an International Symposium on NeUroGastroenterology in Rome, November 9-11, 1995 to discuss five topics which, although they cannot possibly cover the entire field, identify five main areas of human suffering where knowledge integrated from several competences is seen to be greatly needed. The five topics include: functional visceral disorders; visceral disorders of the degenerative nervous diseases; visceral dysfunctions in patients with spinal cord lesions; the congenital nervous and neuromuscular defects affecting children; and the gut-bladder relationships in othotopic bladder and urinary diversions. The researchers who reported on their data and experiences at the Symposium are the contributing authors to this volume. The contents have been organized along two major guidelines; the first to converge on any single topic information derived from several competences so as to offer a comprehensive collection of concepts and data which are either integrated or can be interrelated by the reader; the second to convey and reorganize the above information in such a way that they can be used in the clinical approach and management of the patients.

Functional visceral disorders are among the most prevalent dysfunctions affecting the population at large and, besides the individual suffering involved, they have a tremendous impact on the social and health systems. Nonetheless, very little is known about their pathophysiological mechanisms, and, as a matter of fact, some of their clinical features such as the chronicity, the relapse/remission sequences alternating, and even opposite, patterns of defecation, the degree of severity of the symptoms have not yet satisfactorily been clarified. The first part of this book deals with these disorders which are viewed as the consequence of an altered relationship between visceral motor activity and sensitivity, on the one hand, and psycho/nervous regulation on the other.

The links between the CNS and the viscera are numerous and new evidence is presented to support the interpretation that both CNS and visceral alterations are variably operating and interacting in the origin and maintenance of the functional visceral disorders. Thus, external, environmental factors and, internal, psychological factors and visceral diseases may equally alter brain areas concerned with adaptive response which, in their turn, can affect visceral function as well as other areas of the body. Within this interpretation several issues are newly raised and need to be clarified. Is the disturbance of the brain area the consequence of the deranged activation of a normal nervous loop, of the memory of an adaptive response, or the permanent modification of the neurons in early life? Is visceral hypersensitivity the result of the sensitization of primary visceral attempts or of the central, spinal, neurons? To what degree are the clinical manifestations of functional visceral disorders the expression of the psychosocial status and of the illness behavior? Particular emphasis to the interpretation of pain in functional visceral disorders is given to the presence of an altered visceral perception and/or altered afferent input. Several chapters in fact deal with this issue and a part of the book is specifically devoted to the methods used to assess visceral sensitivity and to the interpretation of these techniques. Pharmacological research has also moved to investigate compounds which, by modifying the visceral afferents, can be employed therapeutically to regulate nociception as well as the triggering thresholds of secretory and motor reflexes. On the basis of the increasing knowledge of the neurotransmitters involved in the regulatory mechanisms distributed along the pathway from CNS, ANS and viscera, several substances have been identified which may influence visceral afferents by acting at one or more levels, peripheral, spinal and supraspinal, along the brain-viscera axis. Likewise, the psychotherapeutical approach may be effective at the level of the higher neuronal levels, acting on the control of adaptive responses and illness behavior. Thus, since excitability of the afferent neurons can be enhanced by the temporal summation of stimuli from the viscera or, alternatively by the facilitatory descending thalamo-spinal pathway, the new therapeutical perspectives of functional gastrointestinal disorders presented in this book refer to substances acting at the different levels of the afferent nervous system and/or to the cognitive-behavioral therapeutical approaches. The extraordinary rapid development in the physiopharmacology of the viscera, testified by several contributions, may be regarded as anticipatory of an era when a proper diagnostic work-up will enable patients to be classified with functional gastrointestinal disorders according to the main neuroregulatory alterations and to be treated by acting specifically on one or more of the identified altered mechanisms with pharmacological and/or psychological therapies.

In neonatal and pediatric age neuronal immaturity and congenital alterations of the neuromuscular apparatus can manifest with visceral dysfunctions. In addition, in the early years of life environmental and psychological factors can more easily influence the organization of the newly forming nervous loop; imprint the memory of adaptive response and even induce permanent modification of the neurons; all the above conditions may profoundly affect the visceral functions and lead to functional disorders in childhood and adulthood.

Contributions to this book present proper diagnostic, possibly non-invasive, strategies which should be employed to investigate visceral dysfunctions presenting immediately after birth and in the early years of life, as they can be the expression of neuronal immaturity, structural congenital neuromuscular alterations or functional disorders. Investigations of the neuromuscular structure and function during embryological development and childhood appear to offer relevant information for understanding congenital disorders affecting the smooth muscle and the enteric nervous system as well as the functional visceral disorders. Among these studies, of interest is the demonstration that Hirschsprung's disease (HSCR) can be the expression of a congenital malformation regarded as a multigenic neurocristopathy. Such data acquisition on the complex genetic etiology of HSCR opened the way to several lines of research: firstly, to have identified a reference model to differentiate polygenic and genetically heterogenous diseases when investigating other multifactorial congenital malformations; secondly, to have increased our knowledge of the embryologic development and migration of the neural crest enteric neurons; thirdly, the RET gene alteration shared by HSCR and the inherited cancer MEN syndrome is a key condition for developing studies on the relationship between cell development and proliferation.

Increasing life expectancy and easier access to improved social health care systems are accompanied by an increasing prevalence of neurological diseases due to congenital, degenerative and traumatic causes. Consequently in clinical practice patients with common neurological diseases such as Parkinson's, multiple sclerosis, cerebrovascular accidents and diabetic automatic neuropathy require proper diagnosis and treatment of the frequently accompanying visceral dysfunctions. Recently developed neurodiagnostic tests have greatly enhanced our knowledge of the structure and function of the CNS but have so far provided very little information on the CNS areas devoted to regulating visceral functions. Also, the diagnostic tests of the ANS which investigate the parasympathetic and the sympathetic systems offer general information on the regulatory mechanisms of the cardiovascular and thermoregulatory functions but very little on the neural control of the gastrointestinal and urinary tract. The development of autonomic tests which could specifically and selectively assess the regulatory mechanisms of the parasympathetic and sympathetic systems at the level of the viscera is thus envisaged as a fundamental step forward in the understanding and management of visceral dysfunctions in patients with structural alterations of the CNS and ANS and even in patients with functional visceral disorders. Evidence is in fact presented that several symptoms and transit dysfunctions referred by patients with functional visceral disorders may be the manifestation of permanent or transient alterations of the ANS, involving either the sympathetic or the parasympathetic system. Knowledge of which part of the ANS is altered appears to be useful in therapeutical planning since preliminary observations would indicate that patients with similar manifestations of functional disorders but with alteration of one of the two ANS regulatory systems responded differently to pharmacological treatment. For the pivotal role of the ANS in the regulation of the visceral functions several contributions of this book deal directly with, or refer indirectly to, this issue, such as the adaptive response and alterations of the ANS in the presence of neuro-degenerative diseases; a comprehensive review of the automatic tests; a synthetic guideline for the diagnostic work-up of the ANS function; the viscero-visceral ANS-mediated effect in response to gastrointestinal and urinary stimuli.

A section of the book is devoted to gastrointestinal and urinary pathophysiology after spinal cord lesions offering relevant information on the role played by the brain centres on the ANS and the visceral function. In clinical practice these basic acquisitions can be usefully employed to guide planning the rehabilitative and pharmacological treatment of the disabling urinary and colorectoanal dysfunctions when they are properly integrated with a diagnostic assessment which should be specifically addressed to evaluate the degree and the severity of the visceral dysfunction in the individual patient.

The lower gastrointestinal and urinary tracts share the same innervation and several, but not all, neuromuscular mechanisms of continence and evacuation. Whenever possible, the physiological and pathophysiological aspects of the neuromuscular function of the lower gastrointestinal and urinary tracts have been presented in close sequence so as to facilitate the exchange of information concerning the two related areas. Contributions by neurologists, urologists and gastroenterologists attempt to enhance an integrated view of the neurological control of the pelvic, visceral and striated, muscles. Another area where interdisciplinary competence between urologists and gastroenterologists should be further integrated is the reconstructive surgery of the bladder with gastrointestinal segments. The use of segments of stomach, colon, and ileum to augment or to replace the bladder has in fact created a unique model which offers comparative information on the intrinsic neuromuscular, absorbitive and secretory regulating functions of the different gastrointestinal tracts. In addition the increasing knowledge of gastrointestinal physiology acquired through this model can be, in its turn, advantageously used by surgeons to improve the reservoir functions of the gastrointestinal tract and the orthotopic bladders.

The ultimate goal of this book is to attempt to reconstitute, through interdisciplinary research and cultural advancement, the unity of the patients, now split up into as many specialties as he/she suffers organ alterations. Although largely and inevitably incomplete, this book on NeUroGastroenterology can be regarded as a new approach to bridge the gap between research and patient care by transferring scientific advances from different competences and disciplines to those entrusted with clinical duties, thus implementing a holistic approach.

Enrico Corazziari

Brain-gut mechanisms of visceral motor activity

L. Buéno

Introduction

The complex relationships between the brain and the gut involve both neural and humoral components. Vagal and splanchnic afferent nerves are involved informing the brain of physiological and pathological events that occur at the periphery. Such information may activate brain structures able to influence gut motility.

The characterization in brain structures of a large number of peptides known to influence gastrointestinal motility has provided new impetus for the evaluation of their role at cerebral and spinal levels in the control of gut motility. The first evidence that a hypothalamic factor may affect gastrointestinal motility by acting primarily on the central nervous system (CNS) was given by Smith et al. [46] (1977) who showed that thyrotropin-releasing-hormone (TRH) administered by ICV route stimulates colonic motility in the anaesthetized rabbit. Furthermore the use of microcannulas directed into nuclei and microiontophoretic deposit of substances has largely contributed to this improvement of our knowledge. We review herein the role of brain structures and neurotransmitters in the course of gut motility not only in physiological conditions but also in experimentally induced pathological states as well as in the modulation of intestino-intestinal inhibitory reflexes.

Gut motor profiles and digestive status

Brain contains highly specific binding sites for many peptides located in areas involved in the control of gut motility. A large number of these peptides have been found to influence gastric emptying and intestinal transit when injected centrally but the physiological relevance of these results has not been confirmed as well as the pathways involved.

Several peptides including bombesin, calcitonin, calcitonin gene-related-peptide (CGRP), cholecystokinin (CCK), neuropeptide Y (NPY), neurotensin, oxytocin, somatostatin, substance P, opioid peptides and corticotropin-releasing-hormone (CRH) influence gastrointestinal transit and the patterns of gastrointestinal motor activity when injected centrally but little information concerning the mechanisms and the sites of action is, at present, available.

The neurohumoral mechanisms involved in the effects of these peptides are different. While the inhibition of gastric emptying elicited by ICV administration of bombesin is reversed by vagotomy [39], that of calcitonin is abolished by ganglionic blockade but not by vagotomy, hypophysectomy, adrenalectomy or by sympathetic blockade [34]. In contrast the effects of CGRP are abolished after adrenalectomy, while bombesin requires an intact pituitary adrenal axis [20]. Slowing of intestinal transit induced by central administration of neurotensin or CGRP is suppressed after vagotomy [39] and the centrally-mediated intestinal motor effects of neurotensin are blocked by antidopaminergic substances acting on D_2 receptor subtype [15].

Finally, the lateral and medial hypothalamus and limbic system are proposed to be the sites of action of TRH for the acceleration of intestinal transit while the periaqueductal grey matter may be responsible for the antitransit effects of neurotensin as for enkephalins. Most of these effects have been shown to be vagally mediated but the nature of the vagal fibres involved remains to be determined.

Hypothalamic CCK and gut motor adaptation

Among the peptides released after feeding CCK_8 induces a "fed-like" pattern when injected centrally. The highest level of binding sites being found in the ventromedial hypothalamic nucleus. Exogenous CCK_8 introduced into the cerebrospinal fluid could reach CCK_8 terminals in the hypothalamic area and act at these sites to affect not only intestinal but also colonic motility [5, 37]. However, CCK_8 applied iontophoretically stimulates neurons of the dorsal vagal nucleus which influence gastrointestinal motility and microinfused into the VMH in rats, CCK_8 disrupts the MMC pattern and stimulates colonic activity while the same amount injected into the LHA is not active [37]. Furthermore, the CCK_A receptor antagonist L364,718 injected bilaterally prior to feeding into the VMH, consistently reduces the duration of the "fed pattern" and suppresses feeding-induced colonic hyperkinesia confirming that CCK_8 is involved at hypothalamic (VMH) level in maintaining the postprandial duodenal motor pattern but also the colonic motor response to the meal [36]. The origin of active CCK_8 is not clear, since CCK_8 released into the blood stream after feeding is supposed not to cross the blood−brain barrier. It is also known that CCK_8 from nerve terminals is released at hypothalamic level after a meal. It is possible, however, that feeding may induce a late CCK_8 release in the CNS. The fact that a CCK_A antagonist injected bilaterally into the VMH prior to feeding abolishes the colonic motor response to feeding strongly supports the hypothesis that CCK_8 is involved as the major CNS component in the adaptation of colonic motility to the fed state by acting through CCK_A receptor subtype in colonic motility. (Fig. 1)

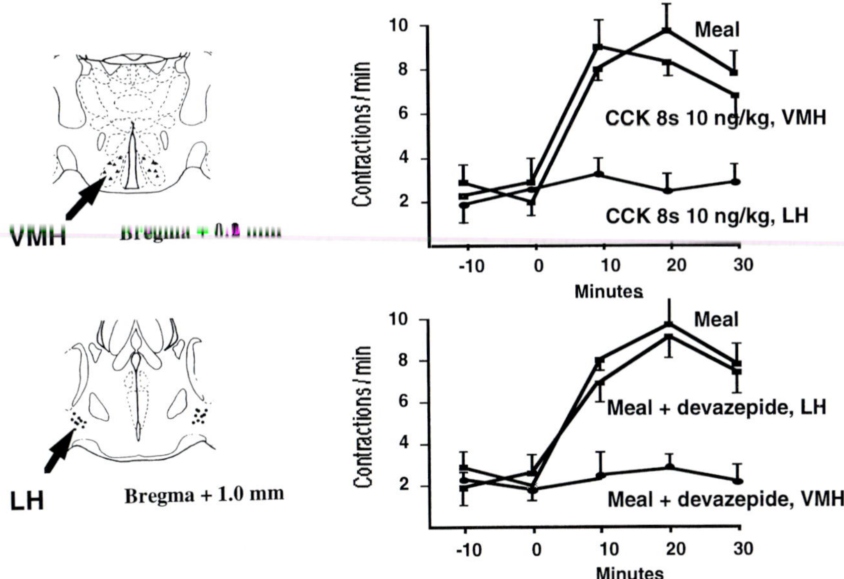

Fig. 1: Upper panel: comparative influence of CCK$_8$ injected into the ventromedian (VMH) or lateral (LH) hypothalamus on the frequency of colonic contractions compared to meal in awake rats.
Lower panel: influence of previous treatment with devazepide (10 µg/kg) injected bilaterally into the VMH or LH on meal stimulated colonic contractions.

Stress and upstream inhibitory reflexes

The role of the brain in the genesis of stress-induced gastrointestinal and colonic motor alterations has been extensively reviewed [10]. The evidence that the CNS release of CRF is directly involved in the initiation of the digestive motor disturbances induced by different stressors was first obtained in rats [51, 35] and in mice [6].

In this last species, pretreatment with ICV administration of antiserum against rat CRF, as well as α-helical-CRF$_{9-41}$ considered to be a CRF antagonist is able to prevent the increase in gastric emptying of a milk meal induced by acoustic and cold stress at doses that block the effects produced by ICV administration of CRF [6].

This result was confirmed in rats on which cerebroventricular administration of α-helical CRF$_{9-41}$, but not of the CRF fragment CRF$_{1-20}$, prevents the gastrointestinal secretory and motor (transit) responses elicited by partial body restraint. Moreover α-helical CRF$_{9-41}$ prevents the abdominal surgery-induced inhibition of gastric emptying [48].

4   L. Buéno

Upper gut
A cascade of hormonal releases and subsequent activation of the autonomic nervous system is associated with the CNS release of CRF such as peripheral adrenergic activation, and release of β-endorphin, release of vasopressin or activation of central cholinergic pathways.

In rats, opioid peptides and more particularly κ-agonists such as dynorphin, act through specific receptors to inhibit CRF release from the hypothalamus. In dogs, intracerebroventricular administration of the selective non peptide κ-opioid agonists, U50488 and ethylketocyclazocine (EKC), blocks acoustic stress-induced gastric hypomotility and hypercortisolemia [24]. These effects, as those of benzodiazepines, are linked to an inhibition of central CRF release rather than a direct action on the pituitary or adrenal glands.

It is important to note that benzodiazepines, GABAergic substances, or κ-opiate agonists also block the autonomic, endocrine and behavioral responses to CRF, that are considered to be an adaptive bodily reaction to stressful situations.

Lower gut
Several substances block both emotional stress-induced increase in colonic motility and CRF-induced colonic hyperkinesia, indicating that they act on the CRF-mediating pathway rather than on the central release of CRF in response to stress.

In rats, emotional stress (ES) produced by conditioned fear to receive electric footshocks, increases dopamine turnover in the mesoprefrontal neurons arising from the ventral tegmental area (A10). Emotional stress also increases colonic motility and central injection of a dopamine D_1 antagonist (SCH 23-390) blocks the emotional stress-induced colonic motor change but dopamine D_2 antagonist (sulpiride) is inactive at the same dosage [8]; when given intraperitoneally, a 10 times higher dose of SCH 23-390 is required to produce the same blocking effect, which suggests that dopamine is involved at CNS level in colonic response to stress.

Vasopressin potentiates the CRF-induced ACTH release [19] and in our model of emotional stress-induced colonic hyperkinesia, a vasopressin (AVP) antagonist injected intracerebroventricularly blocks the emotional stress- and CRF-induced increase in colonic motility in rats. Since vasopressin injected centrally also stimulates colonic motility, it is suggested that release of vasopressin in the central nervous system in response to stressful stimuli is responsible for the colonic motor disturbances [7]. These results point to the following pathway: stress activates the central release of CRF, which activates the central dopaminergic pathway that then activates the vasopressinergic system which stimulates the colonic motility from the peripheral release of vasopressin (Fig. 2).

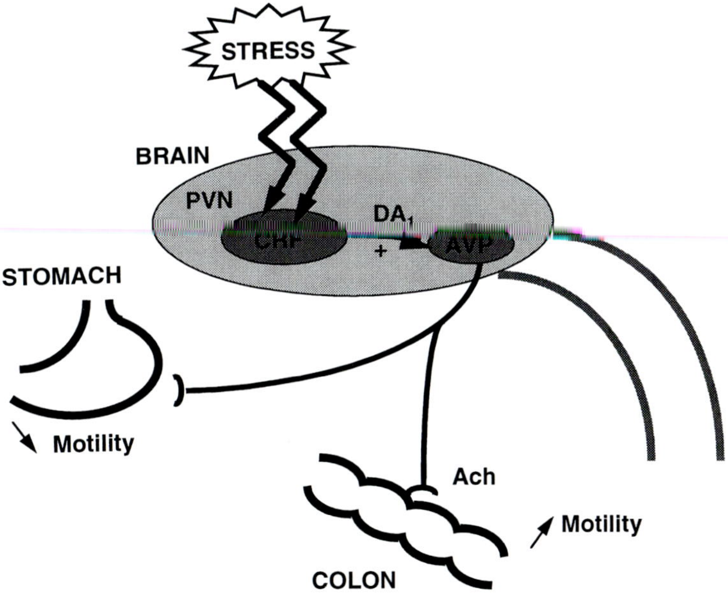

Fig. 2: *Respective role of brain CRF and vasopressin in emotional stress-induced digestive motor disturbances in rats.*

Neuropeptide Y and sigma ligands, such as d-NANM or (IGMESINE) [43], when centrally administered block both stress- and CFR-induced colonic hyperkinesia in rats [26, 29]. Some effects of sigma agonists and $5HT_{1A}$ agonists are linked to the CNS release of CCK and we found that the "visceral" anxiolytic effects of these compounds are blocked by CCK antagonists selective for CCK_A receptor subtype [25]. Moreover CCK_A agonists are also able to block the effects of emotional stress on colonic motility by reducing the activation of central dopaminergic pathways in limbic structures where they are interfering [31].

Finally, these results lead to the conclusion that two kinds of substances can modulate the CRF-induced changes in gastrointestinal motility:

- the first type acts directly at the receptor level; these are substances such as α-helical CRF_{9-41}, dopamine D_1 antagonists, vasopressin antagonists that interfere with CRF, dopaminergic and vasopressin receptors, to block the stress- and CRF-induced gastrointestinal motor disturbances.
- the second type of substances act on pathways that modulate the release of CRF and the mediating pathways through which it stimulates colonic motility. Substances such as NPY act centrally to activate the release of CCK that in turn modulates the dopaminergic system.

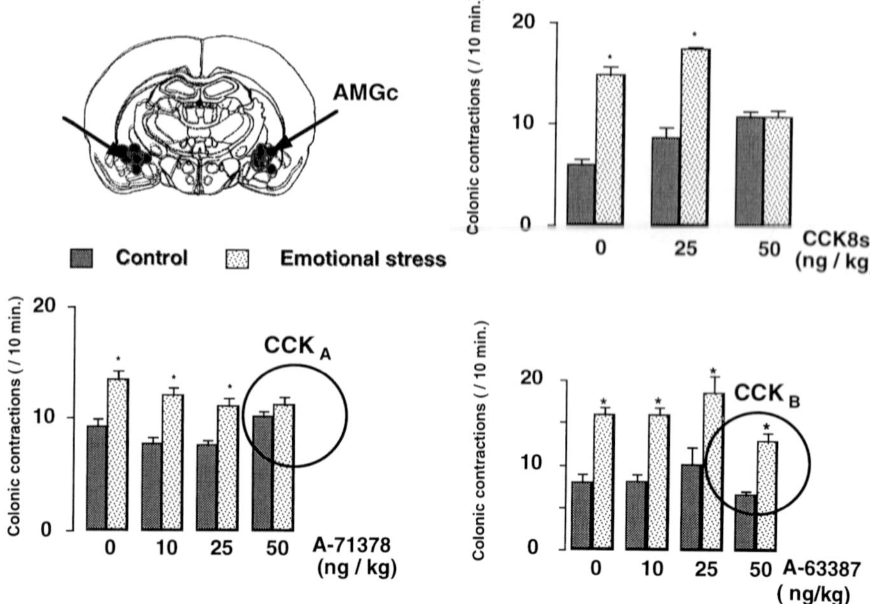

Fig. 3: *Modulation of emotional stress-induced colonic motor stimulation by CCK injected into the central amygdala (AMG$_C$) in conscious rats (upper panel). Comparative influence with selective CCK$_A$ (A-71368) and CCK$_B$ (A-63387) agonists (lower panel) (mean ± SD, n = 8).*

In this issue, the amygdala projects to both the hypothalamus mainly the VMH and to the NTS and appears to be one major modulatory site of hypothalamo-mediated CRF activation of DVC. Consistently CCK agonists such as A 71378 acting mainly on CCK$_A$ receptor subtype microinfused into the central amygdala is able to suppress stress-induced activation of colonic motility while CCK$_B$ agonists such as A 63387, is unable to reproduce such effects [21]. Furthermore destruction of the amygdala by Ibotenic acid suppresses the "visceral" anti-stress effects of CCK$_{8s}$ injected into the central amygdala (Fig. 3).

Intestino-intestinal inhibitory reflex

Numerous studies have shown that afferent fibers from abdominal vagus and splanchnic nerves participate to entero-gastric or recto-colonic inhibitory reflexes induced by local distension. In dogs the afferent pathway involved a nonadrenergic noncholinergic mechanism and in the ferret this inhibitory reflex is mediated by adrenergic pathways [1] and also the vagus [13]. Recently it has been shown that this long reflex which involves brain structures, as evidenced by C-Fos, C-Jun and Krox-24 expressions [17, 4] may be modulated by both

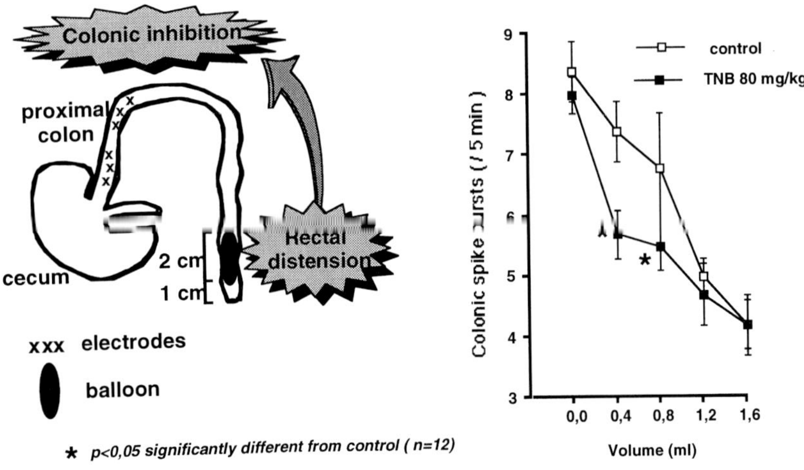

Fig. 4: *Changes in the threshold and amplitude of the recto-colonic inhibitory reflex induced by rectal distension in conscious rats after rectal inflammation induced by TNB. Series of distension were performed before and 3 days after intrarectal instillation of TNB (mean ± SD).*

peripheral and central neuropeptides or mediators. Serotonin appears to be a major candidate to modulate this enterogastric inhibitory reflex through different receptor subtypes. In sheep activation of both $5HT_{1A}$ and $5HT_2$ receptor subtypes are involved at brain level in this enterogastric reflex since the ICV administration of $5HT_{1A}$ (spiroxatrine) and $5HT_2$ (ritanserin) receptor antagonists are able to block the inhibitory reflex while $5HT_3$ receptors are involved only at peripheral level located on afferent sensitive fibers.

Alterations in recto-colonic inhibitory reflex to rectal distension seem to be also important in the genesis of Functional Bowel Disorders since this reflex is enhanced in constipated patients.

In rats this reflex has been recently investigated using electromyographic technique and it was shown that this reflex is enhanced (Fig. 4) 3 days after rectal inflammation with trinitrobenzene sulfonic acid (TNB) [28]. Similarly, repetitive emotional stress during 4 consecutive days also enhanced such recto-colonic inhibitory reflex [4] particularly for low distension volumes (Fig. 5). The mechanism by which stress influences such recto-colonic inhibitory reflex is not known but several peptides may modulate this reflex from a brain site of action. CCK_8 injected centrally attenuates this recto-colonic inhibitory reflex, this effect being linked to stimulation of CCK_A receptor subtype since this effect is mimicked by the CCK_A agonist A-71378 and not the CCK_B agonist A-63387 [21].

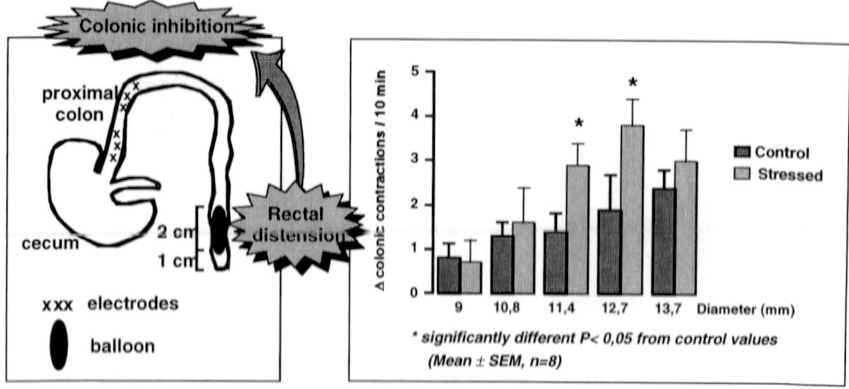

Fig. 5: *Influence of repeated daily emotional stress-session (30 min) during 4 days on the amplitude (Δ colonic contractions/10 min) of colonic motor inhibition induced by gradual rectal distensions. Sessions of distension were performed just before (control) and 1 day (stressed) after the period of stress (mean ± SD).*

Investigations on the nature of mediators involved at both brain and peripheral levels in the mediation of this reflex in normal conditions and in inflamed bowel have shown that NK_1 receptor subtype, a receptor mainly activated by substance P is involved at both CNS level and the periphery [27]. These investigations have identified other mediators responsible for changes related to inflammation corresponding to a lower threshold as well as enhancement of the response. Among them bradykinin is a decisive and primary mediator of such sensitization (Table 1).

Table 1: *Mediators (or receptors) involved in recto-colonic inhibitory reflex in rats.*

	Brain	Periphery
Normal	NK_1; NK_3	NK_1
Inflamed	NK_1	BK_2 CGRP NO

Experimental pathological situations

Prostaglandins mediate the responses at neuroendocrine junctions in the preoptic area at the anterior hypothalamus that are involved in thermoregulation and fever. There is now evidence that prostaglandins are involved in other neuroendocrine responses and ICV administration of prostaglandin E_2 (PGE_2) causes tachycardia and a rise in blood pressure confirming that the pressure response to peripheral PGE_1 and PGE_2 is partially mediated by the central nervous system. This response has been attributed to a prostaglandin-induced activation of adrenergic or cholinergic neurons rather than being considered a reflex reaction to the prostaglandin-induced hyperthermia [12]. Prostaglandins also participate in the regulation of hypothalamic and adenohypophyseal hormone secretions and centrally administered prostaglandins affect gastrointestinal function, injected ICV prostaglandins inhibit forestomach motility in goat [50], insulin-stimulated gastric secretion in rats [40] and cause anorexia in rats [2].

In rats ICV administration of prostaglandin E_2 restores a normal MMC pattern in fasted rats [16] and dogs [9]. These effects are centrally mediated and involve a calcium dependent mechanism. In dogs, oral administration of synthetic prostaglandin E_1 (misoprostol) or prostaglandin E_2 (enprostil) analogues before a meal induces postprandial MMC on the jejunum through a mechanism involving central prostaglandin receptors [47]. Moreover the effects of some peptides injected centrally such as calcitonin, seems related to the central release of PGE_2. Accordingly the effects of calcitonin injected centrally on both feeding behavior (anorexia) and gut motility i. e. MMC recovery, are suppressed after previous ICV administration of indomethacin or piroxicam, two cyclooxygenase inhibitors [16].

Interleukin 1, one of the major cytokines found in brain structures and particularly at hypothalamus level [33], when administered centrally at much lower dose than when administered peripherally, can elicit a number of physiological and behavioral changes similar to that seen following infection, such as fever [14]. It also induces effects characteristic of stress, such as activation of the hypothalamo-pituitary-adrenal axis [3], brain catecholaminergic system, and peripheral sympathetic nervous system [41].

Septic shock produced by endotoxin IV administration was used as a model to trigger abnormal patterns of motility. In rats it has been shown that the intraperitoneal administration of LPS triggers the CNS release of IL-1β. This cytokine released at CNS level is able to modulate gut motility from this site by inhibiting gastric emptying, slowing intestinal transit and motility; in contrast IL-1β stimulates lower gut motility [17]. Several reports have suggested that IL-1β injected ICV induces the release of prostaglandins but also CRF in brain structures involved in the control of motility [44]. Recently it has been shown that the CNS release of PGE_2 is involved in the inhibitory influence of IL-1β on upper gut motility while CRF is responsible for its effects on colonic motility [17]. Moreover both effects depend on catecholaminergic activation through both α1 and α2 receptors for upper gut and through D_2 receptor and $5HT_3$ receptor for the lower gut as represented in Fig. 6 [18].

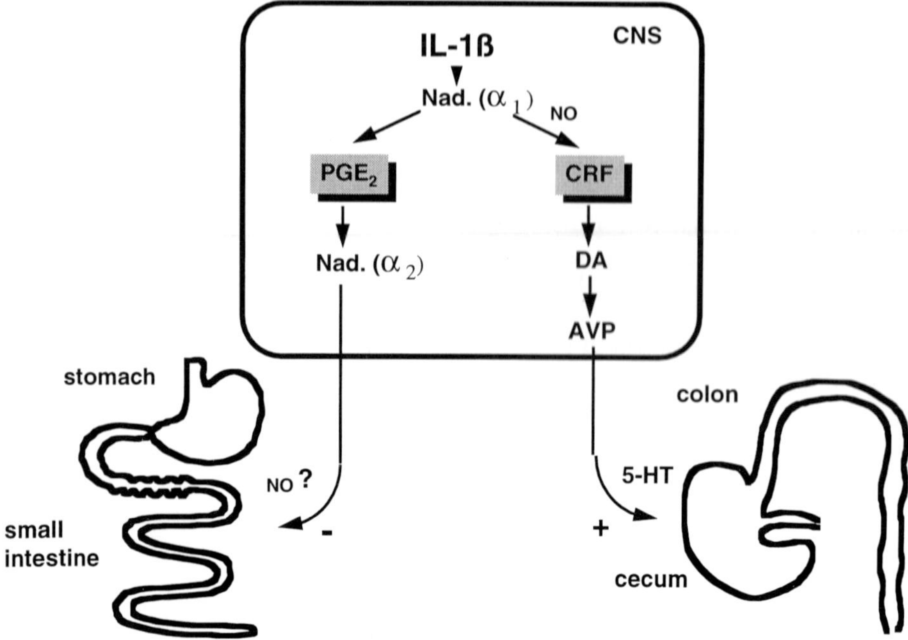

Fig. 6: *Pathways involved in alterations on upper and lower gut motility induced by intracerebro-ventricular administration of IL-1β (adapted from [17, 18]).*

In experimental ileus produced by surgical procedure or peritonitis, the inhibition of gastric activity is also under the control of supraspinal structures and neuromediators. In rats the inhibition of intestinal MMC following laparotomy is suppressed by yohimbine, an α_2 adrenergic blocker; the ratio of the active doses by ICV and IP route is in agreement with a central site of action while the α_1 antagonist, prazosin acts peripherally to suppress such inhibitory reflex [45].

More recently it was shown that gastric and intestinal motor inhibition induced by abdominal surgery involved brain structures and are mediated through the CNS release of CRF since ICV administration of α-helical CRF_{9-41}, a CRF antagonist suppress their effects on gastrointestinal motility. It has also been evidenced that CGRP and NO participate at sympathetic ganglion level in the mediation of nociceptive inputs [48, 42].

Peritonitis induced by IP administration of acetic acid inhibits gastric and intestinal motility in rats. This peritoneo-gastric inhibitory reflex triggered by a chemical substance activates afferent splanchnic nerves involving CGRP and NK_1 receptor subtypes but substance P (or NK_1 receptor) is also involved at CNS level activating efferent vagal fibers through a NANC component to inhibit gastric emptying [28].

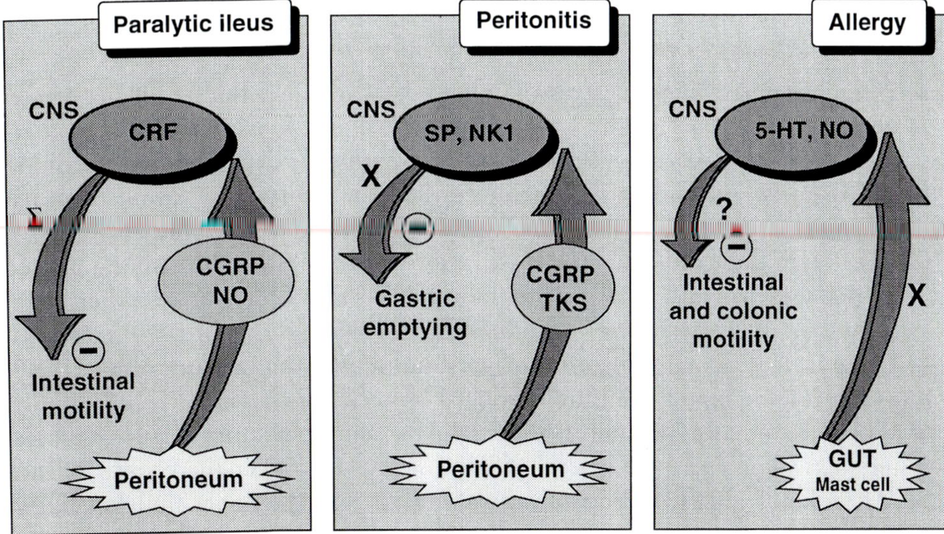

Fig. 7: *Schematic representation of the known pathways and mediators involved in intestinal motor inhibitory reflexes associated with experimental surgical laparotomy (paralytic ileus), intraperitoneal acetic acid (peritonitis) and oral antigenic challenge in sensitized rats.*

Another model of neuro-immune relationships in the gut is represented by alterations in gut motility associated with antigenic challenge in sensitized rats or guinea pigs [49]. The motor alterations are linked to the peripheral release of substance P from mast cells and activation of vagal afferent fibers [11]. The secondary release of 5HT and NO at the level of the nucleus tractus solitarius (NTS) is in part responsible for the observed motor alterations through the brain-gut axis (Fig. 7).

Conclusions

The brain appears to be a major structure controlling not only gut motor patterns but a number of intestino-intestinal reflexes particularly in pathological situations. The hypothalamus and the brainstem are the main targets, modulatory sites but the mechanisms of transduction to the periphery are multiple.

In physiological situations, the central release of neuropeptides such as CCK_8 in response to peripheral stimuli is triggered by the vagus and is of importance in the genesis or in maintaining patterns of gastrointestinal and colonic motility adapted to the digestive status. Our present knowledge suggests a specific participation of some brain hypothalamic nuclei which are able to respond selectively to vagal afferent inputs through the NTS but the efferent route is not well defined as well as the peripheral mediators involved.

- External and/or internal stressors also favor the CNS release of neuropeptides such as CRF, TRH and vasopressin clearly involved in the related alterations of GI motility with selective efferent pathways depending on the digestive segment and motor parameter considered. Central activation of dopaminergic pathways and peripheral release of 5-HT and/or NO are often associated with these induced motor alterations. Pathways can be also modulated by many factors at brain level including NPY and CCK_8 or by other vagal stimuli modulating directly or indirectly the release of hypothalamic factors. These factors also modulate some intestino-intestinal inhibitory reflexes such as the colonic motor inhibition induced by rectal distension.
- Some inflammatory mediators (PGE_2, PAF), neuromediators (5HT) or cytokines activate at peripheral level afferent nerves to trigger the central release of cytokines able to induce motor alterations of the upper and lower gut through the release of either prostaglandins or CRF. These influences participate in many alterations of gut motility observed in different situations such as septic shock while the CNS release of CRF is responsible for the colonic hyperkinesia through an activation of vasopressinergic pathways.
- Inflammation of the gut also alters the afferent inputs to the brain associated with physiological or extraphysiological signals. Rectal inflammation enhances the recto-colonic inhibitory reflex induced by rectal distension associated with sensitization of primary afferents involved in such reflex and depends upon the local release of several neuropeptides like bradykinin, tachykinins (P and CGRP) acting often in cascade. Finally all these alterations in intestino-intestinal reflexes and in the brain modulation of gut motility may contribute to the genesis of symptoms of irritable bowel.

References

1. Andrews, P. L. R., K. L. Wood: Systemic baclofen stimulates gastric motility and secretion via a central action in the rat. Br. J. Pharmacol. 89 (1986) 461–465.
2. Baile, C. A., C. W. Simpson, S. M. Bean et al.: Prostaglandins and food intake of rats. A component of energy balance regulation? Physiol. Behav. 10 (1973) 1077–1079.
3. Berkenbosch, F., J. Van Oers, A. Del Rey et al.: Corticotropin releasing factor-producing neurons in the rat activated by interleukin-1. Science 238 (1987) 524–526.
4. Buéno, L.: CNS control of gastrointestinal motility. In: T. S. Gaginella (Ed.): Handbook of methods in gastrointestinal pharmacology, pp. 294–330. CRC Press Inc., New York 1995.
5. Buéno, L., J. P. Ferré: Central regulation of intestinal motility by somatostatin and cholecystokinin octapeptide. Science 216 (1982) 1427–1429.
6. Buéno, L., M. Gué: Evidence for the involvement of corticotropin-releasing factors in the gastrointestinal disturbances induced by acoustic and cold stress in mice. Brain Res. 441 (1988) 1–4.

7. Buéno, L., M. Gué, C. Delrio: CNS vasopressin mediates emotional stress and CRH-induced colonic motor alterations in rats. Am. J. Physiol. 262 (1992) G427.

8. Buéno, L., M. Gué, C. Fabre et al.: Involvement of central dopamine and D1 receptors in stress-induced colonic motor alterations in rats. Brain Res. Bull. 29 (1992) 135−141.

9. Buéno, L., M. J. Fargeas, J. Fioramonti et al.: Central control of intestinal motility by prostaglandins: A mediator of the actions of several peptides in rats and dogs. Gastroenterology 88 (1985) 1888−1894.

10. Buéno, L.: Stress and upper gut motility disorders: mechanisms involved. In: J. P. Galmiche, R. Jian, M. Mignon (Eds.): Non-ulcer dyspepsia: pathological and therapeutic approaches, pp. 59−67. John Libbey Eurotext, Paris 1991.

11. Castex, N., J. Fioramonti, M. J. Fargeas et al.: C-fos expression in specific rat brain nuclei after intestinal anaphylaxis: involvement of 5-HT$_3$ receptors and vagal afferent fibers. Brain Res. 688 (1995) 149−160.

12. Chiu, K. Y., J. S. Richardson: Effects of central and peripheral prostaglandins on heart rate and blood pressure of rats. Proc. Can. Fed. Biol. Soc. 22 (1979) 48−56.

13. Davison, J. S., M. Hodges, V. Dickson: The enterogastric reflex in the ferret. Dig. Dis. Sci. 29 (1984) 558−562.

14. Dinarello, C. A.: Interleukin 1. Rev. Infect. Dis. 6 (1984) 51−95.

15. Fargeas, M. J., J. Fioramonti, L. Buéno: Involvement of dopamine in the central effect of neurotensin on intestinal motility in rats. Peptides 11 (1990) 1169.

16. Fargeas, M. J., J. Fioramonti, L. Buéno: Prostaglandin E2: a neuromodulator in the central control of gastrointestinal motility and feeding behavior by calcitonin. Science 225 (1984) 1050−1052.

17. Fargeas, M. J., J. Fioramonti, L. Buéno: Central action of interleukin-1β on intestinal motility in rats: mediation by two mechanisms. Gastroenterology 104 (1993) 377−383.

18. Fargeas, M. J., J. Fioramonti, L. Buéno: The role of monoaminergic systems in central IL-1β-induced changes in intestinal motility. Neurogastroenterol. Mot. 6 (1994) 189−195.

19. Gillies, G. E., E. A. Linton, P. J. Lowry: Corticotropin releasing activity of the new CRF is potentiated several times by vasopressin. Nature Lond. 299 (1982) 355−364.

20. Gmereck, D. E., A. Cowan: Pituitary-adrenal mediation of bombesin-induced inhibition of gastrointestinal transit in rats. Reg. Peptides 9 (1984) 299−304.

21. Gué, M., A. Tekamp, N. Tabis et al.: Cholecystokinin blockade of emotional stress- and CRF-induced colonic motor alterations in rats: role of the amygdala. Brain Rrs. 658 (1994) 232−238.

22. Gué, M., C. Alary, C. Delrio et al.: Comparative involvement of 5HT$_1$, 5HT$_2$ and 5HT$_3$ receptors in stress-induced colonic motor alterations in rats. Eur. J. Pharmacol. 233 (1993) 193−201.

23. Gué, M., C. Del Rio, J. L. Junien et al.: Interaction between CCK and opioids in the modulation of the recto-colonic inhibitory reflex in rats. Am. J. Physiol. 269 (1995) 240−245.

24. Gué, M., C. Honde, S. Pascaud et al.: CNS blockade of acoustic stress-induced gastric motor inhibition by K-opiate agonists in dogs. Am. J. Physiol. 254 (1988) G802−G815.

25. Gué, M., J. L. Junien, C. Delrio et al.: Neuropeptide Y and sigma ligand (JO1784) suppress stress-induced colonic motor disturbances in rats through Sigma and cholecystokinin receptors. J. Pharmacol. Exp. Ther. 261 (1992) 850−855.

26. Jimenez, M., L. Buéno: Inhibitory effects of neuropeptide Y (NPY) on CRF and stress-induced caecal motor response in rats. Life Sci. 47 (1990) 205−209.

27. Julia, V., O. Morteau, L. Buéno: Involvement of NK1 and NK2 receptors in viscero-sensitive response to rectal distension in rats. Gastroenterology 107 (1994) 94−102.

28. Julia, V., T. Mezzasalma, L. Buéno: Influence of bradykinin in gastrointestinal disorders and visceral pain induced by acute or chronic inflammation in rats. Dig. Dis. Sci. 40 (1995) 1913−1921.

29. Junien, J. L., M. Gué, L. Buéno: Neuropeptide Y and sigma ligand (JO 1784) act through a GI protein to block the psychological stress and corticotropin-releasing factor-induced colonic motor activation in rats. Neuropharmacology 30 (1991) 1119–1124.

30. Kaneyuki, H., H. Yokoo, A. Tsuda et al.: Psychological stress increases dopamine turnover selectively in mesoprefrontal dopamine neurons of rats: Reversal by diazepam. Brain Res. 557 (1991) 154–161.

31. Lane, R. F., C. D. Blaha, A. G. Phillips: In vivo electrochemical analysis of cholecystokinin-induced inhibition of dopamine release in nucleus accumbens. Brain Res. 397 (1986) 200–204.

32. Lantéri-Minet, M., P. Isnardon, J. de Pommery et al.: Spinal and hindbrain structures involved in visceroception and visceronociception as revealed by the expression of Fos, Jun and Krox-24 proteins. Neuroscience 55 (1993) 737–753.

33. Lechan, R., R. Toni, B. Clark et al.: Immunoreactive interleukin-1β localization in rat forebrain. Brain Res. 514 (1990) 135–140.

34. Lenz, H. J.: Calcitonin and CGRP inhibit gastrointestinal transit via distinct neuronal pathways. Am. J. Physiol. 254 (1988) G920–924.

35. Lenz, H. J., A. Raedler, H. Greten et al.: Stress-induced gastrointestinal secretory and motor responses in rats are mediated by endogenous corticotropin-releasing factors. Gastroenterology 95 (1988) 1510–1517.

36. Liberge, M., M. P. Arruebo, L. Buéno: Role of hypothalamic CCK_8 in the colonic motor responser to a meal in rats. Gastroenterology 100 (1991) 441–449.

37. Liberge, M., P. Arruebo, L. Buéno: CCK_8 neurons of the ventromedial (VMH) hypothalamus mediate the upper gut motor changes associated with feeding in rats. Brain Res. 508 (1990) 118–123.

38. Martinez, J. A., L. Buéno: Buspirone inhibits corticotropin-releasing factor and stress-induced cecal motor response in rats by acting through 5-HT1A receptors. Eur. J. Pharmacol. 202 (1991) 379–383.

39. Porreca, F., T. F. Burks: Centrally administered bombesin affects gastric emptying and small and large bowel transit in the rat. Gastroenterology 85 (1983) 313–317.

40. Purunen, J.: Central nervous system effects of arachidonic acid, PGE_2 PGF_2, PGD_2 and PGI_2 on gastric secretion in the rat. Br. J. Pharmacol. 80 (1983) 255–262.

41. Rivier, C., W. Val: In the rat, interleukin-1α and -β stimulate adrenocorticotropin and catecholamine release. Endocrinology 125 (1989) 3096–3102.

42. Rivière, P. J. M., X. Pascaud, E. Chevalier et al.: Fedotozine reverses ileus induced by surgery or peritonitis: action at peripheral κ-opiod receptors. Gastroenterology 104 (1993) 724–731.

43. Roman, F. J., X. Pascaud, B. Martin et al.: JO 1784, a potent and selective ligand for rat and mouse brain sigma sites. J. Pharm. Pharmacol. 42 (1990) 439–440.

44. Rothwell, N.: Functions and mechanisms of interleukin-1 in the brain. Trends Pharmacol. Sci. 12 (1991) 430–436.

45. Sagrada, A., M. J. Fargeas, L. Buéno: Involvement of alpha-1 and alpha-2 adrenoceptors in the postlaparotomy intestinal motor disturbances in the rat. Gut 28 (1987) 955–959.

46. Smith, J. R., T. R. Lahann, R. M. Chesnut et al.: Thyrotropin-releasing hormone: stimulation of colonic activity following intracerebroventricular administration. Science 196 (1977) 660–661.

47. Staumont, G., J. Fioramonti, J. Frexinos et al.: Oral prostaglandins analogues induce intestinal migrating motor complexes after a meal in dogs: evidence for a central mechanism. Gastroenterology 98 (1990) 888–893.

48. Taché, Y., E. Kolve, R. Stephens et al.: Role of brain CRF in mediating surgical stress induced inhibition of gastric function in the rat. 7th International symposium on gastrointestinal hormones, Shizuoka 1988.

49. Theodorou, V., J. Fioramonti, J. L. Junien et al.: Anaphylactic colonic hypersecretion in cow's milk sensitized guinea-pigs depends upon release on interleukin-1, prostaglandins and mast cell degranulation. Aliment. Pharmacol. Ther. 8 (1994) 301–307.

50. Van Miert, A. S. J., C. T. Van Duick, N. Woutersen-Van: Effects of intracerebroventricular injection of PGE_2 and 5HT on body temperature, heart rate and rumen motility of conscious goats. Eur. J. Pharmacol. 92 (1983) 143–146.

51. Williams, C. L., R. G. Villar, J. M. Peterson et al.: Stress-induced changes in intestinal transit in the rat: a model for the irritable bowel syndrome. Gastroenterology 94 (1988) 611–617.

Brain-gut mechanisms of visceral sensitivity

E. A. Mayer, B. Naliboff, J. Munakata, D. Silverman

Introduction

Symptoms of functional bowel disorders affecting the upper and lower gastrointestinal tract are responsible for a large number of patient visits to gastroenterologists. In addition, functional syndromes with analogous characteristics are observed in patients seeking health care within other medical and surgical specialities (Fig. 1). Yet, despite their prevalence and impact on the healthcare system, the etiology of these syndromes is poorly understood, their diagnosis relies exclusively on symptom criteria and the most commonly prescribed drugs have never been shown to be more effective than placebo in well-designed studies.

The concepts and mechanism(s) put forward to explain the etiology of IBS symptoms cover a remarkably wide spectrum, from mucus colitis to muscle spasms to neuroticism, and decades of investigation have failed to provide a reliable, consistent biological marker of the disorder. In the past decade, a renewed interest in the area of visceral afferent mechanisms, including visceral pain has provided a new perspective of these disorders, which has already produced the first therapeutic compounds in the form of "visceral analgesics."

Chronic intermittent abdominal pain and/or discomfort are present in all patients with IBS, while the prevalence of associated symptoms such as altered bowel habits, passage of mucus and visible abdominal distension greatly vary

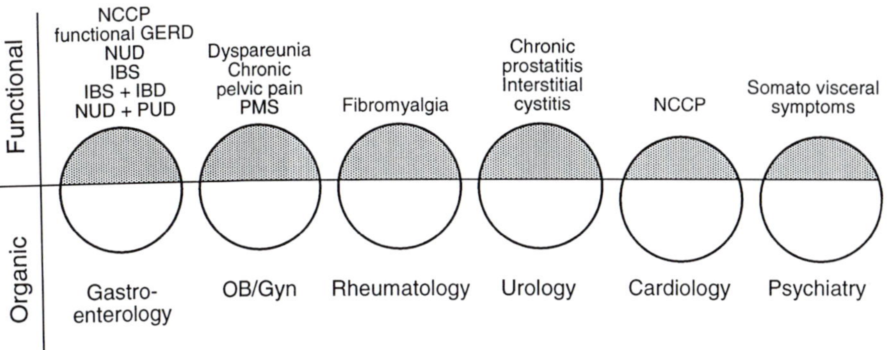

Fig. 1: *Functional syndromes in medical and surgical specialities*

Even though patients with indicated functional disorders consult primarily a particular specialist for their predominant symptom, there is considerable overlap of all listed functional disorders.

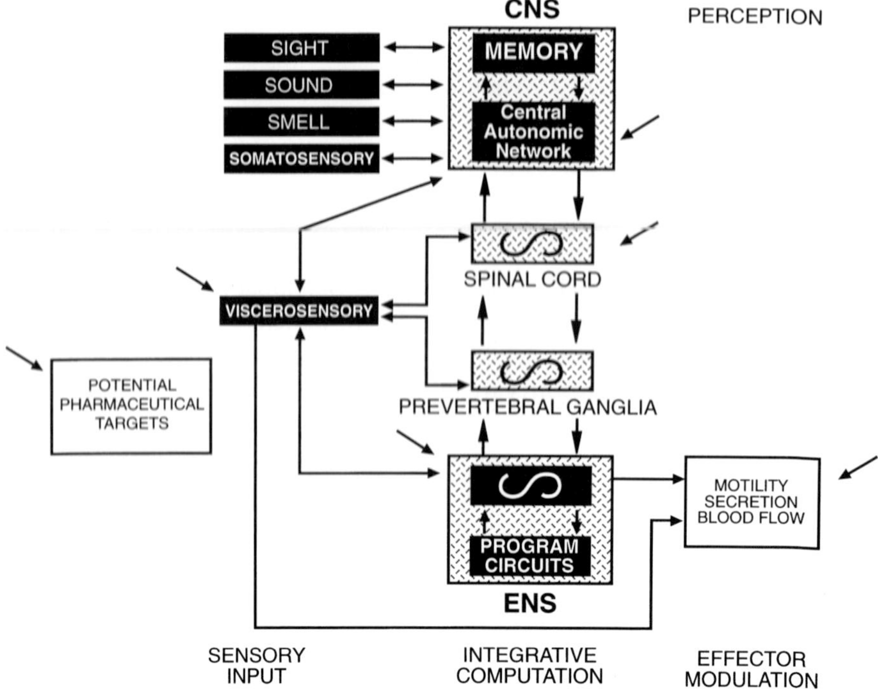

Fig. 2: *Schematic neural circuitry involved in perpetual and autonomic responses to sensory stimulation*

Shown are schematic interactions of different components of the nervous system involved in the processing of visceral sensory stimuli. Both responses can be modulated from the periphery or by the CNS. Modified from Mayer et al. [14]

between patients and even within the same patient over time. Abdominal discomfort includes sensations of gas, fullness, bloating and incomplete evacuation. In the majority of patients, symptoms are exacerbated by food intake and stressful life events, while in some patients symptoms are decreased by distraction and somatic counter irritation. This suggests the action of modulatory influences on visceral perception both from the periphery (special senses, gut) and from the brain (Fig. 2). The fact that IBS patients have no way of validating internal sensations with other sensory modalities (as can be done with somatic sensations) has important consequences for the overall clinical characteristics of IBS patients. The emotional response (anxiety, distress) to the persistent, unexplained sensations, and the anticipatory anxiety related to the unpredictable onset of symptoms may result in significant secondary, autonomic activation, and in the development of a tendency to experience and label sensations arising from the viscera in aversive terms.

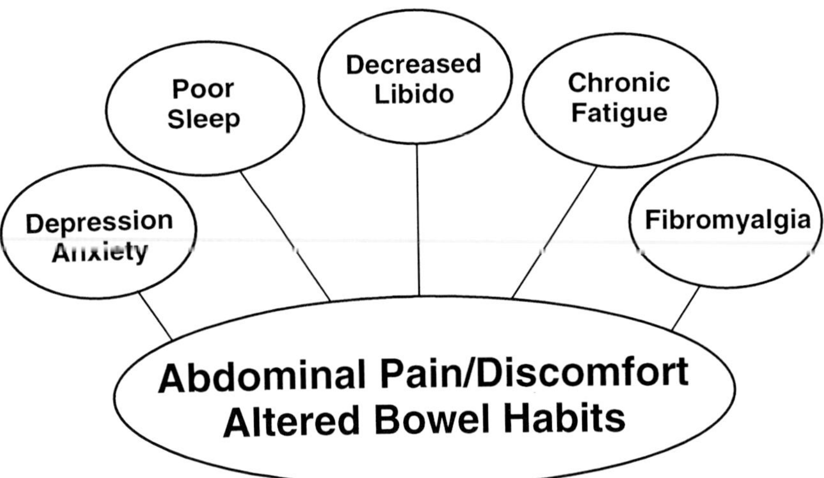

Fig. 3: *Summary of common intestinal and extraintestinal symptoms reported by Functional Bowel Disease (FBD) patients.*

Extraintestinal symptoms are likely to affect perceived symptom severity and overall quality of life of FBD patients.

Evidence for altered CNS mechanisms in IBS

A primary role of the CNS in these disorders is supported by several independent observations: 1) A majority of patients relate the first onset or the exacerbation of symptoms to stressful life events [5, 30]. 2) A majority of patients, when appropriately asked for, give a history of mild functional GI symptoms, typically in form of a "sensitive stomach" or "constipation" dating back to childhood or adolescence. 3) Therapies aimed at the CNS (such as psychotherapy, tricyclic antidepressants or anxiolytics) are frequently effective in symptom relief. 4) Placebo response rates of up to 70% have been reported [9]. 5) Functional symptoms are reported in patients following resection of the suspected target organ (stomach, rectosigmoid), and abdominal symptoms are reported by the majority of patients with high, complete cervical spine lesions [14]. 6) The wide range of symptoms ranging from poor sleep, decreased libido, chronic fatigue and musculoskeletal pain are difficult to explain by a shared peripheral abnormality (Fig. 3).

The fact that IBS patients suffer from a variety of other symptoms in addition to *abdominal* pain and discomfort suggests a more generalized alteration in central processing of sensory information, and associated CNS dysfunction. Associated symptoms include a) altered autonomic regulation of GI function; b) extraintestinal discomfort/pain syndromes and c) generalized CNS dysfunction.

a) Even though incompletely understood, the characteristic symptom of altered bowel habits (ranging from infrequent dry, pebble-like stool to frequent loose bowel movements) is compatible with alterations in autonomic control of intestinal water and electrolyte handling, and in intestinal motility. For example, the extrinsic sympathetic innervation of the gut exerts a powerful inhibitory effect on *intrinsic* reflexes involved in intestinal fluid secretion. Depending on the region of the GI tract (small intestine, left or right colon) sympathetic modulation of epithelial functions would be expected to have markedly different effect on stool consistency. On the other side, the extrinsic parasympathetic innervation mediates both inhibitory and stimulatory effects on gastrointestinal motility and transit. Variations in the relative activity of parasympathetic and sympathetic modulation of intestinal function could explain the inter- and intra-patient variability in stool characteristics, and the inconsistencies in reported colonic motor patterns. b) IBS patients frequently complain of headaches, lower back pain, pelvic pain, dyspareunia, urinary urgency, sensation of incomplete bladder evacuation and fibromyalgia-like symptoms. While some of these symptoms could result from generalized alterations in lumbosacral primary or secondary afferent function, a more general, CNS-based alteration in the processing of sensory information is more plausible. Reports of normal perception thresholds for somatic pain induced by cold temperature or transcutaneous electrical stimulation do not contradict such a concept. Techniques used in these studies were not sensitive enough to detect small threshold differences, and it is well known that pain thresholds are stimulus specific, i. e. the presence of mechanical allodynia does not require the simultaneous presence of temperature-dependent hyperalgesia. c) Poor sleep, chronic fatigue, and decreased sexual drive are reported by the majority of IBS patients, and a large number of patients with chronic fatigue syndrome and post traumatic stress syndrome complain of IBS symptoms.

Functional Bowel Disease (FBD) and chronic visceral hypersensitivity

Does chronic abdominal pain and visceral hyperalgesia explain the symptom complex of functional visceral disorders?

Clinical evidence to suggest the presence of chronic mechanical hyperalgesia in IBS comes from patients' reports of lower abdominal pain, tenderness over the sigmoid colon, and excessive discomfort/pain during sigmoidoscopic examinations. Ritchie first demonstrated with fluoroscopic techniques that sigmoid contractions in IBS patients can be associated with the experience of lower abdominal pain, while healthy subjects do not perceive contractions of much greater amplitude [20]. Kellow and coworkers, using 24 hr ambulatory motility recordings from the small intestine have shown that physiological repetitive contractions of the intestine (such as phase III of the migrating motor complex) can be associated with discomfort in some IBS patients, whereas these events are not perceived by healthy controls [8].

Following the fruitless search for an etiologic role of a gastrointestinal motility disturbance [15, 16], there has been a recent surge of interest to view FBDs as chronic abdominal pain syndromes. From a clinical standpoint, abdominal pain has been identified as the primary outcome measure in the therapy of FBD. Abdominal pain is the strongest predictor of the physician's judgement of severity of disease [3, 4, 23], and epidemiological studies have demonstrated that abdominal pain (presumably as the most threatening GI symptom), is the strongest predictor of physician's visits [27, 28]. The concept of chronic visceral hyperalgesia is attractive since it uses a single, specific symptom (i. e. abdominal pain), rather than a range of poorly quantifiable complaints to explain the pathophysiology, and measure symptom severity and treatment outcome.

However, even though abdominal pain is reported by the majority of patients seen at a tertiary referral center as one of their GI symptoms, only 25% of patients indicated abdominal pain as their primary symptom, while bloating-type symptoms were reported by the majority of patients as the single most bothersome symptom (Lembo, T., Fullerton S., Mayer EA. Is pain the predominant symptom in irritable bowel syndrome (IBS)? Gastroenterology 110: A 705, 1996.). Similarly, when evaluating published studies on altered visceral perception of visceral stimuli, there is not a single report demonstrating the presence of basal visceral hyperalgesia in patients with either functional or inflammatory bowel disorders. In the somatic pain field, the term hyperalgesia has been defined as an increased sensitivity to noxious stimuli, which manifests as a lowered threshold to painful stimuli, a greater response, or a change in the stimulus response curve. However, truly noxious stimuli have not been used in any published study on visceral balloon distension in humans, and alterations in stimulus response curves have not been reported. More appropriately, one may refer to the altered perception of visceral stimuli in IBS patients as allodynia, which refers to a situation where previously non-painful stimuli are experienced as painful. However, true pain thresholds (obtained by unbiased measures of the visceral pain threshold) in IBS patients have not been reported. Until conclusive experimental evidence supports the presence of either hyperalgesia or allodynia, it may therefore be best to refer to reported perceptual alterations in IBS patients as visceral hypersensitivity.

Several laboratories have studied subjective responses to balloon distension of different regions of the GI tract to identify and characterize altered perception of visceral stimuli. When exposed to ascending series of distending stimuli (a paradigm greatly susceptible to response bias), IBS patients tend to report discomfort at lower volumes or pressures during distension of the rectum, descending colon, small intestine and esophagus. In general, this hypersensivity is only seen during rapid distension. Mertz and coworkers have recently shown that close to 100% of IBS patients show evidence for altered perception of rectal distension in the form of lowered discomfort thresholds, increased intensity of discomfort or altered viscerosomatic referral. Even though these findings are consistent with altered spinal processing of rectal afferent signals, true hyperalgesia (as defined above) was not demonstrated in this study.

All published reports are flawed by the use of test paradigms highly subjective to response bias, by the failure to distinguish between primary sensory abnormalities and secondary effects of gut wall compliance on perception thresholds, and by the inappropriate labeling of perception thresholds as pain thresholds, when pressures are used which do not elicit nociceptive cardiovascular responses, and which are significantly below the true pain thresholds of the human GI tract reported in the literature [11]. What we currently know about visceral perception in patients with FBD can be summarized as follows: The majority of patients exhibit one of several alterations in the perception of visceral events, either induced experimentally, or occurring in response to physiological events. Experimental alterations include a lower threshold for the use of the label "discomfort" during distension of small intestine or colorectum, a greater intensity of perception at the discomfort threshold and an aberrant and/or enlarged area of viscerosomatic referral [1, 22]. However, if visceral hypersensitivity is simply defined as a lowered threshold for perception of rectal distention as "discomfort", only about 40−50% of patients can be classified as hypersensitive. Since normo- and hyper-sensitive patients do not differ on a wide range of clinical parameters, the relevance of this perceptual alteration in IBS symptom generation is currently not known.

In contrast to the lack of a consistent alteration in baseline perceptual responses which can be observed in all patients, Munakata et al. have recently demonstrated that virtually all IBS patients will develop rectal hypersensitivity (determined by an unbiased threshold tracking technique) following prolonged noxious mechanical stimulation of the sigmoid colon [17]. This effect seems to be specific for IBS patients, since neither healthy subjects nor patients with inflammatory bowel disease show the same perceptual response. If these preliminary results are confirmed, it would represent the first demonstration of a ubiquitous alteration in the processing of visceral sensory stimuli in IBS patients.

Alternative approaches to characterize altered perception in IBS patients have aimed at eliminating the pitfalls of subjective intensity ratings, and at identifying specific afferent fibers involved in the transmission of intestinal pain.

These approaches have included transmucosal electrical stimulation, and measurement of evoked potentials over the spinal cord and brain [6]. While attractive from a theoretical viewpoint, these studies so far have failed to demonstrate significant differences between normal subjects and IBS patients. However, preliminary results from studies using non-invasive functional brain imaging techniques suggest a potential of this approach to identify quantitative differences in brain activation in response to visceral stimulation, or to the anticipation of visceral pain (see below).

Mechanisms of visceral hyperalgesia

Despite a multitude of modulatory mechanisms, sensory information arising from innocuous stimuli is assumed to be transmitted centrally in direct proportion to the strength and duration of the stimulus. For the great majority of stimuli arising from the viscera, there is no conscious perception of such physiological events as distension and contraction, except for behaviorally relevant sensations such as satiety and the urge to have a bowel movement. In contrast to physiological stimuli, noxious stimuli can alter the gain of the sensory transduction system. The human organism has multiple mechanisms which allow the body to either increase or decrease the nociceptive input, the experience and the reaction to pain and the reflex responses to pain. These mechanisms involve transient functional changes in peripheral and central neuronal activity and long-lasting changes involving neuronal plasticity. Different neurophysiological mechanisms are recruited at the peripheral and central levels depending on the nature, magnitude and time course of the noxious stimulus [12].

Sensitization of afferent pathways by acute tissue irritation in the periphery
Persistent input from irritated or inflamed tissue can involve both low and high threshold afferent fibers. In the periphery, at least two mechanisms, referred to as peripheral sensitization will increase the gain of the transduction system during noxious stimulation: sensitization of mechanically sensitive fibers by inflammatory mediators, and recruitment of so-called silent (mechanically insensitive) afferent fibers. These functional changes will greatly increase the release of neuroactive chemicals (in particular glutamate, substance P and CGRP) at the central synapse of visceral afferents in response to mechanical stimulation of the gut. These neuroactive chemicals increase the excitability of spinal neurons and lead to expansion of peripheral receptive fields. They can also lead to a "memory" of the initiating peripheral insult which can last under experimental conditions for several hours. Mechanisms involved in central hyperexcitability involving the viscera have recently been characterized in urinary bladder, colon, esophagus and gallbladder. An increased excitability of dorsal horn neurons receiving afferent input (referred to as spinal hyperexcitability,

central sensitization or wind-up) can result from repetitive activation of visceral mechanoreceptors, from experimentally induced inflammation, and from chemical irritation.

Arguments against the development of chronic visceral hyperalgesia in response to chronic inflammatory mucosal events
The initial enthusiasm that animal models of acute visceral hyperalgesia may be useful as animal models for functional bowel disorders has not been supported by experimental or clinical data to date. According to this concept, and in analogy to concepts developed for the development of chronic somatic pain, irritation of visceral primary afferent will first result in the sensitization of primary afferents (peripheral sensitization). The resultant dramatic increase in afferent input to dorsal horn neurons in the superficial laminae of the dorsal horn will lead to increased excitabilty of these neurons (central sensitization). It was hypothesized that based on this central sensitization, longlasting hyperalgesia (pain memory) could develop by a mechanism analogous to development of longterm synaptic potentiation (LTP) in the hippocampus [13]. Arguments against a mechanism of spinal LTP in the etiology of visceral syndromes presenting with chronic visceral pain can be made from an evolutionary standpoint. Prolonged somatic pain typically results in behaviorally adaptive responses such as decreased use and protection of the affected body from further injury. In contrast, there is no behavioral response to chronic visceral pain that would give the organism an adaptive advantage. For example, there is little an organism can do in response to persistent visceral pain which would increase the recovery from the initiating event. Furthermore, clinical evidence does not support the concept that in humans, visceral inflammation will result in longlasting mechanical visceral hyperalgesia. For example, the most common inflammatory conditions of the GI tract (H. pylori gastritis, uncomplicated inflammatory bowel disease) are not associated with chronic abdominal pain. Similarly, while in animal models acute mucosal irritation of the esophagus, the colon or the urinary bladder are associated with hypersensitivity in balloon distension [18], perception of colonic distension in patients with inflammatory bowel disease during periods of clinical remission is either normal or attenuated [14], arguing against the development of longlasting visceral hyperalgesia in response to mucosal irritation.

These observations are most consistent with the concept that even though the CNS does react to acute inflammatory visceral events with the initial development of peripheral and central sensitization, this upregulation of afferent transmission is counterbalanced in the healthy organism by the activation of powerful pain inhibitory systems. This counterregulation starts in the periphery with the action of immune cell-derived opioids onto peripheral terminals of primary afferents [25], with the activation of spinal and descending pain inhibitory pathways [13] and with adaptive CNS responses to increased spinothalamic input.

Modulation of perceptual responses to visceral stimulation by the CNS
A series of experimental evidence suggests the involvement of endogenous pain inhibition systems in the modulation of visceral and somatic pain in humans. For example, patients with Crohn's disease have increased somatic pain threshold and increased visceral perception thresholds at sites not affected by the inflammatory process. A painful electrical stimulus applied to the forearm increases the tolerance of gastric and duodenal distension. Repetitive intense sigmoid sensitization increases the perception threshold in the rectum in normal volunteers. Modulation of perceptual responses to physiologic or experimentally induced visceral events can occur by direct descending modulation of the excitability of spinal projection neurons. In addition, such modulation may also occur at the level of the thalamus and cortex.

Spinal pathways originating in nuclei within the medulla (bulbospinal descending systems) have a modulatory effect on perception and autonomic reflexes. Descending modulatory influences onto second order spinal neurons can be excitatory or inhibitory, can be activated acutely and transiently in response to central or peripheral stimuli and can exert a tonic modulatory influence. Changes in dorsal horn excitability by bulbospinal inhibitory pathways are likely to play an important role in determining the size of receptive fields, referral areas and pain thresholds. Under normal conditions, descending bulbospinal pathways are likely to limit the development of increased excitability (i. e. the membrane potential) of dorsal horn neurons in the presence of peripheral tissue irritation. Randic and co-workers have demonstrated in a spinal cord slice preparation that identical trains of tetanic stimulation of afferent rootlets can induce neuroplastic changes consistent with longterm synaptic potentiation (LTP) or longterm depression (LDP), depending on the resting potential of the postsynaptic cell during afferent stimulation [19]. Extrapolating to the in vivo condition, these findings could indicate that the type of synaptic plasticity developing in response to peripheral tissue irritation is conditional on the membrane potential of the projection neuron. By influencing the membrane potential of dorsal horn neuron, the activity of descending systems (bulbospinal, propriospinal) could therefore play an important conditional role in determining the type (LTP vs. LTD), extent and time course of synaptic plasticity.

Activation of specific brainstem areas results in decreased excitability of spinothalamic tract neurons, inhibition of nociceptive input, and inhibition of reflexes evoked by nociceptive stimuli. In addition, various environmental factors including stress, and acute and chronic pain have been demonstrated to activate descending pain modulation systems. The areas in the brainstem are part of the central autonomic network and receive excitatory (and likely inhibitory) inputs from higher centers, including the rostral limbic system (amygdala, prefrontal, insular and cingulate cortices), and also from ascending nociceptive pathways,

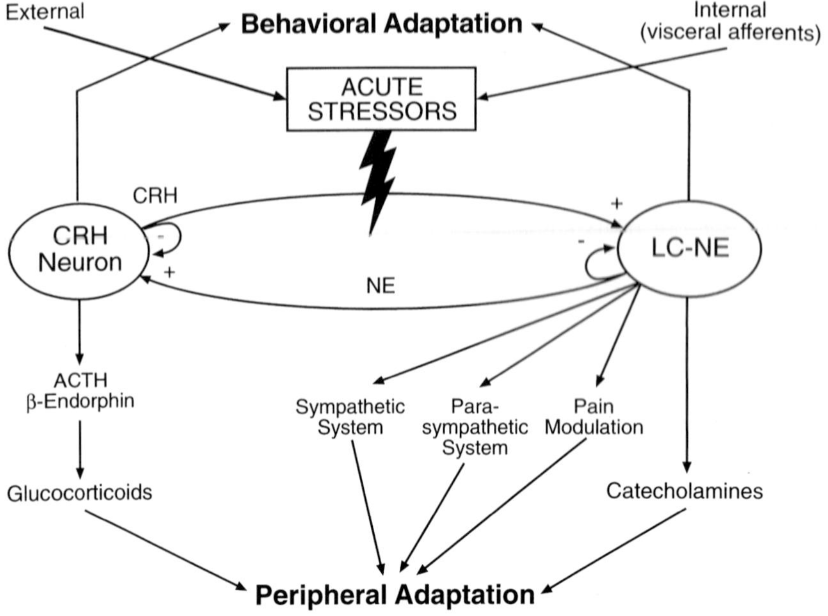

Fig. 4: *Possible role of locus coeruleus (LC) in FBD symptom generation*

LC neurons can be activated in response to stressful life events and by visceral afferent input. LC projections are involved in descending bulbospinal pain inhibition (noradrenergic system), in modulation of parasympathetic output, and in sympathtic activation. Modified from Sternberg et al. [26], with permission of the publisher.

including branches axons of the spinothalamic and spinoreticular tract. Thus, brain areas involved in processing of the affective pain component are integrated into a feedback loop involving ascending tracts and descending bulbospinal tracts. One of the brainstem regions with a particular relevance for IBS etiology is the pontine nucleus locus ceruleus (LC) (Fig. 4). This nucleus provides the primary noradrenergic innervation of the brain, projects extensively to regions giving rise to parasympathetic outflow such as dorsal motor nucleus of the vagus and the sacral spinal cord, and projects to limbic areas such as the amygdala, i. e. brain areas involved in the control of emotions and cardiovascular control. Furthermore, its noradrenergic projections are a major component of the bulbospinal pain modulation systems. Traditionally, the role of the LC has been seen as central "novelty detector" which is activated by a number of environmental sensory stimuli. Its role has been implicated in behavioral functions such as vigilance, alarm and anxiety reactions to novel and especially threatening stimuli.

An alternative mechanism by which perceptual responses to visceral events may be altered is related to the mechanism of visceral learning well-established in animal models of conditioned responses [7]. Animal studies have shown that the amygdala is necessary for the conditioned emotional response. It may be the site where synapses from neurons activated by a conditioned stimulus (i. e. a tone) have attained the ability to fire neurons that produce the conditioned response (i. e. a change in heart rate), after pairing with the unconditioned response [10]. The human amygdala also appears to receive viscerosensory inputs, and stimulation of the amygdala produces visceromotor responses. However, in place of simple sensory inputs, the human amygdala receives highly processed cognitive information. Thus, the human equivalent of the conditioned emotional response may consist of learning to produce visceral responses to external (environmental stimuli), or internal events (thoughts) that have previously been associated with visceral upset. This concept is attractive in view of the high prevalence of abuse history in patients with FBD [2], and in view of the commonly reported history of visceral reactions to external or internal events (in form of a "sensitive stomach" or altered bowel habits) going back to childhood. It may be hypothesized that an associative memory is formed between the strong visceral responses normally associated with traumatic life events and with aversively perceived events in general. Once formed, such a memory — manifested both in visceromotor responses and in images, thoughts and feelings — could be recalled by stimuli arising in the environment, within the viscera or in the form of thoughts and emotions.

Novel experimental approaches to identify CNS alterations underlying altered perceptual responses to visceral stimuli

Positron emission tomography (PET) has evolved as a unique non-invasive technique to quantitate changes in blood flows in man as an index of neuronal activity in response to physiological stimuli, including somatosensory pain and the anxiety associated with expected pain. Patients with functional and organic pain syndromes show differences in their brain activities in response to an acute thermal pain stimulus. While patients with chronic functional facial pain showed exaggerated anterior cingulate responses, patients with rheumatoid arthritis had decreased responses in the thalamus, lentiform nucleus, anterior cingulate and prefrontal cortex, when compared to normal control subjects. However, no differences in the responses of the somatosensory cortex were seen between patients with chronic functional and chronic organic pain.

Regional brain activity correlates to visceral pain have only recently been reported. Electrical vagal stimulation produces increased blood flow localised to the ipsilateral thalamus and cingulate gyrus. Transmucosal esophageal electrical stimulation resulted in changes localised to the sensory cortex as well as to the temporal lobe [29]. Pharmacologically induced anginal pain is associated with rCBF increases in the hypothalamus, periaqueductal gray, bilateral thalamus, prefrontal and cingulate cortex [21].

Our own recent data [24] using $H_2^{15}O$ PET suggest that anticipation of a painful visceral stimulus, as well as actual painful rectal distension, result in specific changes in cerebral blood flow. Significant responses to intestinal pressure stimuli have been measured in several brain regions (most notably anterior cingulate cortex, left prefrontal cortex, right mesiotemporal cortex and thalamus), and some disease-specific differences in activity patterns have already emerged. For example, we have observed significant regional cerebral activation in normal subjects not only in PET images obtained during actual delivery of painful pressure stimuli, but also in PET images obtained during anticipated delivery of such stimuli. During such anticipation, activity of the 'affective' division of the anterior cingulate cortex has been found to correlate with subjective pain intensity, and thalamic activity to correlate with heart rate. IBS patients tend to show greater autonomic and thalamic responses. Failure of the cingulate activation has been a consistent disease-associated feature of IBS patients examined so far. IBS patients, on the other hand, demonstrate significantly greater activation of portions of the prefrontal cortex during anticipation of pain.

Summary and conclusions

In summary, one may speculate from the available published data that FBD patients (and possibly patients suffering from analogous disorders such as interstitial cystitis), exhibit more than one perceptual alteration regarding sensations arising from the viscera. 1) A tendency to label visceral sensations primarily with affective descriptors as aversive, unpleasant or discomfort. These descriptors are used by FBD patients at lower stimulus intensities (for example rectal balloon pressure or volume) than by healthy control subjects. 2) The disease-specific development of visceral hyperalgesia in response to intense visceral stimulation (mechanical, chemical, inflammatory). Symptoms such as bloating, fullness or gas in the majority of FBD patients under baseline conditions may be related to the aversive interpretation of normal physiological events, in the absence of visceral hyperalgesia. In contrast, following prolonged stimulation of visceral afferents (for example stimulation of sigmoid mechanoreceptors) in response to stress or to food intake IBS patients develop transient rectosigmoid hyperalgesia, presenting as abdominal pain. This hypothesis is consistent with both clinical characteristics and reported experimental findings: 1) The characteristic symptomatic presentation of symptoms of chronic abdominal discomfort with associated transient abdominal pain episodes associated with food intake and stressful life events. 2) The inconsistency of baseline rectal hypersensitivity in reported studies. 3) The disease-specific induction of rectal hypersensitivity by repetitive sigmoid stimulation.

The etiology of the perceptual alterations in FBD patients remains unknown. Visceral hypersensitivity could develop as a sequence of events starting at the peripheral nerve endings of primary visceral afferents ("bottom up model"), or evolve as a sequence of events starting in the brain ("top down model").

Bottom-up model: Irritation of primary afferent nerve terminals located in the mucosa or non-mucosal parts of the gut could result in peripheral sensitization and sensitization of mechanically-insensitive C-fibers, followed by the development of central sensitization at the level of the spinal cord. Persistence of dorsal horn neuron hyperexcitability, resulting in prolonged increased afferent input to medullary and hypothalamic nuclei and thalamus could result in the development of increased excitability at these higher levels. In principle, peripheral neuroplastic changes could reverse to their normal state, while central changes may persist. Different regional manifestations of visceral hyperalgesia, such as symptoms referred primarily to the lower or upper abdomen, or even to the chest could result from increased excitability of spinal neurons involving different levels of the spinal cord, or central projection areas. In addition, neuroplastic changes could develop in circuits of the rostral limbic system, resulting in the development of a visceral, context-dependent memory at the level of the amygdala. Such a memory could be recalled later during certain emotional states, even in the absence of peripheral events.

Top-down model: Alterations in the reactivity of autonomic brainstem nuclei, such as the LC, to environmental and/or visceral stimuli could result in alterations in visceral autonomic regulation and in alterations of endogenous pain modulation systems. Such a dysfunction could exist in form of exaggerated activation of LC neurons by normal gastrointestinal events, in form of delayed adaptation of the response to visceral stimuli, or in the lowered threshold for the activation of peripheral sympathetic outflow. For example, longlasting changes in synaptic plasticity in the LC has been implicated as an important etiological factor in patients with the posttraumatic stress syndrome, a disorder commonly associated with functional bowel symptoms.

It is obvious that the two models of IBS are not mutually exclusive, and differ only in the site where the primary abnormality is located. Both share as a central component the development of a positive feedback loop involving visceral afferents, activation of autonomic centers, perceptual responses and modulation of visceral afferents by autonomic pathways (Fig. 2). This integrated concept may explain why symptoms can be initiated or exacerbated by both peripheral and centrally acting events, and why therapies aimed at peripheral *and* central mechanisms appear to be beneficial.

References

1. Accarino, A. M., F. Azpiroz, J.-R. Malagelada: Receptor vs suprareceptor level of gut sensory disfunction in the irritable bowel syndrome (IBS). Gastroenterology 104 (1992) A413.
2. Drossman, D. A., J. Leserman, G. Nachman et al.: Sexual and physical abuse in women with functional or organic gastrointestinal disorders. Ann. Intern. Med. 113 (11) (1990) 828−833.
3. Drossman, D. A., Z. Li, E. Andruzzi et al.: U.S. Householder Survey of Functional GI Disorders: Prevalence, Sociodemography and Health Impact. Dig. Dis. Sci. 38 (1993) 1569−1580.
4. Drossman, D. A., D. C. McKee, R. S. Sandler et al.: Psychosocial factors in the irritable bowel syndrome. A multivariate study of patients and nonpatients with irritable bowel syndrome. Gastroenterology 95 (1988) 701−708.
5. Drossman, D. A., R. S. Sandler, D. C. McKee: Bowel patterns among subjects not seeking health care. Gastroenterology 83 (1982) 529−534.
6. Enck, P. T., Frieling: Human gut−brain interactions. J. Gastrointest. Motility 5 (1993) 77−87.
7. Halgren, E.: Emotional neurophysiology of the amygdala within the context of human cognition. In: J. P. Aggleton (Ed.): The Amygdala, pp. 191−228. Wiley−Liss, New York 1992.
8. Kellow, J. E., C. M. Eckersley, M. P. Jones: Enhanced perception of physiological intestinal motility in the irritable bowel syndrome. Gastroenterology 101 (6) (1991) 1621−1627.
9. Klein, K. B.: Controlled treatment trials in the irritable bowel syndrome: A critique. Gastroenterology 95 (1988) 232−241.
10. LeDoux, J. E.: Emotion and the Amygdala. in: J. P. Aggleton (Ed.): The Amygdala, pp. 339−352. John Wiley & sons, Inc., New York 1992.
11. Lipkin, M., M. H. Sleisenger: Studies of visceral pain: Measurements of stimulus intensity and duration associated with the onset of pain in esophagus, ileum and colon. JCI 37 (1957) 28−34.
12. Mayer, E. A., G. F. Gebhart: Basic and clinical aspects of visceral hyperalgesia. In: Y. Tache, D. Wingate, T. Burks (Eds.): Innervation of the Gut: Pathophysiological Implications, CRC Press, Boca Raton, FL 1993.
13. Mayer, E. A., G. F. Gebhart: Basic and clinical aspects of visceral hyperalgesia. Gastroenterology 107 (1994) 271−293.
14. Mayer, E. A., J. Munakata, H. Mertz et al.: Visceral hyperalgesia and the irritable bowel syndrome. In: G. F. Gebhart (Ed.): Visceral Pain. Progress in Pain Research and Management, Vol. 2, in press. ASP Press, Seattle 1995.
15. McKee, D. P., E. M. M. Quigley: Intestinal motility in irritable bowel syndrome: Is IBS a motility disorder? Dig. Dis. Sci. 38 (1993) 1761−1782.
16. McKee, D. P., E. M. M. Quigley: Intestinal motility in irritable bowel syndrome: Is IBS a motility disorder? Part II. Dig. Dis. Sci. 38 (1993) 1773−1782.
17. Munakata, J., L. Chang, C. An et al.: Repetitive activation of sigmoid mechanoreceptors results in the development of rectal hyperalgesia in IBS patients. Gastroenterology 108 (1995) A653.
18. Ness, T. J., G. F. Gebhart: Visceral pain: a review of experimental studies. Pain 41 (1990) 167−386.
19. Randic, M., M. C. Jiang, R. Cerne: Long-term potentiation and long-term depression of primary afferent neurotransmission in the rat spinal cord. J. Neurosci. 13 (1993) 5228−5241.
20. Ritchie, J.: Mechanisms of pain in the irritable bowel syndrome. In: N. W. Read (Ed.): Irritable bowel syndrome, pp. 163−172. Grune & Stratton, London 1985.
21. Rosen, S. D., E. Paulesu, C. D. Frith et al.: Central nervous pathways mediating angina pectoris. Lancet 344 (1994) 147−150.
22. Routledge, J. H., H. Elliott: Pain studies in pelvic viscera. Am. J. Obst. Gyn. 83 (1962) 701−709.
23. Sandler, R. S., D. A. Drossman, H. P. Nathan et al.: Symptom complaints and health care seeking behavior in subjects with bowel dysfunction. Gastroenterology 87 (1984) 314−318.

24. Silverman, D. H. S., H. Ennes, J. Munakata et al.: Differences in thalamic activity associated with anticipation of rectal pain between IBS patients and normal subjects. Gastroenterology 108 (1995) A1006. (Abstract)
25. Stein, C.: The control of pain in peripheral tissue by opioids. N. Engl. J. Med. 332 (1995) 1685–1690.
26. Sternberg, E. M., G. P. Chrousos, P. W. Gold: The stress response and the regulation of inflammatory disease. Ann. Intern. Med. 117 (1992) 854–866.
27. Talley, N. J., E. A. O'Keefe, A. R. Zinsmeister et al.: Prevalence of gastrointestinal symptoms in the elderly: a population-based study. Gastroenterology 102 (1992) 895–901.
28. Talley, N. J., A. R. Zinsmeister, C. Van Dyke et al.: Epidemiology of colonic symptoms and the irritable bowel syndrome. Gastroenterology 101 (1991) 927–934.
29. Tougas, G., M. V. Kamath, S. Garnett et al.: Mapping of cerebral response to vagal and esophageal stimulation using positron emission tomography (PET) and topographic EEG in humans. Gastroenterology 106 (1994) A486.
30. Whitehead, W. E., M. D. Crowell, J. C. Robinson et al.: Effects of stressful life events on bowel symptoms: subjects with irritable bowel syndrome compared with subjects without bowel dysfunction. Gut 33 (1992) 825–830.

Psychosocial aspects of the functional gastrointestinal disorders

D. A. Drossman

Introduction

Over the last 15–20 years, scientific efforts to study how GI symptoms relate to their physiologic and psychosocial correlates has changed how we conceptualize the gastrointestinal disorders. Until recent years, the assumption was made that symptoms have a causal and linear relationship with the presence and degree of histopathologic disease (the Biomedical Model). However, in one study [22], only about 10% of presenting medical symptoms in an ambulatory internal medicine clinic, when followed up for one year, were given a specific (organic) medical diagnosis.

This study and our clinical observations indicate that there is a complex relationship between symptoms and GI illness. For the functional GI disorders, motility patterns like the discrete clustered contractions in IBS, or high amplitude contraction patterns in the nutcracker esophagus exist as candidate markers for these disorders, but for the most part, these motility patterns relate only incompletely to the symptoms. Even when an organic disease is present like peptic ulcer or inflammatory bowel disease, severe symptoms may occur with little disease activity, and active disease may occur with few symptoms. For example, while heartburn is presumed to result from acid exposure on the esophageal mucosa, we know that many patients with severe reflux, Barret's esophagus and strictures give little history of heartburn, and many patients with acid sensitivity do not have abnormal reflux or esophagitis [10].

The marked variation in symptoms relative to pathologic change or motility can relate to any of three possible factors:

1. individual differences in visceral sensitivity, at the level of the visceral mucosa or afferent neuron

2. CNS modulation of visceral sensory input, via corticofugal effects at the level of the spinal cord, or

3. intrinsic psychological effects on symptom generation [26].

In this presentation I will focus on the contribution of psychosocial factors on the symptom experience and its outcomes.

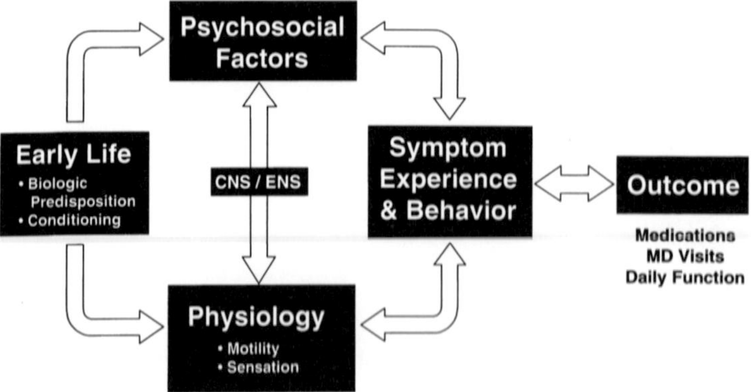

Fig. 1: *Biopsychosocial relationship between early life, psychosocial factors, physiology and symptom experience and behavior. See text for details.*

Biopsychosocial model

The systems or biopsychosocial model [18] proposes that symptoms and consequent behaviors result from interacting systems rather than from a single, linearly determined cause. As shown in Fig. 1, early life factors influence later psychosocial experiences, physiologic functioning or susceptibility to a pathological condition, which in turn affects the symptom experience and behavior and the clinical outcome. Therefore, a psychosocial stressor, interpreted from previous experiences, may produce symptoms as a purely psychological event or indirectly through changes in intestinal physiologic function via the CNS−ENS axis. It may even affect immunity or disease activity through the hypothalamic-pituitary-adrenal axis [8]. Similarly, intestinal dysmotility or a duodenal ulcer will have varying effects on symptoms and the clinical outcome depending on the psychosocial milieu.

Early life

Biological predispositions or conditioning experiences in early life will influence later psychosocial, physiologic or pathologic conditions. Biological predispositions including genetics or congenital events may lead to psychosocial conditions like alcoholism or psychiatric disease, or physiological and pathological conditions like the functional GI disorders, IBD or peptic ulcer. Similarly, certain conditioning experiences early in life such as illness reinforcement, losses and abuse may influence later illness behaviors.

Illness reinforcement

Can the parent's responses toward a child's tummy ache at age 6 affect that person's later attitudes and behaviors around later illness? In a telephone survey of 832 persons, Dr. Whitehead's group identified 8% to have IBS and 10% to have PUD [39]. Those with IBS were more likely than the ulcer group or normals to have abnormal illness behavior manifest as multiple somatic complaints, the perception that colds were more serious, and the receipt of gifts and privileges when they were ill.

Our research group performed interviews of IBS patients, IBS non-patients who had never been to the doctor, and normals [25]. We found that IBS patients when compared to normals perceived themselves to have had poorer general health during childhood, and when ill, to receive greater parental attention, and take more school absences. IBS patients were also more likely than the non-patients with IBS and normals to see physicians more frequently when ill as children.

In a more recent study [38], Dr. Whitehead's group was able to address the specificity of reinforcement of illness behavior. In comparing patients with IBS, with those having dysmenorrhea or cold symptoms, he found that reinforcement of bowel symptoms predicted the later development of IBS.

These data suggest that early experiences may affect either the susceptibility to developing the condition, or one's attribution to it. So, if as a child, you had a tummy ache and stayed home from school and saw the doctor, then you would be more likely to do the same as an adult.

Sexual and physical abuse

A history of sexual or physical abuse has recently been shown to affect later symptom behavior and outcome in gastrointestinal disorders [12, 17]. As shown in Fig. 2, when using the same question items [12], the frequency of abuse reporting progressively increases from normals to those with mild and severe IBS in a primary care setting or HMO [24], and it is highest in a referral center where the prevalence can reach 50% in some studies. Furthermore, independent of diagnosis, a history of abuse is associated with greater symptom reporting, such as pelvic pain and other GI and non-GI symptoms, more doctor visits and more operations [12, 14, 17, 24, 33]. So, while these early life experiences are not etiologic for GI disorders, they do influence the symptom experience and subsequent behaviors including doctor visits. Stated another way, regardless of diagnosis, patients referred with refractory symptoms are at risk for having an abuse history.

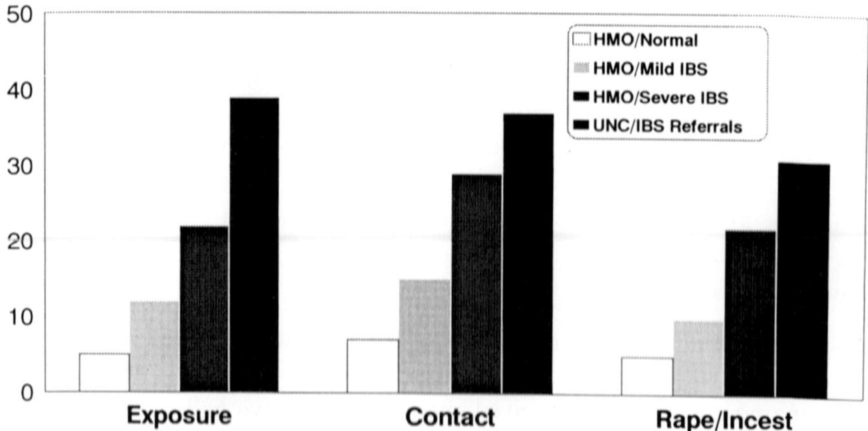

Fig. 2: *Comparison of frequencies of sexual abuse history (for sexual exposure, contact abuse and rape/incest) between HMO members without bowel symptoms, mild IBS, severe IBS, and patients seen at a university referral GI clinic [12, 24]. The progressive rise in frequency supports a relationship of abuse history with IBS, its severity, and primary care vs referral status. (With permission[9]).*

Psychosocial factors, physiology, pathology and symptoms

The association between psychosocial factors, physiology/pathology symptoms and behavior are delineated by several observations:

1. There is an incomplete relationship between symptoms and motility
While psychological stress can produce both symptoms [2, 16] and dysmotility in normals and patients with functional GI disorders [19, 23, 28, 35], the symptoms are not fully explained by the dysmotility. In a study involving patients with IBS, ulcerative colitis, and a normal control group [23] abnormal contractions in the jejunum in response to stress were found most commonly among patients with IBS. Of the 18/22 IBS patients with these abnormal contractions, only 8 reported pain. In a later study by Kellow [21] most but not all of the IBS patients studied who developed prolonged propagated contractions in response to CCK or neostigmine experienced symptoms, and this occurred more in IBS patients than normal subjects.

Therefore, these abnormal contraction patterns are seen more often in IBS than normals, though they are not specific for the disorder. Furthermore, the partial correlation of symptoms with the contraction abnormalities occur to a greater degree in IBS patients than in normals, suggesting greater sensitivity. However, patients can also have symptoms without associated contraction abnormalities [1, 20, 23]. These observations support the idea that patients with functional GI disorders may have an abnormal sensory response to normal motility as well as abnormal motility.

2. Psychosocial disturbances are common in functional GI disorders
A number of studies have shown that persons with functional GI disorders
when compared to normals or other medical control groups have a higher frequency of psychosocial disturbances [6, 11, 12, 27, 34, 39, 40]. When standardized diagnostic criteria are used to evaluate the frequency of psychiatric diagnoses, about 40−60% of IBS patients will have a major psychiatric diagnosis,
compared to 20% or less for patients with other medical conditions or normals [11].

3. Psychosocial factors relate to patient status
The high frequency of psychosocial disturbances reported in patients with functional GI disorders actually overestimate the psychosocial nature of most persons with IBS, since the data are drawn from patients who are selectively referred to medical centers. In fact, persons with IBS who do not see physicians
are psychologically similar to normal subjects [15, 29, 36], and conversely, frequent clinic attenders regardless of medical diagnosis have a high frequency of
psychosocial disturbances [31]. Therefore, psychosocial factors are not a part
of the IBS *per se*, but they influence the individual's illness behavior including
the clinical outcome [7]. This may be manifest as increased pain reporting,
physician visits or medication use, the seeking of alternative medical treatments
[30] and requests for unneeded surgery [5].

4. Psychosocial factors may influence visceral sensation
This may occur through descending pathways on the dorsal horn of the spinal
cord, where there is corticofugal modulation of visceral sensation via the opiate
mediated analgesic system [26]. Serotonin is an important neurotransmitter in
this system, so there is at least a theoretical basis for the using antidepressants
or the newer 5HT agents in helping control visceral pain.

5. Psychosocial factors may independently produce symptoms
There are several examples. Individuals may be hypnotized to have pain. Patients with somatization disorder will complain of GI (and other) symptoms,
yet may not have GI physiologic dysfunction. In one study [32], patients with
esophageal motor disorders when compared to controls reported lower sensation thresholds from balloon distension, but there were no differences in the
distension related amplitude and quality of cerebral evoked potentials [32].
Therefore, the chest pain seemed to be related to abnormal central processing
of normal afferent information.

6. Psychosocial factors may "buffer" adverse effects
Social support and coping style are modifying factors that can improve a patient's adjustment to an illness by "buffering" the adverse effects of stress [8].
Patients with functional GI disorders may have less effective social support and
coping strategies than comparison groups. In one study [3], the authors found

that "less-mature" coping strategies, and less availability of emotional support through social relationships was significantly associated with functional dyspepsia. Similarly, in another study [4] patients with functional chest pain reported significantly greater use of maladaptive (emotional-based) coping strategies (praying and hoping) than did a control group of patients with IBS or coronary artery disease. They also reported a significantly lower sense of ability to control their pain.

Outcome

Outcome research identifies the impact of a medical condition through "hard" endpoints obtained by external verification, such as physician visits, disability, number of procedures and costs, or "soft", patient related endpoints, including physical and psychological symptoms and daily function, and health related quality of life. One example of "hard" endpoints are the data from the U.S. Householder Epidemiologic Survey [13] which found that persons with functional GI disorders had 2–3 times more disability, work or school absences and physician visits.

Finally an important "soft" outcome is health related quality of life (HRQOL). It differs from "hard" outcomes because it evaluates patient perceptions of illness rather than external measures. HRQOL assessments can evaluate the influence of psychosocial factors. Few studies have been reported that evaluate HRQOL in the functional GI disorders. One study, published in abstract form [37], found that when using a generic measure of HRQOL, the SF-36, IBS patients had a poorer quality of life compared to nonpatients with IBS and normals, and the nonpatients with IBS were intermediate.

Final comments

These observations provide evidence that psychosocial factors have a role in: 1) early life conditioning experiences, 2) modulation of symptoms and behavior, and 3) affecting clinical outcome. An appreciation of the interactive role of psychosocial factors with physiological disturbances (e. g., motility and visceral sensitivity) is needed in order to provide optimal care to patients with functional GI disorders.

References

1. Achem, S. R., J. Crittenden, B. Kolts et al.: Long-term clinical and manometric follow-up of patients with nonspecific esophageal motor disorders. Am. J. Gastroenterol. 87 (1992) 825–830.

2. Almy, T. P., F. J. Kern, M. Tulin: Alteration in colonic function in man under stress: II. Experimental production of sigmoid spasm in healthy persons. Gastroenterology 12 (1949) 425−436.

3. Bennett, E., J. Beaurepaire, P. Langeluddecke et al.: Life stress and non-ulcer dyspepsia: a case-control study. J. Psychosom. Res. 35 (1991) 579−590.

4. Bradley, L. A., J. E. Richter, I. C. Scarinci et al.: Psychosocial and psychophysical assessments of patients with unexplained chest pain. Am. J. Med. 92 (1992) 65S−73S.

5. Burns, D. G.: The risk of abdominal surgery in irritable bowel syndrome. South Afr. Med. J. 70 (1986) 91.

6. Craig, T. K. J., G. W. Brown: Goal frustration and life events in the aetiology of painful gastrointestinal disorder. J. Psychosom. Res. 28 (1984) 411−421.

7. Drossman, D. A.: Illness behaviour in the irritable bowel syndrome. Gastroenterology International 4 (1991) 77−81.

8. Drossman, D. A.: Psychosocial Factors in the Care of Patients with Gastrointestinal Disorders. In: T. Yamada (Ed.): Textbook of Gastroenterology, pp. 620−637. J. B. Lippincott Co., Philadelphia 1995.

9. Drossman, D. A.: Sexual and physical abuse and gastrointestinal illness. Scand. J. Gastroenterol. Suppl. 208 (1995) 90−96.

10. Drossman, D. A.: Importance of the psyche in heartburn and dyspepsia. Scand. J. Gastroenterol. Suppl. (In Press).

11. Drossman, D. A., F. H. Creed, G. A. Fava et al.: Psychosocial aspects of the functional gastrointestinal disorders. Gastroenterology International, 8 (1995) 47−90.

12. Drossman, D. A., J. Leserman, G. Nachman et al.: Sexual and physical abuse in women with functional or organic gastrointestinal disorders. Ann. Intern. Med. 113 (1990) 828−833.

13. Drossman, D. A., Z. Li, E. Andruzzi et al.: U.S. Householder Survey of Functional Gastrointestinal Disorders: Prevalence, Sociodemography and Health Impact. Dig. Dis. Sci. 38 (1993) 1569−1580.

14. Drossman, D. A., Z. Li, J. Leserman et al.: Frequency of abuse history by GI diagnosis and effect on health status. Gastroenterology 108 (1995) 593 (Abstract).

15. Drossman, D. A., D. C. McKee, R. S. Sandler et al.: Psychosocial factors in the irritable bowel syndrome. A multivariate study of patients and nonpatients with irritable bowel syndrome. Gastroenterology 95 (1988) 701−708.

16. Drossman, D. A., R. S. Sandler, D. C. McKee et al.: Bowel patterns among subjects not seeking health care. Use of a questionnaire to identify a population with bowel dysfunction. Gastroenterology 83 (1982) 529−534.

17. Drossman, D. A., N. J. Talley, K. W. Olden et al.: Sexual and physical abuse and gastrointestinal illness: Review and recommendations. Ann. Intern. Med. 123 (1995) 782−794.

18. Engel, G. L.: The need for a new medical model: A challenge for biomedicine. Science 196 (1977) 129−136.

19. Kellow, J. E., P. M. Langeluddecke, G. M. Eckersley et al.: Effects of acute psychologic stress on small-intestinal motility in health and the irritable bowel syndrome. Scand. J. Gastroenterol. 27 (1992) 53−58.

20. Kellow, J. E., S. F. Phillips: Altered small bowel motility in irritable bowel syndrome is correlated with symptoms. Gastroenterology 92 (1987) 1885−1893.

21. Kellow, J. E., S. F. Phillips, L. J. Miller et al.: Dysmotility of the small intestine in irritable bowel syndrome. Gut 29 (1988) 1236−1243.

22. Kroenke, K., M. E. Arrington, A. D. Mangelsdorff: The prevalence of symptoms in medical outpatients and the adequacy of therapy. Arch. Intern. Med. 150 (1990) 1685−1689.

23. Kumar, D., D. L. Wingate: The irritable bowel syndrome: A paraxysmal motor disorder. Lancet 2 (1985) 973−977.

24. Longstreth, G. F., G. Wolde-Tsadik: Irritable bowel-type symptoms in HMO examinees. Prevalence, demographics and clinical correlates. Dig. Dis. Sci. 38 (1993) 1581−1589.

25. Lowman, B. C., D. A. Drossman, E. M. Cramer et al.: Recollection of childhood events in adults with irritable bowel syndrome. J. Clin. Gastroenterol. 9 (1987) 324–330.
26. Mayer, E. A., G. F. Gebhart: Basic and clinical aspects of visceral hyperalgesia. Gastroenterology 107 (1994) 271–293.
27. Palmer, R. L., A. H. Crisp, E. Sonehill et al.: Psychological characteristics of patients with the irritable bowel syndrome. Postgrad. Med. J. 50 (1974) 416–419.
28. Richter, J. E.: Stress and psychologic and environmental factors in functional dyspepsia. Scand. J. Gastroenterol. Suppl. 182 (1991) 40–46.
29. Sandler, R. S., D. A. Drossman, H. P. Nathan et al.: Symptom complaints and health care seeking behavior in subjects with bowel dysfunction. Gastroenterology 87 (1984) 314–318.
30. Smart, H. L., J. F. Mayberry, M. Atkinson: Alternative medicine consultations and remedies in patients with the irritable bowel syndrome. Gut 27 (1986) 826–828.
31. Smith, R. C., D. S. Greenbaum, J. B. Vancouver et al.: Psychosocial factors are associated with health care seeking rather than diagnosis in irritable bowel syndrome. Gastroenterology 98 (1990) 293–301.
32. Smout, A. J. P. M., M. S. DeVore, C. B. Dalton et al.: Cerebral potential evoked by oesophageal distension in patients with non-cardiac chest pain. Gut 33 (1992) 298–302.
33. Talley, N. J., S. L. Fett, A. R. Zinsmeister et al.: Gastrointestinal tract symptoms and self-reported abuse: A population-based study. Gastroenterology 107 (1994) 1040–1049.
34. Walker, E. A., P. P. Roy-Byrne, W. J. Katon et al.: Psychiatric illness and irritable bowel syndrome: a comparison with inflammatory bowel disease. Am. J. Psychiatry 147 (1990) 1656–1661.
35. Welgan, P., H. Meshkinpour, M. Beeler: Effect of anger on colon motor and myoelectric activity in irritable bowel syndrome. Gastroenterology 94 (1988) 1150–1156.
36. Whitehead, W. E., L. Bosmajian, A. B. Zonderman et al.: Symptoms of psychologic distress associated with irritable bowel syndrome. Comparison of community and medical clinic samples. Gastroenterology 95 (1988) 709–714.
37. Whitehead, W. E., C. K. Burnett, E. Cook, III et al.: Health related quality of life in IBS: patients compared to IBS non-consulters and asymptomatic individuals. Am. J. Gastroenterol. 89 (1994) 1700 (Abstract).
38. Whitehead, W. E., M. D. Crowell, B. R. Heller et al.: Modeling and reinforcement of the sick role during childhood predicts adult illness behavior. Psychosom. Med. 6 (1994) 541–550.
39. Whitehead, W. E., C. Winget, A. S. Fedoravicius et al.: Learned illness behavior in patients with irritable bowel syndrome and peptic ulcer. Dig. Dis. Sci. 27 (1982) 202–208.
40. Young, S. J., D. H. Alpers, C. C. Norland et al.: Psychiatric illness and the irritable bowel syndrome. Practical implications for the primary physician. Gastroenterology 70 (1976) 162–166.

Functional esophageal disorders

R. E. Clouse

Introduction

The esophagus is involved in several syndromes that have no recognized structural or metabolic causes, a requisite for a functional diagnosis. Two of the disorders, functional globus and rumination, are sufficiently distinct from the remainder to be discussed separately. Functional disorders arising from the distal, smooth-muscle region of the esophagus (e. g., chest pain, dysphagia) commonly overlap, may share pathogenetic mechanisms, and are discussed together. Except in the case of rumination, the events responsible for the functional esophageal disorders are poorly understood. However, clinical observations have identified common associations that have both mechanistic and treatment implications.

Functional globus

Definition and clinical features

The globus sensation (globus pharyngis, globus hystericus) is the feeling of a lump or tightness in the throat. The discomfort is sensed in the midline over the thyroid cartilage in more than three-quarters of the patients with slight deviation to other sites in the anterior neck in the remainder [7]. Dysphagia and odynophagia are distinctly absent, and swallowing liquids or solid foods may actually improve the symptom.

The globus sensation commonly leads to referral to subspecialists, including otolaryngologists and gastroenterologists, to complete the important exclusionary evaluation for esophageal and cervical disorders which may produce the symptom [26]. The principal conditions leading to the complaint are esophageal motility disorders involving the distal esophagus, gastroesophageal reflux disease, and structural esophageal and extra-esophageal cervical lesions (Fig. 1). Once these processes have been excluded, the functional diagnosis is established. At present there are insufficient data to determine if functional globus can be differentiated from the others based on symptom presentation alone [21].

Epidemiologic studies indicate that functional globus is a female predominant disorder, but these data are confounded by the fact that disorders mimicking functional globus may be included in the study populations [7, 22, 33, 47].

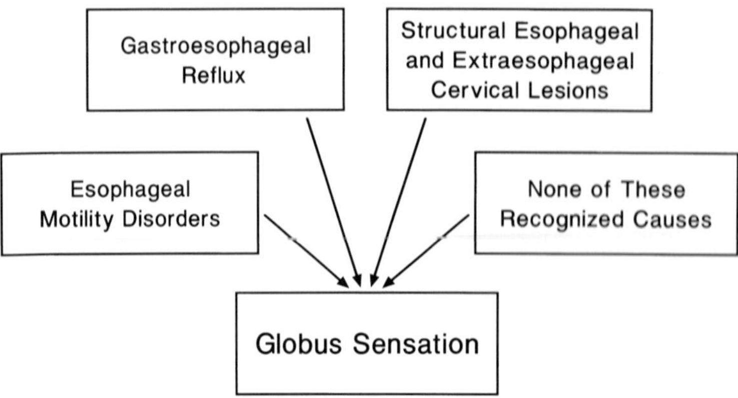

Fig. 1: *The globus sensation is produced by esophageal and extraesophageal disorders. A functional diagnosis cannot be given until a careful exclusionary evaluation is completed.*

Intermittent symptoms occur in nearly half the population, whereas chronic persistent globus is reported by 12.5% of surveyed individuals [24]. Only a third of these seek medical attention. Chronicity appears to be the rule in patients who see physicians and are ultimately diagnosed with the functional disorder.

Potential pathogenetic mechanisms

Physiologic studies have not provided a satisfactory explanation for the symptom. Because of its location, globus sensation is thought to arise from the region of the cricopharyngeus muscle. However, consistent abnormalities in motor function in this region have not been demonstrated. The types of abnormalities sought in cricopharyngeus muscle behavior are listed in Tab. 1. Two reports have demonstrated a high prevalence of *bona fide* distal esophageal disorders (including achalasia and esophageal spasm) in patients referred for evaluation of persistent globus sensation [25, 34]. In at least a subset of these patients, the referred symptom resolved with treatment of the distal motor abnormality. Nevertheless, larger series have failed to show that alterations in distal esophageal motor activity are sufficiently prevalent to provide an explanation for functional globus [19, 47].

Very limited information is available concerning visceral sensory abnormalities in these subjects (Tab. 1). Two types of sensory provocation tests have been employed in an attempt to reproduce the symptom − acid perfusion and esophageal distention. Studies using acid perfusion in patients with functional globus have produced equivocal results [13, 18]. Preliminary data show that the symptom can be reproduced with proximal esophageal distention in some subjects [18]. Consequently, visceral hypersensitivity may be a relevant component

Table 1: *Esophageal abnormalities of potential pathogenetic relevance to functional globus.*

Finding or abnormality	Strength and direction of evidence	References
Motor abnormalities		
Increased resting UES pressure	Favors against	[19, 47]
Hyperreactive UES to stimulation	Favors against	[4, 18, 19, 47]
Exaggerated after-contraction of the UES	Limited data in favor	[47]
Referred symptom of distal motor disorders	Favors against	[19, 47]
Sensory abnormalities		
Symptom production with acid perfusion	Equivocal	[13, 18]
Symptom production with esophageal distention	Preliminary data in favor	[18]

UES = upper esophageal sphincter.

of the pathogenetic process for globus as it is for distal esophageal functional syndromes. Better characterization of sensory abnormalities in functional globus is needed.

There are insufficient data to indicate that a distinct central process is involved in globus sensation. No specific central neurologic disorder is suspected, and neurologic abnormalities have not surfaced in longitudinal observation. Although psychiatric disturbances had long been suspected as having importance in the production of this syndrome, studies reproducibly identifying specific psychiatric disorders or psychological characteristics as common markers are remarkably absent [22]. In particular, contemporary studies demonstrating a high rate of somatization disorder (the disease hysteria for which the symptom was originally named) are not available. The elusive quality to the pathophysiology suggests that multiple mechanisms are involved in the production of the functional globus syndrome that vary from patient to patient.

Management approaches

Management begins with a careful exclusionary evaluation that usually is accomplished rapidly considering the location of the symptom and limited differential diagnosis. Unlike the case with distal functional esophageal syndromes, an invasive evaluation for visceral, extra-esophageal causes is unnecessary. The outcome of functional globus is restricted to symptoms, but long-term follow-up studies demonstrate the chronic and persistent nature of symptoms without some type of intervention [46]. The certainty of the functional diagnosis gives confidence to a benign prognosis. Consequently, reassurance is attended by a

Table 2: *Response to treatments for presumed functional globus*.*

Treatment	All subjects	Males	Females
Reassurance	59%	47%	68%
Anxiolytic therapy	39%	29%	50%
Antireflux therapy	4–12%	8–14%	0–8%
Overall success	77%	72%	80%

* Percentage response in 64 patients without symptoms of reflux disease; data from [33].

fairly high success rate (Tab. 2). Antireflux therapy may seemingly help as many as 15% of patients, even for those who have had a reasonable evaluation for gastroesophageal reflux disease [33].

Despite lack of evidence for the relevance of psychiatric disorder in symptom production, psychoactive agents have been used in a nonspecific manner for symptom control [9, 10]. In the occasional patient with a co-morbid anxiety disorder, anxiolytic therapy may reduce globus symptoms [9]. Anxiolytic therapy may have a role in other subjects by reducing fears of a serious disorder or through nonspecific pharmacologic effects. Formal treatment trials of psychopharmacologic agents for this disorder have not been reported. At present, the data are too limited to conclusively identify a specific management approach that is helpful for all patients. Because of the nature and clinical course of the symptom, it may be reasonable to consider functional globus a chronic pain syndrome using nonspecific treatment strategies that are effective in such situations.

Rumination syndrome

Definition and clinical features

Rumination is the remastication and swallowing of regurgitated, recently ingested food. The symptom is not accompanied by nausea or vomiting and generally is a nonbothersome or even satisfying experience [36]. The pattern ceases in most instances once the gastric contents become acidic and unpleasant. These symptoms are sufficiently unique to rumination that the diagnosis is commonly established on clinical grounds. A limited evaluation of the upper gastrointestinal tract is required to exclude a regurgitant disorder mimicking rumination, especially gastroesophageal reflux disease. Other processes that truly mimic rumination are rare.

Rumination occurs in two principal patient groups − in mentally retarded children and in normally developed children and adults. The more severe cases are encountered in the former, whereas rumination has little medical consequence in the latter. A recent household survey suggested that as many as 11% of adult respondents may fulfill criteria for the disorder, yet in this group the complaint is rarely brought to medical attention [24]. In contrast, rumination occurs at a similar rate in institutionalized retarded children, but life-threatening complications (e.g., malnutrition, aspiration pneumonia) are important causes of morbidity and mortality [45].

Potential pathogenetic mechanisms

The mechanism of rumination is better understood than the mechanisms of other functional esophageal disorders. Although classified as esophageal, rumination actually occurs through a complex set of events involving the entire esophagogastric region and abdominal wall [3, 41]. Antiperistaltic esophageal motor events as identified in ruminant animals have not been observed in humans with this syndrome. However, initiating events are similar to those occurring in ruminant animals, including reduction of lower esophageal sphincter pressure and brisk contraction of the abdominal wall [3, 41]. The latter produces synchronous pressure spikes throughout the esophagogastric region on manometric recordings (Fig. 2). Contraction of the abdominal wall muscles and diaphragm appears to be the primary maneuver responsible for the spike configurations, and regurgitation is not the result of a visceral motor aberration [3]. Identifying spike events is not possible nor necessary for diagnosis in the majority of subjects [35].

As the regurgitant forces are provided by coordinated contraction of voluntary muscles, rumination unquestionably results from a central abnormality. The syndrome is suspected as being a learned behavior pattern, and hypotheses regarding the development of this behavior have derived primarily from studies in developmentally normal children. Two principal theories have evolved: one suggesting that rumination is a self-stimulatory behavior pattern resulting from inadequate external gratification (primarily from the mother) and the other presuming a conditioned response maintained by parental attention and the gratifying taste of food [45]. Similar theories may apply to adults with this syndrome, as most indicate that the "habit" has extended from childhood.

Management approaches

A variety of behavioral treatments have been used successfully to stop rumination [38, 42, 44, 45]. Treatment strategies are influenced by both the age of the patient and the degree of mental retardation, if present at all. Aversive, dietary, and differential reinforcement approaches are used in the mentally retarded but not in patients of normal intelligence. Other behavioral approaches successfully

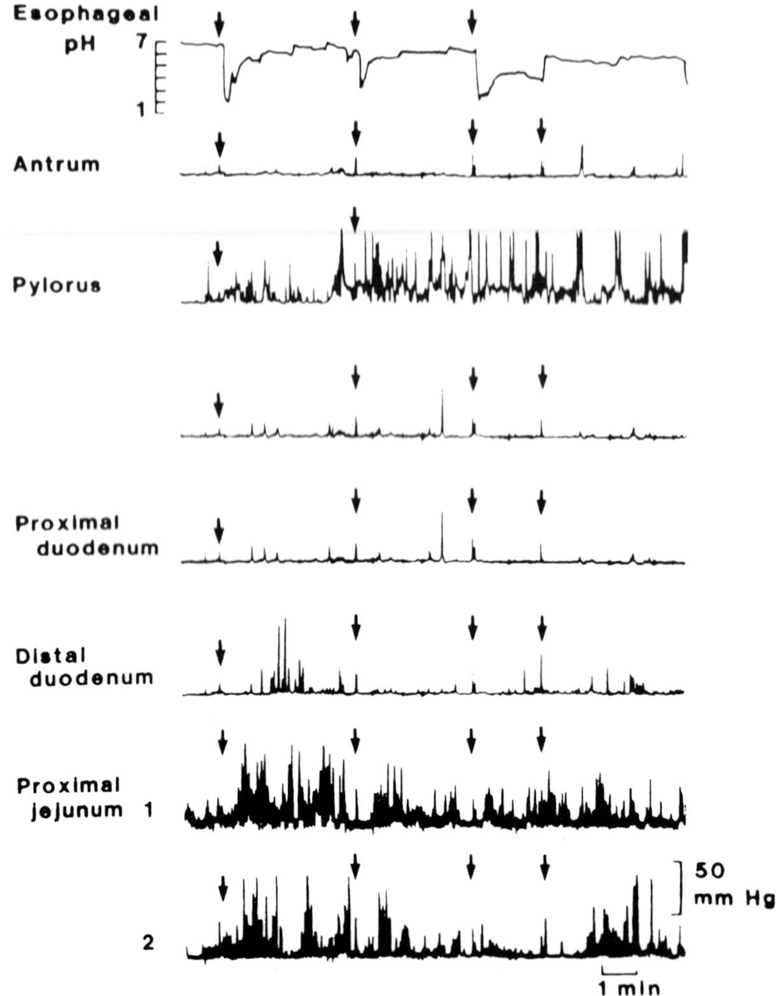

Fig. 2: *Motility recording from the stomach and proximal small intestine in a patient with rumination syndrome. Arrows indicate the synchronous occurrence of pressure spikes on all manometry leads associated with precipitous decreases in esophageal pH. The spikes corresponded with rumination events. From [3].*

improve or eliminate the symptom in the latter groups. For example, biofeedback therapy can be very effective when aimed at stopping postprandial abdominal wall contraction or specific pharyngeal movements that accompany initiation of events [45]. Most of the limited ongoing investigation relates to the appropriate treatment approach in the developmentally retarded.

Functional distal esophageal disorders

Definition and clinical features

Three symptoms arc included under this heading: chest pain, dysphagia, and heartburn. Although each is classified as a distinct functional disorder by the international committee that established current nosology [36], the overlap in presentation is apparent (Tab. 3). Definition for each depends fully on comprehensive exclusion of esophageal and nonesophageal (e. g., cardiac) diseases that produce similar symptoms, as presently there are no characteristic symptom features that establish dependably and reliably a functional basis. The best described within this group is functional esophageal chest pain, as the other disorders occur less commonly as dominant isolated complaints.

Table 3: *The overlapping occurrence of symptoms in patients with functional distal esophageal disorders and nonspecific esophageal manometric abnormalities*.*

	Symptom (% of patients)		
Nonspecific manometric finding	Chest pain	Dysphagia	Heartburn
Increased wave amplitude	79	64	41
Increased wave duration	73	70	56
Double-peaked contraction waves	76	60	44
Triple-peaked waves	71	65	45

* Data extracted from Reidel, W. L., R. E. Clouse: Variations in clinical presentation of patients with esophageal contraction abnormalities. Dig. Dis. Sci. 30 (1985) 1065–1071.

Functional distal esophageal disorders are identified exclusively by symptoms. No physiologic or other clinical test is useful in positively diagnosing subjects other than to exclude confounding disorders with similar presentation. Pathology-based motor disorders (e. g., achalasia, diffuse esophageal spasm) and gastroesophageal reflux disease should be systematically excluded in patients with chest pain, and exclusion of the latter is essential in establishing the diagnosis of functional heartburn. Before establishing the diagnosis of functional dysphagia, structural lesions and pathology-based motility disturbances must be carefully sought. When patients with functional distal esophageal disorders are defined in this fashion, a female predominant group will be identified – at least in the case of functional chest pain where more data are available for establishing the gender ratio [36].

Potential pathogenetic mechanisms

Three types of measurable abnormality are prevalent: (1) disturbances of esophageal motor and sensory function (but not the pathology-based disorders), (2) acid reflux events in association with symptoms (but not gastroesophageal reflux disease), and (3) psychiatric abnormalities. All three have been identified in the chest pain patients, the group in which many studies have been performed examining these assocaitions. The other symptom groups have not been sufficiently studied, but similar associations are likely.

Identified esophageal motility disturbances include the entire group of nonspecific motility disturbances associated with exaggerated contraction [28]. Abnormalities are found in up to 50% of the patients, a rate 2–3 times that present in asymptomatic subjects or comparable controls. An elevation of mean distal contraction amplitude (the "nutcracker esophagus") is the most common manometric diagnosis within the group [28]. The clinical significance of these findings remains debated, but data directly supporting their pathogenetic importance are meager. Some evidence exists that transit of semi-solid liquids may be impaired with these disturbances, and motor disturbances induced with balloon distention in patients with functional dysphagia have seemingly produced symptoms in some subjects at the time of the test [23]. However, the manometric abnormalities correlate poorly with symptoms in cross-sectional and longitudinal studies, and their pharmacologic manipulation has not had a significant impact on symptom reporting [32].

Provocative testing using intraluminal acid perfusion, edrophonium chloride injection, and intraluminal balloon distention as painful stimuli provides evidence for visceral sensory dysfunction in these subjects [30]. Balloon distention studies have been the most productive, with nearly half of chest pain patients reporting symptom reproduction with a low-volume distention stimulus. Less than 10% of matched, asymptomatic control subjects will develop chest pain with the same stimulus [37]. The observation has been reproduced with intragastric distention in subjects with functional dyspepsia and rectal distention in subjects with irritable bowel syndrome [17]. These findings indicate that regional visceral hyperalgesia is a shared feature of many functional gut disorders.

Important data are missing to confirm that visceral hyperalgesia as identified by distention sensitivity is more than an epiphenomenon of the syndromes. For example, a good intrasubject correlation between change in distention sensitivity and change in symptoms has not been demonstrated. Consequently, the reproduction of chest symptoms with intraesophageal balloon distention is not sufficiently sensitive nor specific for the functional esophageal syndromes to be useful as a diagnostic test or to direct therapeutic approaches. The same is true for the nonspecific motility disturbances mentioned above. Refinements in techniques used to measure visceral hyperalgesia may alter these conclusions. From a mechanistic standpoint, the observations may indicate that alterations in motor or sensory physiology within the esophagus participate in an indirect or intermittent fashion in producing the functional symptoms.

The second type of observation with potential pathogenic relevance, particularly for functional chest pain and functional heartburn, is the association of symptoms with acid reflux events. Discrete episodes of chest pain that are distinct from typical reflux symptoms are recognized as an atypical presentation of reflux disease. Consequently, acid reflux events may be important symptom triggers in patients with functional chest pain who have no evidence of reflux disease. In one important study that addressed this issue, Hewson et al. found a potential relationship of chest pain to acid reflux in 60% of subjects who had pain during ambulatory pH monitoring [27]. In the 50% of patients who had normal esophageal acid exposure times and no other evidence of reflux disease, chest pain and acid reflux events were at least partially associated in more than half. Response by this latter group to anti-reflux treatment would strongly support the pathogenetic role of reflux events in functional chest pain, but therapeutic studies are meager [1].

Information regarding the relationship of reflux to other functional distal esophageal disorders is very limited. Also using ambulatory pH monitoring, Baldi and colleagues examined the association of acid reflux events to heartburn episodes in patients with and without evidence of reflux disease [6]. They found a reduction in the percent association as evidence of reflux disease diminished (from overt esophagitis to abnormal acid exposure time to neither of these). Although patients with overt esophagitis had a nearly uniform association of reflux with heartburn, less than 40% of heartburn episodes were preceded by acid reflux in patients with the functional complaint (i. e., no pH-monitoring or endoscopic evidence of reflux disease) [3, 36]. As for functional chest pain, data suggest that acid reflux is an intermittent or partial contributor to functional heartburn but is insufficient to fully explain the genesis of the symptom.

The third type of association established primarily in patients with functional chest pain is with psychiatric disorder. At least 7 studies using defined psychiatric diagnostic criteria demonstrate up to a three-fold increase in psychiatric disorders in patients with noncardiac chest pain compared with control subjects (Tab. 4). The principal increases have been in anxiety and affective disorders. Panic disorder is found in one-third to one-half of patients; major depressive disorder is found in up to 40% of subjects. A psychiatric diagnosis can be established in fully 60−80% [14]. When subjects with nonspecific motility disorders are studied separately, the psychiatric diagnosis rates are similar to those of the entire group that had been unselected by any physiologic marker (Tab. 4) [14]. These observations are paralleled in irritable bowel syndrome, although the rate of panic disorder may be higher in chest pain patients [43]. The psychiatric disorders when present likely have important mechanistic implications and probably participate in bringing the patient to medical attention. Anxiety, affective, and somatization disorders have in common an accentuated aware-

Table 4: *The prevalence of psychiatric diagnoses in patients with functional chest pain[1]).*

Subject group primary enrollment requirement [reference]	Study type[3])	N[4])	Panic disorder	GAD	Major depressive disorder	Any psychiatric diagnosis
					Diagnosis rates, %[2])	
Non-cardiac chest pain patients						
— At time of stress test or cardiac catheterization with no prior heart disease history [20]	Controlled, blinded	49	47 (6)	—	39 (8)	80 (26)
— Following coronary arteriography with no prior heart disease [29]	Controlled, blinded	28	43 (6)	—	36 (4)	79 (26)
— Emergency room visit for chest pain [15]	Uncontrolled	112	47	—	14	—
— Within 24 hours of normal coronary arteriography [8]	Uncontrolled	94	34	—	25	—
— Within 72 hours of emergency room visit for chest pain [48]	Uncontrolled	35	31	23	23	60
— Urgent first admissions for chest pain [31]	Controlled, blinded	19	11 (2)	14 (2)	21 (7)	47 (27)
— In-patient males in India [2]	Controlled, blinded	28	50 (10)	4 (3)	25 (3)	68 (27)
Non-cardiac chest pain patients with esophageal and/or cardiac physiologic abnormalities						
— Vigorous esophageal contraction wave abnormalities [16]	Controlled, blinded	25	36 (8)	—	52 (17)	84 (33)
— Vigorous esophageal contraction wave abnormalities [15]	Uncontrolled	35	3	46	31	71
— Cardiac microvascular dysfunction [39]	Uncontrolled	15	40	33	53	73
— Mitral valve prolapse [12]	Controlled, blinded	10	40 (0)	—	60 (19)	80
— Cardiac microvascular dysfunction, sensitivity to ventricular pacing, and/or esophageal motor dysfunction [11]	Uncontrolled	60	43	—	33	63

[1]) Selected studies in which a structured diagnostic interview was used in conjunction with DSM-III or DSM-IIIR criteria; data from [14].
[2]) Rates for the comparison group are provided in parentheses.
[3]) From the standpoint of psychiatric diagnosis.
[4]) Number subject group.
GAD = generalized anxiety disorder; — = rate not reported.

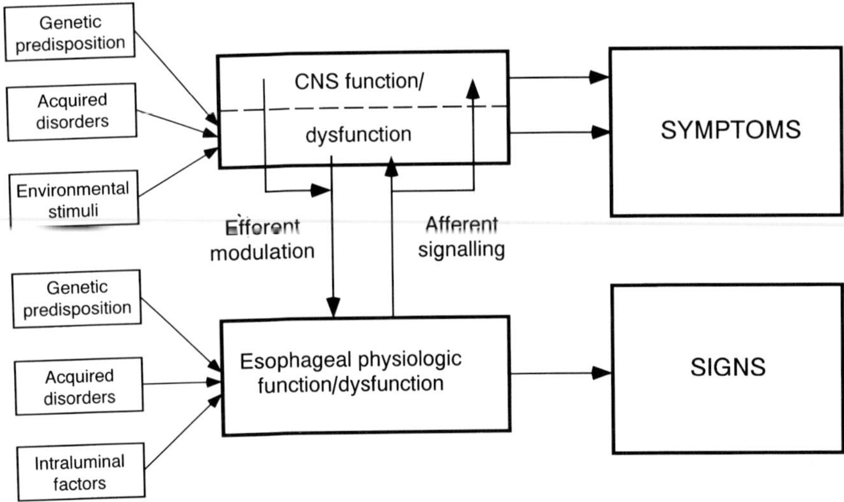

Fig. 3: *A clinical model demonstrating pathways of symptom production that appear operational in functional distal esophageal syndromes. Symptoms presented to the physician derive from the normal reporting of abnormal sensations from the esophagus and from the dysfunctional interpretation and reporting of normal and abnormal visceral signals. Various factors (e. g., genetic, environmental) may be triggers to the types of psychiatric dysfunction encountered in these patients. Visceral triggers include acid reflux and distention events.*

ness of and concern about normal bodily function (as well as minor physical problems) and a tendency to deny or overlook a psychological basis for symptoms or concerns. Long-term outcome in patients with functional chest pain also appears strongly related to psychosocial outcome [14].

Any mechanistic model that is sufficiently comprehensive to include the above associations and additional clinical observation must allow for symptom production from several different paths. The model shown in Fig. 3 indicates that symptom production may result from two important mechanisms: the normal interpretation and reporting of non-pathologic sensations from the esophagus or the abnormal interpretation and reporting of these events. CNS dysfunction from psychiatric disorder can be provoked by a variety of factors and may result in misinterpretation, exaggerated focusing, and enhanced reporting of visceral input.

Management approaches

The management approaches that emanate from clinical investigation and observation are conspicuous. Treatment outcome data are only available presently for chest pain patients. Antireflux therapy provides partial benefit in many patients but complete resolution of symptoms is probably restricted to those with some evidence of reflux disease [1, 40]. Manipulation of nonspecific motility disturbances has been disappointing, and motility-acting agents appear to have limited benefit [32]. Management directed at active co-morbid psychiatric illness results in improvement in chest pain symptoms and functional outcome but not complete symptom resolution. However, because physiologic triggers are often unidentifiable, psychological manipulations move to forefront in many contemporary treatment algorithms.

Treatment strategies aimed specifically at reducing visceral hyperalgesia have not yet been reported for these patients. Two studies have used low-dose antidepressant therapy with positive outcomes [11, 15]. One used the heterocyclic antidepressant trazodone in patients with chest pain and nonspecific motility disorders [15]; the other used a low-dose tricyclic agent (imipramine) in chest pain patients, some of whom had nonspecific cardiac and/or esophageal physiologic abnormalities [11]. Both double-blind studies showed therapeutic efficacy of the antidepressant for chest symptoms, a benefit that was independent of psychiatric effects. Although the findings have been interpreted as indicating a potential reduction in visceral hyperalgesia, physiologic demonstration of this suspicion has not been documented. In fact, symptom response did not correlate with a change in esophageal intraluminal distention sensitivity in the imipramine study [11]. Low-dose antidepressant therapy appears to be one important therapeutic approach in patients with functional distal esophageal disorders, but the mechanism of action remains uncertain.

The most effective treatment undoubtedly varies from patient to patient. It is up to the physician interpreting the patient's complaints to contemplate the paths shown in Fig. 3 when developing a treatment strategy. Attention to active psychiatric disorder or its precipitating factors may be helpful for some patients. For others, treatment of visceral symptom triggers, particularly acid reflux, may be the most satisfying approach. Nonspecific reduction in symptoms using antidepressant therapy in a low-dose range appears useful in a large percentage of the remainder. A similar biopsychosocial treatment approach has been suggested for irritable bowel syndrome. Antidepressant therapy is equally useful in these patients; as many as 80% of patients referred to subspecialists will respond to open-label treatment [17].

Summary

The functional esophageal disorders are a heterogeneous group of syndromes for which, in most cases, the mechanisms remain poorly understood. One uniform concept is that different mechanistic paths may result in expression of the same clinical syndrome. Consequently, versatility in management strategies is important. The distal esophageal syndromes are the most common disorders encountered, wherein both esophageal and central nervous system factors appear important in symptom production. Pharmacologic research directed toward interfering with the projection of visceral input into the cognitive symptom realm provides an exciting prospect for new management approaches.

References

1. Achem, S. R., B. E. Kolts, R. Wears et al.: Chest pain associated with the nutcracker esophagus: a preliminary study of the role of gastroesophageal reflux. Am. J. Gastroenterol. 88 (1993) 187–192.
2. Alexander, P. J., S. G. Prabhu, E. S. Krishnamoorthy et al.: Mental disorders in patients with noncardiac chest pain. Acta Psychiatr. Scandinav. 89 (1994) 291–293.
3. Amarnath, R. P., T. L. Abell, J. R. Malagelada: The rumination syndrome in adults. A characteristic manometric pattern. Ann. Intern. Med. 105 (1986) 513–518.
4. Andreollo, N. A., D. G. Thompson, G. P. Kendall et al.: Functional relationships between cricopharyngeal sphincter and oesophageal body in response to graded intraluminal distension. Gut 29 (1989) 161–166.
5. Ayuso Mateos, J. L., C. Bayon Perez, J. Santo-Domingo Carrasco et al.: Atypical chest pain and panic disorder. Psychother. Psychosom. 52 (1989) 92–95.
6. Baldi, F., F. Ferrarini, A. Longanesi et al.: Acid gastroesophageal reflux and symptom occurrence. Analysis of some factors influencing their association. Dig. Dis. Sci. 34 (1989) 1890–1893.
7. Batch, A. J. G.: Globus pharyngeus (Part I). J. Laryngol. Otol. 102 (1988) 152–158.
8. Beitman, B. D., V. Mukerji, J. W. Lamberti et al.: Panic disorder in patients with chest pain and angiographically normal coronary arteries. Am. J. Cardiol. 63 (1989) 1399–1403.
9. Bishop, L. C., W. T. Riley: The psychiatric management of globus syndrome. Gen. Hosp. Psychiatry 10 (1988) 214–219.
10. Brown, S. R., J. M. Schwartz, P. Summergrad et al.: Globus hystericus syndrome responsive to antidepressants. Am. J. Psychiatry 143 (1986) 917–918.
11. Cannon, R. O., A. A. Quyyumi, R. Mincemoyer et al.: Imipramine in patients with chest pain despite normal coronary angiograms. N. Engl. J. Med. 330 (1994) 1411–1417.
12. Carney, R. M., K. E. Freedland, P. A. Ludbrook et al.: Major depression, panic disorder, and mitral valve prolapse in patients who complain of chest pain. Am. J. Med. 89 (1990) 757–768.
13. Cherry, J., C. I. Siegel, S. I. Margulies et al.: Pharyngeal localization of symptoms of gastroesophageal reflux. Ann. Otol. Rhinol. Laryngol. 79 (1970) 912–914.
14. Clouse, R. E., R. M. Carney: The psychologic profile of non-cardiac chest pain patients. Eur. J. Gastroenterol. Hepatol. 1995, in press.
15. Clouse, R. E., P. J. Lustman, T. C. Eckert et al.: Low-dose trazodone for symptomatic patients with esophageal contraction abnormalities. Gastroenterology 92 (1987) 1027–1036.
16. Clouse, R. E., P. J. Lustman: Psychiatric illness and contraction abnormalities of the esophagus. N. Engl. J. Med. 309 (1983) 1137–1342.
17. Clouse, R. E.: Antidepressants for functional gastrointestinal syndromes. Dig. Dis. Sci. 39 (1994) 2352–2363.
18. Cook, I. J. et al.: Role of mechanical and chemical stimulations of the esophagus in globus sensation. Gastroenterology 96 (1989) A99.
19. Cook, I. J., J. Dent, S. M. Collins: Upper esophageal sphincter tone and reactivity to stress in patients with a history of globus sensation. Dig. Dis. Sci. 34 (1989) 672–676.

20. Cormier, L. E., W. Karon, J. Russo et al.: Chest pain with negative cardiac diagnostic studies. Relationship to psychiatric illness. J. Nerv. Mental Dis. 176 (1988) 351−358.
21. Deary, I. J., J. A. Wilson, M. B. Harris et al.: Globus pharyngis: development of a symptom assessment scale. J. Psychosom. Res. 39 (1995) 203−213.
22. Deary, I. J., J. A. Wilson, L. Mitchell et al.: Covert psychiatric disturbance in patients with globus pharyngis. Br. J. Med. Psychol. 62 (1989) 381−389.
23. Deschner, W. K., K. A. Maher, E. L. Cattau Jr. et al.: Manometric responses to balloon distention in patients with nonobstructive dysphagia. Gastroenterology 97 (1989) 1181−1185.
24. Drossman, D. A., Z. Li, E. Andruzzi et al.: U.S. Householder survey of functional gastrointestinal disorders: prevalence, sociodemography, and health impact. Dig. Dis. Sci. 38 (1993) 1569−1580.
25. Farkkila, M. A., L. Ertama, H. Katila et al.: Globus pharyngis, commonly associated with esophageal motility disorders. Am. J. Gastroenterol. 89 (1994) 503−508.
26. Fraser, A. G.: Review article: gastro-oesophageal reflux and laryngeal symptoms. Aliment Pharmacol. Ther. 8 (1994) 265−272.
27. Hewson, E. G., J. W. Sinclair, C. B. Dalton et al.: Twenty-four hour esophageal pH monitoring: the most useful test for evaluating non-cardiac chest pain. Am. J. Med. 90 (1991) 576−583.
28. Kahrilas, P. J., R. E. Clouse, W. J. Hogan: American Gastroenterological Association technical review on the clinical use of esophageal monometry. Gastroenterology 107 (1994) 1865−1884.
29. Katon, W., M. L. Hall, J. Russo et al.: Chest pain: relationship of psychiatric illness to coronary arteriographic results. Am. J. Med. 84 (1988) 1−9.
30. Katz, P. O., C. B. Dalton, J. E. Richter et al.: Esophageal testing of patients with noncardiac chest pain or dysphagia, results of three years experience with 1161 patients. Ann. Intern. Med. 106 (1987) 593−597.
31. Kisely, S. R., F. H. Creed, L. Cotter: The course of psychiatric disorder associated with non-specific chest pain. J. Psychosom. Res. 36 (1992) 329−335.
32. McCord, G. S., A. Staiano, R. E. Clouse: Achalasia, diffuse spasm and non-specific motor disorders. Bailliere's Clin. Gastroenterol. 5 (1991) 307−335.
33. Moloy, P. J., R. Charter: The globus symptom. Incidence, therapeutic response, and age and sex relationships. Arch. Otolaryngol. 108 (1982) 740.
34. Moser, G., G. V. Vacariu-Granser, C. Schneider et al.: High incidence of esophageal motor disorders in consecutive patients with globus sensation. Gastroenterology 101 (1991) 1512−1522.
35. O'Brien, M. D., B. K. Bruce, M. Camilleri: The rumination syndrome: clinical features rather than manometric diagnosis. Gastroenterology 108 (1995) 1024−1029.
36. Richter, J. E., F. Baldi, R. E. Clouse et al.: Functional esophageal disorders. Gastroenterol. Internat. 5 (1992) 3−17.
37. Richter, J. E., C. F. Barish, D. O. Castell: Abnormal sensory perception in patients with esophageal chest pain. Gastroenterology 91 (1986) 845−852.
38. Rogers, B., P. Stratton, J. Victor et al.: Chronic regurgitation among persons with mental retardation: a need for combined medical and interdisciplinary strategies. Am. J. Mental Retard. 96 (1992) 522−527.
39. Roy-Byrne, P. P., P. Schmidt, R. O. Cannon et al.: Microvascular angina and panic disorder. Int. J. Psych. Med. 19 (1989) 315−325.
40. Singh, S., J. E. Richter, E. G. Hewson et al.: The contribution of gastroesophageal reflux to chest pain in patients with coronary artery disease. Ann. Intern. Med. 117 (1992) 824−830.
41. Smout, A. J., R. Breumelhof: Voluntary induction of transient lower esophageal sphincter relaxations in an adult with the rumination syndrome. Am. J. Gastroenterol. 85 (1990) 1621−1625.
42. Starlin, S. P., R. W. Fuqua: Rumination and vomiting in the developmentally disabled: a critical review of the behavioral, medical, and psychiatric treatment research. Res. Developmental Disabilities 8 (1987) 575−605.

43. Walker, E. A., P. P. Roy-Byrne, W. J. Katon: Irritable bowel syndrome and psychiatric illness. Am. J. Psychiatry 147 (1990) 565−572.
44. Whitehead, W. E., V. M. Drescher, E. Morrill-Corbin et al.: Rumination syndrome in children treated by increased holding. J. Ped. Gastroenterol. Nutr. 4 (1985) 550−556.
45. Whitehead, W. E., M. M. Schuster: Rumination syndrome, vomiting, aerophagia, and belching. In: W. E. Whitehead, M. M. Schuster (Eds.): Gastrointestinal disorders: behavioral and physiological basis for treatment, pp. 67−90. Academic, Orlando Fl. 1985.
46. Wilson, J. A., I. J. Deary, A. G. Maran: The persistence of symptoms in patients with globus pharyngis. Clin. Otolaryngol. 16 (1991) 202−205.
47. Wilson, J. A., A. Pryde, J. Piris et al.: Pharyngoesophageal dysmotility in globus sensation. Arch. Otolaryngol. Head Neck Surg. 115 (1989) 1086−1090.
48. Wulsin, L. R., L. M. Arnold, J. R. Hillard: Axis I disorders in ER patients with atypical chest pain. Int. J. Psych. Med. 21 (1991) 37−46.

Functional dyspepsia

F. Azpiroz

Functional dyspepsia: definition

Functional upper gut diseases are a very common problem in gastroenterology. These patients complain of abdominal symptoms presumably related to the stomach and/or small intestine, but no organic cause can be found by conventional tests. Some of these syndromes are clearly related to a motility disorder. For instance, in the gastroparesis syndrome the stomach is unable to accomplish emptying, which results in gastric stasis [2]. Another syndrome related to a motility disorder is the chronic intestinal pseudoobstruction syndrome. These patients present chronic or recurrent symptoms, chiefly abdominal pain and distension, that resemble a mechanical intestinal obstruction. Here, the intestine is affected by either a myopathy or a neuropathy, and produces a defective propulsion of chyme [20]. There are other functional syndromes related to the upper gut, with clear-cut clinical features, such as the idiopathic cyclic nausea and vomiting syndrome, the rumination syndrome and the aerophagia/belching syndrome, in which the relationship to a motility disorder is unclear [12]. Apart from these relatively well defined syndromes, there is a vast majority of functional patients, usually with less intense and rather unspecific manifestations, categorized as functional dyspepsia. Functional dyspepsia is a common condition characterized by episodic or persistent abdominal symptoms referrable to the upper gut and without any demonstrable structural abnormality by conventional radiological or endoscopic tests [22]. The symptom complex is usually related to feeding and includes epigastric pain, early satiety, fullness, bloating, belching, nausea and vomiting. It is not possible to demonstrate whether the symptoms originate in the upper or lower gut, but dyspeptic symptoms are more suggestive of upper gut dysfunction. Patients with symptoms related to mid/lower gut dysfunction are usually included in the "irritable bowel syndrome" category, although overlaps and mixed upper and lower gut syndromes are relatively frequent.

The motor dysfunction hypothesis

Although functional dyspepsia probably constitutes the symptomatic expression of a heterogeneous group of disorders, there was widespread belief during the past decade that an underlying gastrointestinal motility disturbance was responsible for its manifestations. In these patients evaluation of gastric motility and emptying can be performed by manometric and scintigraphic tests, respectively. The indication of these tests has changed over the past few years as experience has been gained. Patients with functional symptoms, that is, without organic cause, presumably arising from the upper gut, are evaluated when: a) gastric statis is suspected, for instance, when food retention has been evidenced in previous endoscopies, b) in the evaluation of processes that may affect the stomach, such as diabetes, or c) in the presence of severe, chronic and refractory symptoms. The value of these tests in the routine evaluation of other categories of patients with functional dyspepsia is debatable and basically depends on the interpretation of the possible findings. Overall both tests are complementary, and the order of application may depend on the clinical impression. In case of suspected gastroparesis, gastric emptying may be evaluated first, and in other cases, particularly when intestinal motor dysfunction is searched, gastrointestinal manometry seems more appropriate.

Gastrointestinal manometry

Gastrointestinal manometry is performed by means of multilumen tube introduced through the mouth into the intestine. Each lumen of the tube has a terminal opening into the gut at a different level and is connected to a pressure transducer to monitor the intraluminal pressure changes produced by gut contractions. Antrointestinal pressure activity is recorded for 3 hours during fasting. Then the patient ingests a standard solid/liquid meal, and the fed pattern is recorded for the subsequent two postcibal hours [11]. During fasting the upper gut exhibits a cyclical motility pattern, alternating periods of quiescence and periods of activity. The episodes of activity usually originate in the antrum and migrate down into the intestine. However, they may also originate in the proximal intestine, and thus, the antral component may be absent. During the three hours fasting observation period in healthy individuals a complete motor cycle is recorded in most cases, but due to the variability of these events, either more or none may be seen. After the ingestion of the test meal in healthy individuals the cyclic interdigestive activity is interrupted and converted into a fed pattern. The antrum generates phasic pressure waves at a three per minute rhythm, and the intestine develops continuous phasic pressure activity with irregular rhythm for the entire two-hour postcibal study period. Special attention has to be paid to the type of manometric tube used, because antral activity is usually recorded only in the most distal segment of the antrum, close to the pylorus. Hence, reliable assessment of antral activity requires multiple and closely spaced recording sites, for instance 5 ports at 1 cm intervals, located at the antroduodenal junction. Otherwise, oral displacement of the manometric tube will reflect a silent activity and may induce a false impression of hypomotility.

Scintigraphic gastric emptying measurement

Radioscintigraphic measurement of gastric emptying remains the gold standard of quantitative assessment of the emptying function of the stomach [8, 12, 24]. This test consists in the administration to the patients of a meal in which one or several components (usually the aqueous phase and one of the solid components) have been labelled each with a different radioisotopic gamma-emitting marker. An external gamma camera quantifies simultaneously the disappearance of each marker from the stomach. A commonly employed combination of isotopes are ^{99m}Tc to label one of the solid components of the meal and ^{113m}In dissolved into the liquid phase. Once the patient has eaten the meal, images are taken at regular intervals during the postprandial period. There are several technical requisites that must be fulfilled to obtain a reliable evaluation. These include the use of large field of view gamma camera equipment, that obtains radioscintigraphic images encompassing a broad field over the abdomen. It is important also to obtain simultaneously (or sequentially by asking the patient to turn) anterior and posterior images. Taking the geometric average between anterior and posterior activity adequately corrects potential errors caused by posteroanterior motion of the isotope, as material progesses from proximal to distal stomach. Computerized methods for correction of posteroanterior motion, based on a lateral image of the stomach, have been also developed. Corrections for the decay and crossover of the isotopes should be also carefully performed in each detection.

Manometric-scintigraphic findings and interpretation

A considerable proportion of dyspeptic patients, between twenty and forty percent depending on the specific population studied, exhibit postprandial antral hypomotility [4, 21]. Antral hypomotility in these patients is usually characterized by reduced frequency of normal amplitude contractions. Antral motility has to be specifically evaluated during the postprandial period, because postprandial antral hypomotility in dyspeptic patients usually coexists with a normal antral activity during fasting. Normally, the stomach liquefies the meal and empties into the intestine a liquid chyme [10, 13]. Therefore, ingested liquids empty rapidly from the stomach, but solid constituents of the meal are retained by the pyloric sieve until the grinding process is completed. In normal conditions peristaltic antral contractions produce the liquefaction of meal solids. As the peristaltic contraction progresses along the antrum it concentrates solid particles. When the contraction reaches the terminal antrum, the pylorus closes, and the terminal antral contraction against pyloric closure results in a retrograde jet ejection that produces solid fragmentation. Therefore, postprandial antral hypomotility is associated with impaired grinding of solids. The correlation of gastrointestinal motility and gastric emptying in dyspeptic patients shows that antral hypomotility is associated to a certain delay in solid emptying, but with a normal emptying of liquids [8, 18, 24]. The clinical features of functional dyspepsia overlap with the gastroparesis syndrome. However, the patients with grossly abnormal gastric emptying of both solids and liquids demonstrated by scintigraphy fall in the category of true gastroparesis and should not be considered as functional dyspepsia.

Very infrequently patients with dyspeptic-type symptoms, usually with intense and refractory manifestations, may exhibit specific patterns of disorganized motor activity that suggest the existence of a neuropathy of the gut. These intestinal dysmotility patterns are multimorphic and include features such as an abnormal configuration or propagation of the interdigestive period of activity (i. e., simultaneous appearance or retrograde propagation over long intestinal segments), aberrant hypermotility patterns (i. e., bursts of intestinal contractions or sustained activity of an intestinal segment uncoordinated with the rest of the gut), and failure to develop a fed pattern after the meal [11, 20]. Again, once the diagnosis of gut neuropathy is established, the patient should not be considered any longer as functional dyspepsia.

In most patients with functional dyspepsia both manometric and scintigraphic studies are normal. Hence, after extensive series of studies performed over the past decade it has become apparent that the clinical manifestations of functional dyspepsia may not be caused by a motor dysfunction of the gut, because in many patients gastric motility, secretion and emptying are normal [4, 18, 24].

Gastrointestinal responses to stress

As we have seen, gastrointestinal manometry may identify some motility abnormalities in patients with dyspeptic symptoms, but still in most patients the symptoms cannot be explained on the basis of a motor dysfunction. For instance, a discrete antral hypomotility and a slight delay in solid emptying, which are frequent features in dyspepsia, hardly explain the development of epigastric discomfort or even frank pain immediately after ingestion of the meal. A possible explanation for this lack of objective abnormalities could be that gut motor activity in dyspeptic patients is normal during basal conditions, but certain conditions would produce aberrant motor responses. Dyspeptic patients frequently relate their symptoms to stress. Indeed, mental or somatic stress relay at a central level and induce, through a variety of pathways, changes in gastrointestinal motility [19]. Therefore, it has been postulated that these effects of stress may be exaggerated in functional dyspepsia. Subacute stress by transcutaneous nerve stimulation inhibits postprandial antral activity in healthy individuals and induces a picture of antral hypomotility similar to that found in dyspeptic patients. In dyspeptic patients with normal antral motility transcutaneous nerve stimulation produces the same effect, and in those dyspeptic patients with antral hypomotility, transcutaneous nerve stimulation does not induce any further change in antral activity [4]. Hence, antral motility during stress is similar in dyspeptic patients and in healthy subjects. Further studies have shown that other gastric responses to stress are also normal in functional dyspepsia [15].

Gastric tone and accommodation to distension

Manometry exclusively evaluates the phasic motility of the antrum and upper small bowel, but does not evaluate other functions, such as the tonic contraction of the proximal stomach. This type of activity, named gastric tone, has a very important physiological function, because it determines the capacity of the stomach [10, 13]. Indeed, changes in gastric tone accomplish the reservoir function of the stomach, that is, meal reception, temporal storage and progressive intestinal delivery. During ingestion the stomach relaxes to accommodate the meal, and subsequently, a progressive contraction gently squeezes gastric content and produces gastric emptying [16]. Postprandial gastric tone is finely regulated, so that meal-distension of the stomach during gastric accommodation and the gastric emptying process are unperceived. A distortion of this regulation may result in symptomatic perception. Particularly, since dyspeptic symptoms are usually related to meals, they may originate in the process of gastric accommodation, so that physiological distension of the stomach by food ingestion may produce symptomatic perception. This hypothesis was experimentally tested by distending the stomach with an air-filled bag [9, 15]. It was shown that gastric compliance, that is, the response of the stomach to distension, was similar in dyspeptic patients and in healthy controls. However these studies were performed during fasting, and hence, did not exactly reproduce the conditions of meal accommodation. Interestingly these studies found heightened perception of gastric distension in dyspeptic patients: while gastric distension was largely unperceived by healthy individuals, dyspeptic patients developed significant symptoms, similar to those elicited by meals. These data suggested that the symptoms in functional dyspepsia could be related to altered gastric sensitivity, rather than to gastric motor dysfunction.

The visceral hypersensitivity hypothesis

The hypothesis of altered visceral perception as a mechanism of functional gut symptoms spread out in the early nineties and prompted the study of visceral sensitivity, that was so far practically unexplored [14]. The initial results in dyspepsia were confirmed by subsequent studies. Furthermore it was shown that hypersensitivity was not related to Helicobacter pylori. The sensory dysfunction in patients with functional dyspepsia seems restricted to the gut, because somatic sensitivity, both to the cold pressure test and to transcutaneous electrical nerve stimulation, is normal in these patients [5, 15]. However it still remains unclear whether the small intestine is also affected. Increased gastric but normal duodenal sensitivity was shown in a specific subset of dyspeptic patients predominantly complaining of postcibal bloating, i. e., the bloating syndrome [5]. These patients invariably recognized that gastric distension, but not duodenal distension, reproduced their customary symptoms. By contrast, other studies have reported increased perception of intestinal distension in patients with functional dyspepsia [6, 7]. Patients with functional dyspepsia are heterogeneous and different criteria for definition and selection of the patients could possibly explain the conflicting data. Many dyspeptic patients also manifest symptoms of the irritable bowel syndrome, and it has been shown that patients with the irritable bowel syndrome exhibit hypersensitivity of the small intestine [1].

Some data indicate that altered perception in dyspepsia is associated to a dysfunction of gut reflexes. Duodenal distension in healthy subjects induces perception and stimulus-related gastric relaxation. Both responses are independently induced by specific mechanisms [3]. In dyspeptic patients both duodenal sensitivity and compliance are normal, but duodenal distension induces impaired relaxation of the stomach [5]. Canine studies have shown that this is a vagal reflex mediated by a nonadrenergic, noncholinergic mechanism similar to the reflexes that control gastric tone by the nutrient composition of chyme in the small intestine [10, 13]. It has been also reported that other reflexes, such as sympathetic intestinointestinal reflexes, that inhibit intestinal motor activity in response to distension, may be also impaired in dyspepsia [6, 7]. The concomitant dysfunction of sensory and reflex pathways in patients with dyspepsia may be due to a process that affects the stomach wall, and produces both hypersensitivity and hyporeactivity without disturbing central efferent pathways or compliance. Alternatively, the sensory and reflex dysfunctions may be explained on the basis of a multifocal or diffuse gut neuropathy.

Putative clinical implications of sensory-reflex dysfunctions

The clinical relevance of these sensory-reflex disturbances is still unclear. Dyspeptic patients with significant symptoms after meals exhibit discomfort at lower levels of gastric distension than healthy controls, but the differences are relatively small. Meal ingestion involves a larger number of intraluminal stimuli, which may recruit a pool of altered signals in dyspeptic patients, and thus, produce symptomatic perception. Furthermore, ingestion induces a relaxation of the proximal stomach to accommodate the meal without increments in intragastric pressure [16]. A gastric hyporeactivity to enterogastric reflexes would predictably result in a defective accommodation of the proximal stomach and antral overload. Indeed, reduced fundal residency and increased antral filling has been reported in patients with functional dyspepsia [23].

Inpaired meal accommodation could potentiate the hypersensitivity to distension, because the stomach tolerates smaller volumes when not properly relaxed [17]. Distension of the stomach with an air-filled bag in healthy subjects produces symptoms that resemble those reported by dyspeptic patients after meal ingestion. At the same intragastric volumes, the intragastric pressures and the intensity of perception are lower when the stomach is relaxed, for instance by intravenous glucagon, than when the stomach is contracted. Further experimental data indicate that increased intragastric pressure after a meal, simulating a defective gastric accommodation, produces dyspeptic-type symptoms without disturbing gastric emptying [16], a condition that resembles most patients with functional dyspepsia [8, 18, 24]. Hence, it is plausible that the gastric hyporeflexia exacerbates the poor tolerance of dyspeptics to intragastric volumes, and thus, contributes to generation of clinical symptoms in the absence of major motor dysfunctions. Altered reflex activity and altered conscious perception of gut stimuli may combine to different degrees, and this may explain the heterogeneity of dyspepsia.

Conclusion

Functional dyspepsia includes an heterogeneous group of patients. In some patients manometric abnormalities can be found, but still in most cases the cause of the symptoms remains obscure. Recent data suggest that dyspeptic symptoms may be related to subtle forms of gastric dysfunction, such as visceral hypersensitivity and abnormal reflex reactivity, that still remain to be characterized.

References

1. Accarino, A. M., F. Azpiroz, J.-R. Malagelada: Selective dysfunction of mechanosensitive intestinal afferents in the irritable bowel syndrome. Gastroenterology 108 (1995) 636−643.
2. Azpiroz, F., J.-R. Malagelada: Gastric tone measured by an electronic barostat in health and postsurgical gastroparesis. Gastroenterology 92 (1987) 934−943.

3. Azpiroz, F., J.-R. Malagelada: Perception and reflex relaxation of the stomach in response to gut distention. Gastroenterology 98 (1990) 1193−1198.

4. Camilleri, M., J.-R. Malagelada, P. C. Kao et al.: Gastric and autonomic responses to stress in functional dyspepsia. Dig. Dis. Sci. 31 (1986) 1169−1177.

5. Coffin, B., F. Azpiroz, J.-R. Malagelada: Selective gastric hypersensitivity and reflex hyporeactivity in functional dyspepsia. Gastroenterology 107 (1994) 1345−1351.

6. Greydanus, M. P., M. Vassalo, M. Camilleri et al.: Neurohormonal factors in functional dyspepsia: insights on pathophysiological mechanisms. Gastroenterology 100 (1991) 1311−1318.

7. Holtmann, G., J. Hüber, H. Fisher et al.: Functional dyspepsia: a sensory duodenal defect with impaired intestinointestinal reflexes. Gastroenterology 106 (1994) A511.

8. Jian, R., F. Ducrot, A. Ruskone et al.: Symptomatic, radionuclide and therapeutic assessment of chronic idiopathic dyspepsia. A double-blind placebo-controlled evaluation of cisapride. Dig. Dis. Sci. 34 (1989) 657−664.

9. Lémann, M., J. P. Dederding, B. Flourie et al.: Abnormal perception of visceral pain in response to gastric distension in chronic idiopathic dyspepsia. The irritable stomach. Dig. Dis. Sci. 36 (1991) 1249−1254.

10. Malagelada. J.-R., F. Azpiroz: Determinants of gastric emptying and transit in the small intestine. In: S. G. Schultz, J. D. Wood, B. B. Rauner (Eds.): Handbook of Physiology. Section 6: The Gastrointestinal System. Vol. 1: Motility and Circulation, 2nd ed, pp. 909−937. Bethesda MD, Am. Physiol. Soc. 1989.

11. Malagelada, J.-R., M. Camilleri, V. Stanghellini: Manometric diagnosis of gastrointestinal motility disorders. Thieme−Stratton, New York 1986.

12. Malagelada, J.-R., F. Azpiroz, F. Mearin: Gastroduodenal motor function in health and disease. In: M. H. Sleisenger, J. S. Fordtran (Eds.): Gastrointestinal Disease: Pathophysiology, Diagnosis, Management. Vol. 4, 5th ed, pp. 486−508. PA Saunders, Philadelphia 1993.

13. Mayer, E. A.: The physiology of gastric storage and emptying. In: L. R. Johnson (Ed.): Physiology of the Gastrointestinal Tract, Vol. 1, 3rd ed, pp. 929−976. Raven, New York 1994.

14. Mayer, E. A., H. E. Raybould: Role of visceral afferent mechanisms in functional bowel disorders. Gastroenterology 99 (1990) 1688−1704.

15. Mearin, F., M. Cucala, F. Azpiroz et al.: The origin of symptoms on the brain-gut axis in functional dyspepsia: Gastroenterology 101 (1991): 999−1006.

16. Moragas, G., F. Azpiroz, J. Pavía et al.: Relations among intragastric pressure, postcibal perception and gastric emptying. Am. J. Physiol. 264 (1993) G1112−G1117.

17. Notivol, R., B. Coffin, F. Azpiroz et al.: Gastric tone determines the sensitivity of the stomach to distension. Gastroenterology 108 (1995) 330−336.

18. Scott, A. M., J. E. Kellow, B. Shuter et al.: Intragastric distribution and gastric emptying of solids and liquids in functional dyspepsia. Dig. Dis. Sci. 38 (1993) 2247−2254.

19. Stanghellini, V., J.-R. Malagelada, A. R. Zinsmeister et al.: Effect of opiate and adrenergic blockers on the gut motor response to centrally acting stimuli. Gastroenterology 87 (1984) 1104−1113.

20. Stanghellini, V., M. Camilleri, J.-R. Malagelada: Chronic idiopathic intestinal pseudoobstruction: clinical and intestinal manometric findings. Gut 28 (1987) 5−12.

21. Stanghellini, V., C. Ghidini, M. R. Maccarini et al.: Fasting and postprandial gastrointestinal motility in ulcer and non-ulcer dyspepsia. Gut 33 (1992) 184−190.

22. Talley, N. J., B. Colin-Jones, M. Koch et al.: Functional dyspepsia: A classification with guidelines for diagnosis and management. Gastroenterol. Int. 4 (1991) 145−160.

23. Troncon, L. E. A., R. J. M. Bennett, N. K. Ahluwalia et al.: Abnormal intragastric distribution of food during gastric emptying in functional dyspepsia. Gastroenterology 102 (1992) A528.

24. Tucci, A., R. Corinaldesi, V. Stanghellini et al.: Helicobacter pylori infection and gastric function in patients with chronic idiopathic dyspepsia. Gastroenterology 103 (1992) 768−774.

Functional bowel disorders:
are they independent diagnoses?

W. E. Whitehead

International consensus committees have defined a variety of functional bowel disorders (e. g., irritable bowel syndrome, functional constipation, functional diarrhea, functional bloating, chronic abdominal pain) and functional anorectal disorders (e. g., functional incontinence, levator ani syndrome, proctalgia fugax, and pelvic floor dyssynergia) [9]. However, it remains controversial whether these are distinct syndromes or disorders. This paper will summarize the diagnostic criteria, epidemiology, and pathophysiological mechanisms for each of these functional bowel and anorectal disorders. Following these brief descriptions, the evidence for and against these being distinct disorders will be discussed.

Irritable bowel syndrome (IBS)

Diagnosis: According to the Rome definition [25], the symptom criteria for IBS are abdominal pain which is relieved by defecation or associated with a change in the frequency or consistency of stools, plus two or more of a list of 5 other symptoms: altered stool frequency, altered stool form, dyschezia or urgency, passage of mucus, and bloating. The symptoms which make up this list are derived from the early study by Manning and colleagues [19], who identified 6 symptoms which were significantly more common in patients with a clinical diagnosis of IBS than in patients with organic gastrointestinal disorders. The utility of the Manning criteria was supported by a number of subsequent investigations [26, 4, 22, 23]. However, the diagnosis of IBS also requires the exclusion of alternative diagnoses which could explain the symptoms, in addition to the presence of the symptoms enumerated above.

Epidemiology: Using the Rome criteria [25], the prevalence of IBS is estimated to be 9.4% of U.S. adults [7]. In Western countries, it is more common in women than in men by approximately 2 : 1, although the gender difference may be reversed in some Asian societies. In the United States, the prevalence is similar in Caucasian and African-American ethnic/racial groups [24].

Possible mechanisms: None is proved. Suggestions include (a) altered small bowel motility (discrete clustered contractions, giant ileal contractions) [15, 14], (b) increased reactivity (i. e. exaggerated stimulation of contractions in both small [16] and large intestines [31] to stress, eating, or other provocative stimuli; (c) visceral hyperalgesia [20]; and (d) somatization disorder (i. e., a psychological tendency to interpret normal somatic sensations as symptoms of disease).

Functional bloating

Diagnosis: This diagnosis may be made on the basis of symptoms of abdominal fullness, bloating, or distension unrelated to obvious maldigestion or other gastrointestinal disease, in patients not meeting criteria for IBS, functional dyspepsia, or any other functional disorder [25]. In Great Britain, bloating is regarded as a hallmark symptom of IBS [13], although in the United States and Canada, it is less frequently associated with IBS. Factor analytic studies [24] suggest that, in the U.S. at least, bloating is a syndrome which is distinct from IBS.

Epidemiology: In the U.S. Householder study [7], 32.1% met the symptom criteria for functional bloating. This is far too high to be meaningful as an estimate of morbidity and suggests that the diagnostic criteria require refinement.

Possible mechanisms: None is proved. Suggestions include: (a) slowed intestinal transit [17], (b) hyperalgesia, and (c) increased intestinal gas attributable to carbohydrate malabsorption or aerophagia [12].

Functional constipation

Diagnosis: The Rome criteria [25] define functional constipation as two or more of three symptoms (straining, passing hard stools, or feeling of incomplete evacuation on 25% of bowel movements), or a stool frequence of ≤ 2/week, in patients not meeting criteria for IBS. This definition does not make any distinction between colonic inertia and pelvic floor dyssynergia although they are believed to be distinct types of constipation based on physiological investigations. Moreover, pelvic floor dyssynergia appears to be included in the definition of functional constipation even though the Rome criteria treat it as a distinct functional disorder [30]. As a consequence, there is an almost complete overlap between type of functional constipation and pelvic floor dyssynergia.

Epidemiology: Three percent of adults [7], but a much higher proportion of elderly people meet criteria for functional constipation. In young adults, the prevalence is much greater in women than in men [11].

Possible mechanisms: Constipation may be due to any of three factors: decreased numbers of peristaltic contractions in the colon (colonic inertia) [2], increased numbers of non-peristaltic contractions in the sigmoid colon [5], or failure of the pelvic floor muscles to relax during defecation (pelvic floor dyssynergia) [21]. Good physiological data support the existence of each of these subtypes of constipation, but the extent to which different subtypes of constipation covary is not known.

Functional diarrhea

Diagnosis: The Rome criteria [25] are two or more of three symptoms, unformed (mushy or watery) stools more than ¾ of the time, ≥ 3 BMs per day, or increased stool weight, in patients who do not meet criteria for IBS. Other causes of diarrhea (e.g., carbohydrate malabsorption, bacterial or parasitic infection, secretory disorders) should be excluded.

Epidemiology: Two to 4% of adults [7] meet the criteria for functional diarrhea. It is slightly more common in males than in females.

Possible mechanisms: None is proved. Increased numbers of peristaltic contractions throughout the colon [3] and decreased numbers of segmental (non-peristaltic) contractions in the sigmoid region of the colon have been suggested.

Functional abdominal pain

Diagnosis: All of the following symptom criteria must be met, according to the Rome criteria [25]: frequent or continuous abdominal pain for at least 6 months, incomplete or no relationship of pain to physiological events such as eating or defecation, impairment of daily functioning, absence of any organic disease explanation, and failure to satisfy criteria for other functional gastrointestinal diagnoses.

Epidemiology: Approximately 1.2% of adults [7]. Women outnumber men 2:1.

Possible mechanisms: These are primarily psychological rather than physiological. Contributing psychological factors may include (a) a history of psychosocial trauma often including physical or sexual abuse [8], (b) inadequate social support, (c) Axis I psychiatric disorder or Axis II personality disorder, and (d) a pattern of abnormal illness behavior characterized by preoccupation with illness and disability disproportionate to physical findings [29].

Functional incontinence

Diagnosis: Functional fecal incontinence may be defined [30] as uncontrolled passage of fecal material in an individual over 3 years of age, associated with fecal impaction, megarectum, or megacolon. This definition excludes fecal incontinence which is due to weakness of the external anal sphincter, loss of ability to perceive rectal distension, decreased rectal compliance, and incontinence secondary to diarrhea.

Epidemiology: In adults, the overall prevalence of fecal incontinence is 6.9% for soiling and 0.3% for gross incontinence [7]. Functional fecal incontinence (as defined above) is rare in young adults but affects 1.5% of children and a significant number of elderly people. Functional fecal incontinence associated with constipation accounts for 96% of the fecal soiling seen in children [18] and for a significant but undefined proportion of fecal incontinence in elderly patients.

Possible mechanisms: Constipation with the development of a fecal impaction and subsequent overflow around a fecal mass is believed to be the cause of functional fecal incontinence [18]. Pelvic floor dyssynergia (anismus) may be responsible for the constipation in 30–50%.

Levator ani syndrome

Diagnosis: Chronic or recurrent rectal pain or aching, with episodes lasting 20 min or longer, in the absence of organic disease which could account for the pain [30]. The pain is usually worse with sitting. It is typically described as a dull ache or as muscle soreness. A sensation of burning or stinging suggests a different etiology.

Epidemiology: Levator ani syndrome occurs in 6.0% of adults, and is more common in women than in men [7].

Possible mechanisms: None is proven, but chronically tense pelvic floor muscles are believed to be responsible for the pain [30].

Proctalgia fugax

Diagnosis: Anal or rectal pain lasting for seconds to minutes and then disappearing for days to months, in the absence of organic disease to account for these symptoms [30]. *Epidemiology*: It is present in 7.9% of the population [7], but very few people with this syndrome consult physicians. *Possible mechanisms*: None is proved, but speculations have included tense pelvic floor muscles and rectal spasm [30].

Pelvic floor dyssynergia

Diagnosis: The Rome criteria for this diagnosis [30] are straining or feeling of incomplete evacuation or digital facilitation on at least 25% of bowel movements (i. e. dyschezia), plus EMG, manometric, or radiological evidence for inappropriate contraction or failure to relax the pelvic floor muscles during attempts to defecate. Organic disease explanations for these symptoms should be excluded.

Epidemiology: The estimated prevalence of dyschezia is 13.1% [7], but the prevalence of pelvic floor dyssynergia in the community is unknown because the diagnosis requires physiological investigations. It is estimated that this disorder accounts for 30−50% of patients with chronic constipation, although there is concern that there may be many false positive diagnoses due to the reluctance of patients to risk passing fecal material or flatus in the examining room [10].

Mechanism: Paradoxical contraction (or failure to relax) the pelvic floor muscles during defecation is believed to be a learned maladaptive response, which may have been motivated initially by a desire to avoid painful defecation of large, hard stools [30]. Increased pelvic floor muscle tension secondary to generalized anxiety has also been suggested, but not proven, to contribute to the etiology of pelvic floor dyssynergia [27]).

Are the functional bowel and anorectal disorders distinct syndromes?

This question has been approached from two perspectives: The first is to look at the extent to which people receive overlapping diagnoses, e. g., both functional dyspepsia and irritable bowel syndrome (IBS). The second approach is factor analysis.

Symptom covariation

Table 1 shows the co-occurrence of the functional bowel disorders in the U.S. Householder Survey [7]. As expected, the distinction between functional constipation and dyschezia is not supportable since 96.5% of people with chronic constipation also satisfied criteria for dyschezia. The proportion of people with IBS who satisfy criteria for functional anorectal pain (34.3%) and dyschezia (42.4%) is also greater than what would be expected by the base rates of these disorders in the community, but approximately ⅔ of IBS patients do not have these functional anorectal disorders. The three major types of functional anorectal disorders, incontinence, proctalgia, and dyschezia, appear to be relatively

Table 1: *Overlap in diagnoses of functional bowel disorders and anorectal disorders: diagnostic criteria based on [25] and [30]. Data from the U.S. Householder Survey [7].*

	Irritable bowel syndrome	Fecal incontinence	Anorectal pain	Dyschezia
Irritable bowel syndrome	–	21.1	34.3	42.4
Functional constipation	–	12.2	23.4	96.5
Fecal incontinence	30.2	–	27.6	26.2
Functional anorectal pain	33.1	18.6	–	37.0
Dyschezia	38.9	16.8	35.3	–
Population prevalence	11.6	7.8	11.6	13.8

independent. Although not shown in Table 1, the proportion of people meeting symptom criteria for dyspepsia who also satisfy criteria for IBS was 37.6%, and the proportion of people with IBS who satisfy criteria for dyspepsia was 28.4%. These rates are higher than the population prevalence of these disorders, but they suggest that there is a useful distinction to be made between these symptom syndromes.

One must interpret data on overlapping diagnoses cautiously since there may be logical reasons for symptom co-occurrence. For example, watery diarrhea and the type of fecal incontinence which is associated with sphincter weakness tend to covary (see Table 1) even though the physiological mechanisms for these two disorders are quite different. The explanation in this case is that a weak sphincter muscle will be adequate in a constipated patient, and conversely, a strong external anal sphincter may be overwhelmed by large-volume secretory diarrhea, leading to fecal incontinence. In the gastrointestinal tract, there is literally only one common pathway, and this fact can lead to symptom covariation.

Factor analysis

Factor analysis is a statistical technique which allows one to determine whether symptoms cluster together in distinct patterns when large numbers of people are asked to report on their gastrointestinal symptoms. The definition of a factor is very similar to the definition of a syndrome in clinical medicine or psychiatry: a syndrome is a cluster of symptoms and signs which tend to covary across individuals. Such covariation may suggest a common underlying mechanism where none has been identified. Based on the similarity between the definition of a factor and a syndrome, we (Whitehead, Crowell, et al. 1990) have argued that factor analysis can be used: (a) to identify symptom syndromes

	Students				Adults	
	Males	Fems	Caucas	Afro Am	Church	P. P.
Manning symptoms						
Loose BM, pain onset	X	X	X	X	X	X
Frequent BM, pain onset	X	X	X	X	X	X
Pain relieved by BM	X	X	X	X	X	X
Bloating	X				X	
Incomplete evacuation						
Mucus						
Other symptoms						
Food reactions		X	X		X	X
Rectal bleeding	X					
Abdominal pain						X
Diarrhea						X
Reaction to milk					X	

Fig. 1: *Replicability of the IBS factor in multiple samples of subjects differing in age, race, and gender. Undergraduate students from the University of Alabama at Birmingham (average age 21.3 years) were divided into groups of 516 males and 828 females which were analyzed separately. The students were separately divided into groups of 982 caucasians and 362 African Americans which were analyzed separately. The adult samples consisted of 149 women (average age 46.7 years) recruited from church women's groups and 351 young women (average age 25.9 years) recruited from Planned Parenthood Clinics in Baltimore and Annapolis, Maryland. A core set of three symptoms loaded on the IBS factor in each subsample studied. Gastrointestinal reactions to eating also loaded on the IBS factor in most of these samples.*

constituting functional gastrointestinal disorders, and (b) to identify which symptoms can best be used to diagnose these disorders. If the same symptoms cluster together in several different samples of subjects, it is reasonable to assume that there is a common underlying pathophysiological or psychological mechanism to explain these symptoms.

Our group has conducted multiple factor analytic studies [28, 24, 6, 32] which allowed us to look at the stability of symptom clusters across different gender and socioeconomic groups. The first two studies were based on a questionnaire containing 22 bowel symptoms. We found distinct symptom clusters representing IBS, functional constipation, and functional bloating across multiple samples (Fig. 1), but we did not see clusters corresponding to the anorectal disorders because the symptom questionnaire used in this study did not include symptoms relevant to these disorders. However, when we applied factor analysis to the data from the U.S. Householder study [32], which included a more comprehensive symptom questionnaire, we found 12 separate factors with eigenvalues greater than 1.0. The data for factors corresponding to functional bowel disorders and functional anorectal disorders may be summarized as follows:

1. The Rome criteria for IBS include a block of 3 symptoms which loaded strongly on one factor, plus 9 other symptoms which load uniformly low on this factor and were distributed among several other factors. The first 3 symptoms are nearly identical to the three Manning symptoms which consistently formed an IBS factor in our other factor analysis studies [28, 24, 6]. Thus, factor analysis supports the first three symptoms listed by the Rome committee [25] as diagnostic of IBS, but suggests that the remaining 9 symptoms are so strongly associated with other syndromes as to be of limited diagnostic value.

2. The symptoms making up the Rome criteria [25, 30] for the diagnoses of functional constipation, functional diarrhea, chronic abdominal pain, bloating, and fecal incontinence formed separate factors which generally agree well with and therefore support the categories set up by the Rome committees.

3. Functional anorectal pain was represented by two symptoms both of which loaded strongly on a single factor. This represents good agreement with the Rome criteria. However, levator ani and proctalgia fugax did not form independent factors, in part because each was represented by only a single question in the survey questionnaire.

4. The Rome criteria for dyschezia were represented by two symptoms, straining and incomplete evacuation, both of which loaded with other symptoms of constipation. The Rome working team recognized that there was overlap between the criteria for functional constipation and the criteria for dyschezia, but nevertheless created separate diagnoses. The factor analysis results demonstrate that this decision is untenable.

A recently published paper by Agreus and colleagues [1] reports a failure to replicate our finding of a distinct IBS factor in two published and two unpublished studies. However, there are differences in experimental design and data analysis which may explain this inconsistency. Agreus and colleagues did not include two of the three symptoms which we found to consistently cluster together to form the IBS factor. Moreover, they did not report the details of their analyses (i. e., the eigenvalues and factor loadings) to allow the reader to judge for himself whether there was a meaningful clustering of symptoms into syndromes.

Summary and conclusions

Committees of experts have defined 5 distinct functional bowel disorders [25] and 4 distinct functional anorectal disorders [30], along with symptom criteria for their diagnosis. These disorders are prevalent and are economically important since they account for a substantial number of physician visits each year. Physiological mechanisms have been suggested for some of these disorders, but there continues to be controversy about whether they are distinct syndromes. A careful examination of the overlap in diagnoses suggests that the co-occurrence of these functional gastrointestinal disorders is 2−3 times what would be expected by chance, but in most cases, the overlap is not strong enough to suggest that the disorders have a common etiology. However, there is too much overlap between dyschezia and functional constipation to suggest that these are distinct entities. Studies employing factor analysis generally lead to similar conclusions: Distinct clusters of symptoms corresponding to IBS, functional bloating, and functional constipation have been found in multiple independent samples, and a study using a more comprehensive questionnaire also found separate clusters of symptoms corresponding to functional diarrhea, fecal incontinence, and proctalgia.

References

1. Agreus, L., K. Svardsudd, O. Nyren et al.: Irritable bowel syndrome and dyspepsia in the general population: Overlap and lack of stability over time. Gastroenterology 109 (1995) 671−680.
2. Bassotti, G., M. Gaburri, B. P. Imbimbo et al.: Colonic mass movements in idiopathic chronic constipation. Gut 29 (1988) 1173−1179.
3. Bazzocchi, G., J. Ellis, J. Villanueva-Meyer et al.: Effect of eating on colonic motility and transit in patients with functional diarrhea. Simultaneous scintigraphic and manometric evaluations. Gastroenterology 101 (1991) 1298−1306.
4. Bolin, T. D., A. E. Davis, V. M. Duncombe: A prospective study of persistent diarrhoea. Australian & New Zealand J. Med. 12 (1981) 22−26.
5. Connell, A. M.: The motility of the pelvic colon. II. Paradoxical motility in diarrhoea and constipation. Gut 3 (1962) 342−348.
6. Cook, E. W. III., E. Taub, J. L. Cuevas et al.: Factor analysis of bowel symptoms: replication in 2,045 students. Gastroenterology 104 (1993) A492.
7. Drossman, D. A., Z. Li, E. Andruzzi et al.: U.S. Householder Survey of Functional Gastrointestinal Disorders: Prevalence, Sociodemography, and health impact. Dig. Dis. Sci. 38 (1993) 1569−1580.
8. Drossman, D. A., J. Leserman, G. Nachman et al.: Sexual and physical abuse in women with functional or organic gastrointestinal disorders. Annal Int. Med. 113 (1990) 828−833.
9. Drossman, D. A., J. E. Richter, N. J. Talley et al. (Eds.): The Functional Gastrointestinal Disorders. Little, Brown, & Co, Boston 1994.
10. Duthie, G. S., D. C. C. Bartolo: Anismus: The cause of constipation? Results of investigation and treatment. World J. Sur. 16 (1992) 831−835.
11. Everhart, J. E., V. L. W. Go, R. S. Johannes et al.: A longitudinal survey of self-reported bowel habits in the United States. Dig. Dis. Sci. 34 (1989) 1153−1162.
12. Haderstorfer, B., W. E. Whitehead, M. M. Schuster: Intestinal gas production from bacterial fermentation of undigested carbohydrate in irritable bowel syndrome. Am. J. Gastroenterol. 84 (1989) 375−378.
13. Heaton, K. W., L. J. D. O'Donnell, F. E. M. Braddon et al.: Symptoms of irritable bowel syndrome in a British urban community: Consulters and nonconsulters. Gastroenterology 102 (1992) 1962−1967.

14. Kellow, J. E., R. C. Gill, D. L. Wingate: Prolonged ambulant recordings of small bowel motility demonstrate abnormalities in the irritable bowel syndrome. Gastroenterology 98 (1990) 1208–1218.
15. Kellow, J. E., S. F. Phillips: Altered small bowel motility in irritable bowel syndrome is correlated with symptoms. Gastroenterology 92 (1987) 1885–1893.
16. Kellow, J. E., S. F. Phillips, L. J. Miller et al.: Dysmotility of the small intestine in irritable bowel syndrome. Gut 29 (1988) 1236–1243.
17. Lasser, R. B., J. H. Bond, M. D. Levitt: The role of intestinal gas in functional abdominal pain. N. Engl. J. Med 293 (1975) 524–526.
18. Levine, M. D.: Children with encopresis: A descriptive analysis. Pediatrics 56 (1975) 412–416.
19. Manning, A. P., W. G. Thompson, K. W. Heaton et al.: Towards positive diagnosis of the irritable bowel. Br. Med. J. 2 (1978) 653–654.
20. Mertz, H., B. Naliboff, J. Munakata et al.: Altered rectal perception is a biological marker of patients with irritable bowel syndrome. Gastroenterology 109 (1995) 40–52.
21. Preston, D. M., J. E. Lennard-Jones: Anismus in chronic constipation. Dig. Dis. Sci. 30 (1985) 413–418.
22. Smith, R. D., D. S. Greenbaum, J. B. Vancouver et al.: Gender differences in Manning criteria in the irritable bowel syndrome. Gastroenterology 100 (1991) 591–595.
23. Talley, N. J., S. F. Phillips, L. J. Melton et al.: Diagnostic value of the Manning criteria in irritable bowel syndrome. Gut 31 (1990) 77–81.
24. Taub, E. et al.: Gastrointestinal syndromes defined by factor analysis: Gender and race comparisons. Dig. Dis. Sci., in press.
25. Thompson, W. G., F. Creed, D. A. Drossman et al.: Functional bowel disease and functional abdominal pain. Gastroenterology International 5 (1992) 75–91.
26. Thompson, W. G., K. W. Heaton: Functional bowel disorders in apparently healthy people. Gastroenterology 79 (1980) 283–288.
27. Whitehead, W. E.: Illness behaviour. In: M. A. Kamm, J. E. Lennard-Jones (Eds.): Constipation, pp. 95–100. Wrightson Biomedical Pub. Ltd., Petersfield, UK 1994.
28. Whitehead, W. E., M. D. Crowell, L. Bosmajian et al.: Existence of irritable bowel syndrome supported by factor analysis of symptoms in two community samples. Gastroenterology 98 (1990) 336–340.
29. Whitehead, W. E., M. D. Crowell, B. R. Heller et al.: Modeling and reinforcement of the sick role during childhood predicts adult illness behavior. Psychosomatic Medicine 56 (1994) 541–550.
30. Whitehead, W. E., G. Devroede, F. I. Habib et al.: Functional disorders of the anorectum. Gastroenterol. Int. 5 (1992) 92–108.
31. Whitehead, W. E., B. Holtkotter, P. Enck et al.: Tolerance for rectosigmoid distention in irritable bowel syndrome. Gastroenterology 98 (1990) 1187–1192.
32. Whitehead, W. E., Z. Li, D. Drossman et al.: Factor analysis of GI symptoms supports Rome criteria for functional GI disorders. Gastroenterology 106 (1994) A589.

Functional bladder disorders

R. J. Opsomer

Introduction

The lower urinary tract comprises the distal part of the ureters, the urinary bladder, the bladder neck and the urethra. While the ureters, bladder, bladder neck and proximal urethra have an autonomic innervation (sympathetic and parasympathetic fibres), the distal urethra and the pelvic floor have a somatic innervation. The sympathetic fibres arise from the Th10−L2 ganglions. The parasympathetic and the somatic fibres arise from the S2−S4 cord segments. Somatic fibres emerge from Onuf's nucleus located in the sacral cord and travel in the pudendal nerve. The pudendal nerve consists of sensory and motor fibres: the dorsal nerve of the penis provides for sensory innervation of the penile shaft and the glans penis and the motor branch of the pudendal nerve innervates the pelvic floor musculature including the periurethral striated sphincteric mechanism, the anal sphincter and the bulbocavernosus muscles [5].

The lower urinary tract is "well balanced" if the urethral sphincter (striated muscle) and the detrusor (bladder musculature-smooth muscle) behave in synergy: a good coordination between the detrusor and the urethral sphincter is mandatory to ensure urinary continence during the filling phase along with the complete emptying of the bladder during micturition under the voluntary control of the subject.

Urinary bladder disorders are divided into morphological abnormalities, neurogenic bladders and functional urinary disorders. Functional disorders constitute a large series of pathologies that urologists usually cannot categorize into either morphological abnormalities or neurogenic disorders. By definition, a functional voiding disorder is characterized by complaints referred to the genitourinary tract in the absence of a precise organic (urologic or neurologic) substratum. Functional bladder disorders are listed in Table 1. Patients with functional urinary disorders have by definition intact neurological control over the lower urinary tract. Some of them may, however, partially lose the coordination between the detrusor muscle and the pelvic floor and so present with neurological-like symptoms and/or pseudoinfravesical obstruction.

Patients suspected of a functional urinary disorder need a complete work-up in order to rule out a subclinical organic pathology: a careful history and physical examination, lab tests (blood and urine samples), urodynamic investigations

Table 1: *Classification of functional bladder disorders.*

Functional bladder disorders in adults

- Urethral syndrome
- Prostatodynia
- Urgency/frequency syndrome
- Idiopathic urinary retention

Functional bladder disorders in children

- Uninhibited pediatric bladder syndrome
- Lazy bladder syndrome
- Enuresis
- Non-neurogenic neurogenic bladder

(free flowmetry and videourodynamics), neurophysiological tests (evoked potentials and sacral reflex latency) and urinary tract imaging are mandatory. Oriented tests will be performed if any abnormality is observed in these tests.

Evaluation of functional bladder disorders

History and physical examination

A careful history is taken in order to rule out a (clinical or sub-clinical) neurological disorder. The physical examination includes a testing of perineal and lower-limb reflexes, a rectal (and vaginal) examination, and a testing of the sensations in the genitourinary area (Table 2).

Table 2: *Neuro-urological physical examination.*

Testing of reflexes	Segments tested
Achilles reflex	S1
Bulbocavernosus reflex	S3−S4
Anal reflex	S4−S5
Plantar reflex	corticospinal tracts

Rectal examination
Prostate
Tonus of the anal sphincter
Voluntary control to the pelvic floor

Testing of sensibility
Superficial sensation
Deep sensation

Laboratory tests

The patient will be subjected to blood and urine analyses: glycemia, urea, creatinine, urine sediment and culture, and, in some patients, fractioned urine samples.

Urodynamic investigation

The urodymanic investigation is the cornerstone of the evaluation of functional urinary disorders to check the filling (continence) and the emptying (micturition) phases of the bladder. A free flowmetry and a videourodynamic investigation are conducted.

Free flowmetry
This is a non-invasive test for which the patient is asked to pass water in the funnel of a flowmeter that records several parameters such as the voided volume, the peak and the mean urinary flows, and the micturition time. After micturition, the residual urine is measured either by ultrasound or by urethral catheterization. The pattern of the micturition is important: bell-shaped curve, staccato micturition.

Video-urodynamics
This test consists of a combination of a voiding cystourethrography and a pressure-flow study. It allows on-line morphological and manometric data to be superimposed. The urinary bladder is infused with diluted contrast medium either transurethrally or suprapubically. The intravesical pressure is recorded continuously during filling and micturition. The rectal pressure, measured by the use of a rectal balloon, is electronically subtracted from the intravesical pressure to obtain the true detrusor pressure. The activity of the periurethral sphincteric mechanism is recorded via a concentric EMG needle electrode (Fig. 1). Filling and micturition are repeated 3 times consecutively to gather reliable parameters: cystometric bladder capacity, absence or presence of unstable bladder contractions during filling, voluntary detrusor contraction during micturition, pattern of micturition, and residual urine [3].

Urinary tract imaging

Intravenous pyelography provides information about the morphology and function of the entire urinary tract. This test is advisable when a functional disorder is first investigated.

Kidney ultrasound is recommended for the follow-up of a functional micturition disorder [3].

Cystourethrography is useful for evaluating the morphology of the lower urinary tract when looking for possible infravesical obstruction (Fig. 2).

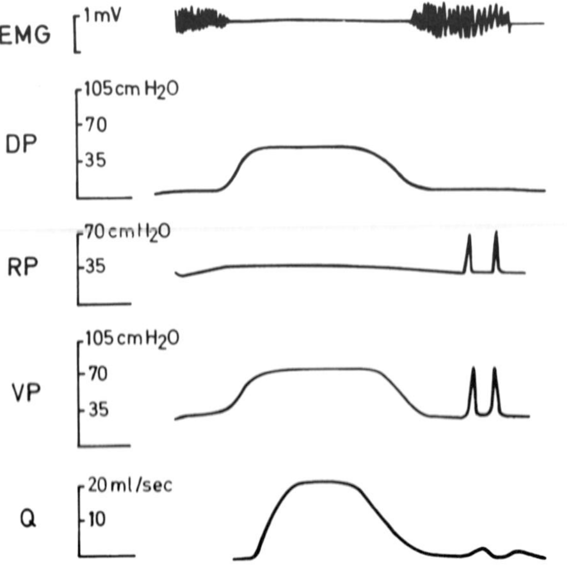

Fig. 1: *Pressure-flow-EMG study: simultaneous recording of the EMG activity from the periurethral striated musculature, detrusor (DP), rectal (RP) and vesical (VP) pressures, and urinary flowmetry (Q).*

Neurophysiological testing

Sacral reflex latency
Testing of the sacral reflexes is useful as it provides information about the integrity of the somatic innervation to the genital tract. The test consists of stimulating the dorsal nerve of the penis/clitoris and recording the reflex response from the periurethral sphincteric mechanism, the anal sphincter, or the bulbocavernosus muscles [4, 5].

Genital somatosensory evoked potentials
The test consists of stimulating the dorsal nerve of the penis/clitoris and recording the response 2 cm behind the vertex. It explores the entire afferent somatic volley from the genital tract to the brain [4, 5].

Functional bladder disorders in adults

We will review briefly two of the most common functional urinary disorders.

The urethral syndrome

Definition
The urethral syndrome is characterized by a combination of irritative symptoms (urgency, frequency), occasional dysuria and pathological findings on micro-

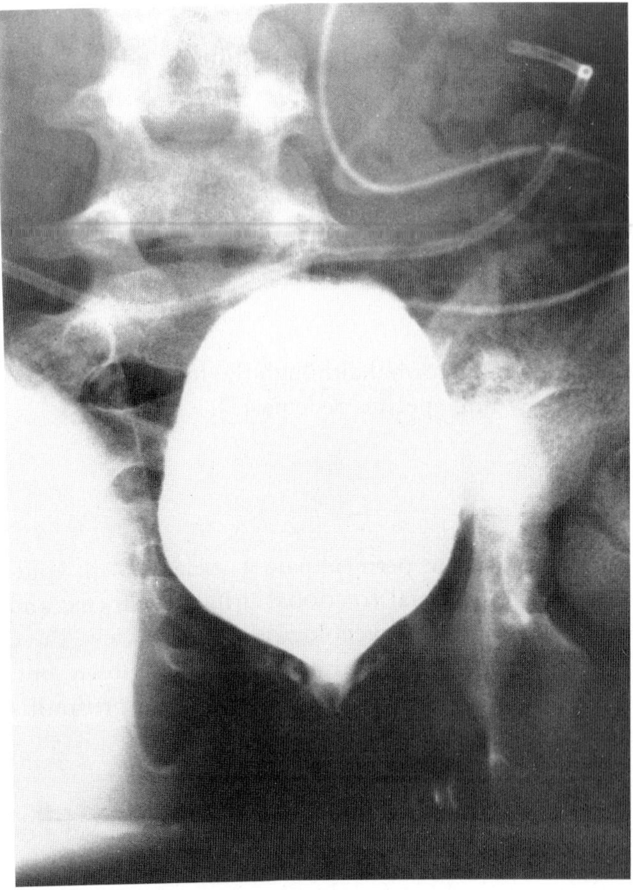

Fig. 2: *Voiding cystourethrography in a child presenting with detrusor-sphincter dyssynergia. Note the "opacification" of the proximal urethra above the closed urethral sphincter.*

scopic evaluation of fractionated urine samples. Fractionated samples are essential in order to isolate the initial urinary stream considered as a "urethral washout" from the mid-urinary stream reflecting the bladder content. The initial urinary stream may show leucocytes with the presence of $< 10^3$ microorganisms on culture. Midstream urine will be negative in patients complaining of urethral syndrome. Carbon dioxide-dependent organisms and chlamydia trachomatis have to be excluded by specific bacteriological techniques [1, 7].

Physical examination and routine investigations
Palpation of the urethra during bi-manual examination may reveal mild tenderness of the organ and surrounding musculature. Frequency/volume charts will demonstrate frequent voidings during the day while at night symptoms seem to subside temporarily.

Urodynamics
Pressure-flow studies demonstrate a stable bladder during filling and a reduced bladder capacity. Micturition is frequently generated by a poor detrusor contraction. The maximum flow rate is usually reduced when compared with the flow rates from controls.

Urethral sensitivity tests
Patients with a urethral syndrome usually have a low urethral sensitivity threshold (hypersensitivity) following electrical stimulation [1, 2].

Urethroscopy
Urethral and bladder mucosa are usually normal although the folds of the proximal urethra may occasionally show non specific oedema [1].

Prostatodynia

Definition
The syndrome is characterized by persistent perineal pain associated with voiding disturbances (urgency, frequency), normal fractional urine specimens, and sterile expressed prostatic secretion. From a psychological point of view, these patients are frequently anxious. The etiology of prostatodynia is unknown, but, in a high percentage, patients have a history of acute and/or chronic prostatitis combined with non-medical factors [6].

Physical examination and routine investigations
Perineal and prostatic tenderness are detected on rectal examination in most of these patients. This has been attributed to an increase in tension of the puborectalis muscles. Routine investigations include fractional urines, prostatic fluid analysis, serology, and imaging of the lower urinary tract. Frequency/volume charts in prostatodynia resemble those found in the female urethral syndrome: they demonstrate frequent voidings during the day, but at night most patients do not get up more than once or twice [6].

Urethrocystoscopy
Urethroscopic examination will usually be normal. In some patients, hyperemia of the proximal urethra may be found along with some degree of bladder neck obstruction.

Urodynamics
Videourodynamics will demonstrate a stable bladder during filling. Bladder capacity is usually reduced. Urinary flow rates are low. The etiology of the low flow is attribuable to a poor (non sustained) detrusor contraction during micturition.

Functional bladder disorders in children

We review here two functional disorders of the children.

The uninhibited pediatric bladder syndrome (UPB)

Definition
The uninhibited pediatric bladder syndrome corresponds to the persistence of a "pediatric type" of bladder behaviour. The child will present with incontinence, nocturia and pollakiuria. He will try to suppress the urge to void by contracting the pelvic floor (Vincent's Curtsey Sign). This may lead to more or less severe problems. If the child attempts to hold urine, he/she may develop sphincteric hypertonia. Bladder capacity will increase and frequency of micturition will finally decrease, which may lead to a lazy bladder. Symptoms of uninhibited bladder may lead to bladder trabeculation, recurrent cystitis, and vesico-ureteral reflux. The etiology of this syndrome remains unclear, but psychological and social factors have to be taken into account in addition to infraclinical neurological factors [3].

Urodynamics
Urodynamic investigations will show detrusor instability with or without detrusor-sphincter dyssynergia. Later on the child may develop a large bladder capacity with an acontractile detrusor.

The lazy bladder syndrome

Definition
The lazy bladder syndrome is characterized by a large bladder capacity with persistent, post-void residual urine. The distended urinary bladder is frequently palpable. The condition is often observed in girls and occurs between the ages of 5 to 10. Complaints consist of infrequent voluntary voidings, overflow incontinence, urinary infection [3].

Urodynamic findings
Micturition is usually generated by a weak detrusor contraction or by abdominal straining. Usually there is no detrusor-sphincter dyssynergia.

Urinary tract imaging
The upper urinary tract remains normal because the bladder distends without an increase in intravesical pressure.

Neurophysiological testing
Evoked potentials and the sacral reflex latency have to be performed to rule out a possible infraclinical neurological disorder.

Treatment modalities of functional bladder disorders

The treatment modalities are determined by the information gathered from the physical examination and urodynamic tests: cystometric bladder capacity, urinary continence or incontinence and the absence or presence of uninhibited detrusor contractions during the filling phase, the pattern of micturition, the presence of residual urine, combined with the results of the other paraclinical investigations: presence of a urinary infection, upper urinary tract dilation. We will briefly list the most accepted treatment modalities [1, 3, 6, 7, 8].

Adults

Urethral syndrome: antibiotics, pharmacotherapy (diazepam, alpha-blocking agents), bladder training, urethral dilatation? neuromodulation?

Prostatodynia: reassurance, physiotherapy, antibiotics, pharmacotherapy (central anxiolytic agents, peripheral muscle relaxants, alpha-blocking agents), neuromodulation?, prostatic massage?

Urgency-frequency syndrome: frequency/volume charts, biofeedback, videourodynamics (= visual biofeedback with the help of the X-ray screen: repeated bladder fillings while increasing stepwise the amount of fluid injected into the bladder), pelvic floor exercises, perhaps psychotropic drugs?

Idiopathic retention: suprapubic catheter with bladder reeducation, clean intermittent self-catheterization, pharmacotherapy (alpha-blocking drugs).

Children

Uninhibited pediatric bladder syndrome (UPB): bladder training, biofeedback with pelvic floor exercises, antiseptics, pharmacotherapy (anticholinergic drugs).

Lazy bladder syndrome: suprapubic catheter with bladder reeducation, clean intermittent (self-)catheterization.

Enuresis: no treatment is required before the age of 7. The best results are obtained after the age of 7 with reinforcement behavioral methods, pharmacotherapy (anticholinergics, desmopressin) and electric alarms.

Non-neurogenic−neurogenic bladder syndrome: bladder training, biofeedback with pelvic floor exercises, pharmacotherapy, clean intermittent catheterization and treatment of potential secondary complications (urinary tract infection, vesicoureteral reflux, and encopresis).

References

1. George, N. J. R.: Urethral syndrome − Clinical features. In: N. J. R. George, J. A. Gosling (Eds.): Sensory disorders of the bladder and urethra, pp. 91−102. Springer-Verlag, Berlin 1986.
2. Opsomer, R. J., T. C. Gerstenberg, P. Klarskov et al.: The electric sensibility threshold in the bladder and the urethra. Abstract 196, Proceedings 2. Joint meeting of the International Continence Society and Urodynamics Society, Aachen, September 1983.
3. Opsomer, R. J., F. X. Wese: Lower urinary tract and genital pathology in children. Acta Urol. Belg. 57 (1989) 251−680.
4. Opsomer, R. J., M. D. Caramia, F. Zarola et al.: Neurophysiological evaluation of central−peripheral sensory and motor pudendal fibres. Electroenceph. clin. Neurophysiol. 74 (1989) 260−270.
5. Opsomer, R. J., J. M. Guérit, P. J. Van Cangh et al.: Electrophysiological assessment of somatic nerves controlling the genital and urinary functions. In: P. M. Rossini, F. Mauguière (Eds.): New Trends and Advanced Techniques in Clinical Neurophysiology (EEG Clin. Neurophysiol. Supp. 41), pp. 298−305. Elsevier Science Publishers, Amsterdam 1990.
6. Osborn, D. E.: Prostatodynia − Clinical aspects. In: N. J. R. George, J. A. Gosling (Eds.): Sensory disorders of the bladder and the urethra, pp. 139−147. Springer Verlag, Berlin 1986.
7. Siroky, M. B., R. J. Krane: Functional voiding disorders in women. In: R. J. Krane, M. B. Siroky (Eds.): Clinical Neurourology, pp. 445−457, 2nd edition. Little Brown and Co, Boston 1991.
8. Wein, A., D. M. Barrett: Voiding function and dysfunction, a logical and practical approach, pp. 326−328. Year Book Medical Publishers, Chicago 1988.

Pharmacotherapy of altered brain-gut interactions

H. Mönnikes

Introduction

Considerable evidence has been obtained in recent years suggesting that symptoms reported in functional gastrointestinal disorders, i.e. patients without apparent lesions identifiable in conventional diagnostic tests, are the outcome of alterations in the interaction between the central nervous system (CNS) and the gastrointestinal (GI) tract. This basic assumption allows to integrate data from various directions of research in the field of functional GI disorders (epidemiology, psychology, pathophysiology, pharmacology), as well as to achieve a better understanding of the complex interaction of biological, psychological and social aspects of the disease in the individual patient [36, 66, 124].

Experimental studies in humans and animals show that altered brain-gut interactions can be caused by primarily altered sensorial responses along afferent gut-brain axis pathways and/or by primarily altered activity in efferent brain-gut pathways; for example, changes in efferent brain-gut activity are well established for experimental stress conditions. In addition, these alterations may induce secondary changes of gut-CNS-gut and CNS-gut-CNS reflex mechanisms [17, 71, 116, 117].

Clinical experience shows that commonly used drugs like antispasmodics often relieve some of the symptoms, i.e. symptomatic treatment, but leave other manifestations of the diseases unimproved since they fail to tackle the mechanisms inducing symptoms. One main obstacle for an effective pharmacotherapy of functional gastrointestinal disorders was the lack of consistent findings of altered gastrointestinal function or other pathophysiological mechanisms underlying the generating of symptoms in these disorders.

However, alterations of visceral perception in a large proportion of patients suffering from non-cardiac chest pain (NCCP), functional dyspepsia (NUD) and irritable bowel syndrome (IBS) have recently been reported by various groups, suggesting that visceral hypersensitivity may be the key mechanism in all of these functional GI disorders, and might even be a biological marker in IBS [66, 71, 99].

Therefore, compounds that directly influence visceral nociception as well as substances that indirectly modify visceral sensation or perception of visceral events by acting along the brain-gut axis could be beneficial in the therapy of these patients. Despite the fact that the mechanisms underlying visceral hypersensitivity in patients with functional GI disorders like IBS are yet unknown, these findings have drawn attention to substances which may influence visceral perception by acting at peripheral, spinal, supraspinal or even several levels of brain-gut interaction [8].

Mechanisms of modulation and alteration of visceral sensitivity

Data in animal models of chronic hyperalgesia suggest that spinal hyperexcitability as a result of peripheral and central sensitization and/or alterations in the endogenous pain modulating systems (descending modulation of spinal afferents in the periphery by local effector cells and of dorsal horn neurons by bulbospinal pathways) may play a critical role in the mediation of visceral hypersensitivity observed in patients with functional GI disorders under experimental conditions [70, 71]. This hypothesis is especially tempting since alterations in the thresholds of visceral afferents could mediate the altered perception of visceral sensation as well as alterations in motor and secretory (reflex) activity of the gut often observed in patients with functional GI disorders [70, 97].

Peripheral and central sensitization

The main mechanisms believed to be involved in chronic visceral pain are the processes of so called peripheral and central sensitization and of corticalization [8, 125, 128, 131].

Peripheral sensitization at noxious tissue irritation induces a decrease in thresholds of mechanosensitive fibers as well as the development of mechanosensitivity of previously mechanoinsensitive fibers, so called 'silent nociceptors'. This is induced by action of inflammatory mediators (e. g. bradykinin, prostaglandin, cytokines, serotonin) or peripheral nerve damage (axotomy, peripheral neuropathy) [125, 128].

Central sensitization might develop in consequence of peripheral sensitization. Peripheral sensitization causes an increased C-fiber input at the dorsal horn neuron, i. e. an increased release of transmitters with excitatory effect on dorsal horn neurons (Fig. 3). This results in increased excitability but also in neuroplastic changes in dorsal horn neurons, a phenomenon called 'wind-up'. Due to neuroplastic changes the spinal hyperexcitability persists even after complete reversal of the noxious stimulation-induced tissue alterations in the periphery [125, 128]. The 'wind-up' is mainly due to additive effects of substance P acting on the neurokinin (NK)-1 receptor, and glutamate which acts on NMDA (N-methyl-D-aspartat) as well as on AMPA (α-amino-3-hydroxy-5-methylisoxazole) receptors [125, 138, 131]. This process may be modulated by other transmitters (opioids, CCK, CGRP, somatostatin, and others) (Fig. 3).

Descending modulation of sensory transmission in the dorsal horn

Descending bulbospinal projections onto sensory neurons in the dorsal horn or via spinal interneurons modulate visceral sensation by excitatory or inhibitory influences. For example, noxious stimuli or stressful conditions can activate inhibitory bulbospinal pathways, thereby reducing excitability of spinal sensory neurons and causing nociceptive hypoalgesia. In contrast, spinal excitability can be increased by bulbospinal pathways mediating pain facilitation. This system can for example be activated by anticipatory anxiety [125, 128].

Thus, brain areas involved in descending modulation of sensory pathways and pain transmission, especially the pontine locus coeruleus, the periaqueductal grey in the midbrain, raphe nuclei and lateral nuclei of the reticular formation in the brain stem could be sensitive drug targets to modify perception (Fig. 1, 2).

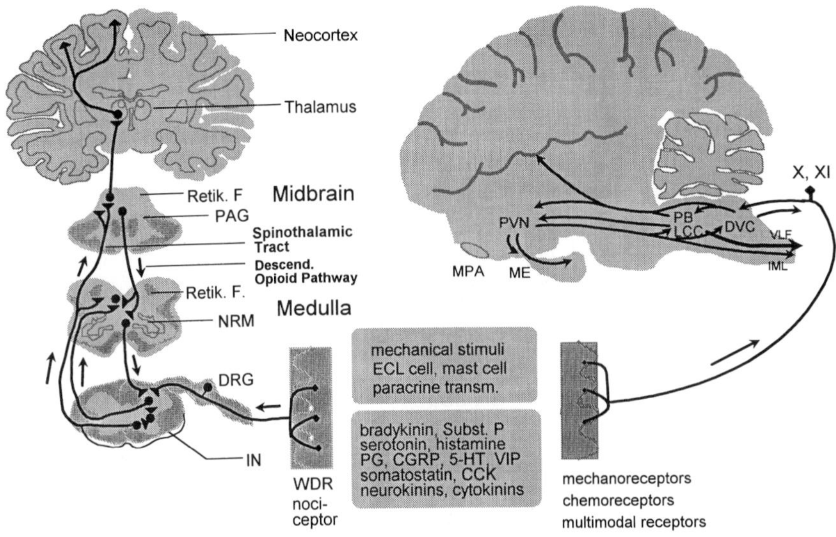

Fig. 1: *Left: Schematic diagram illustrating the regulation of spinal afferent mechanism by bulbospinal pathways.*
PAG: periaqueductal grey; Retik. F.: reticular formation; NRM: nucleus raphe magnus; DRG: dorsal root ganglion; IN: interneuron.
(Redrawn from Jessel and Kelley, 1991)
Right: Schematic diagram about the interaction of afferent vagal pathways, pontine areas and hypothalamic nuclei.
PVN: Paraventricular nucleus of the hypothalamus; ME: median eminence; MPA: medial preoptic area; PB: parabrachial nucleus; LCC: locus coeruleus; DVC: dorsal vagal complex.

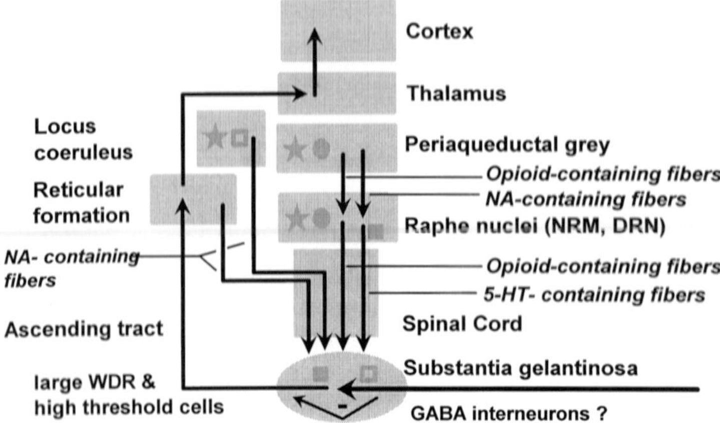

Fig. 2: *A schematic diagram illustrating the descending noradrenergic (NA), serotonergic (5-HT) and opioid pathways of the bulbospinal inhibitory pain modulating system. (□: alpha-2 adrenergic receptors; ●: mu-opioid receptors; ☆: kappa-opioid receptors).*

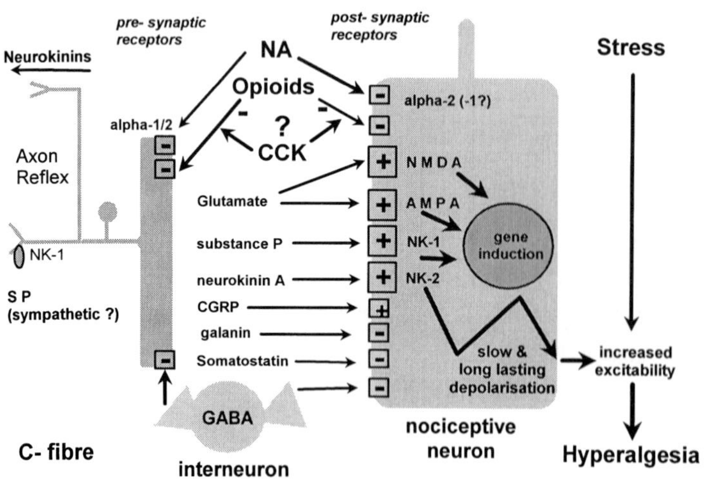

Fig. 3: *Schematic diagram illustrating the release of neurotransmitters from sensory C-fibres, the effects of these substances on the excitability of sensory dorsal horn neurons (+ increase; − decrease), and receptors involved in neuroplastic changes at central sensitization.*

The main neurotransmitters implicated in the descending pain control system are serotonin (5-HT), noradrenaline (NA) and endogenous opiates [125, 128] (Fig. 2). However, spinal opiod receptors are the key site of antinociceptive action of bulbospinal pathways. The level of opioid effectiveness is modulated at spinal sites by cholecystokinin (CCK) from spinal interneurons, which reduces the analgesic action of e.g. morphine, and by descending noradrenergic (NA) influences from the brain stem (Fig. 2, Fig. 3). CCK reduces the analgesic action of opioids in the spinal cord. In contrast, increases in descending nor-adrenergic outflow enhances spinal morphine analgesia, independently of direct antinociceptive effects of NA [125, 128, 131].

Modulation of sensory transmission by vagal pathways

It has been shown that, besides input by spinal pathways, also vagally mediated visceral-afferent information plays a role in conscious perception of sensations related to gastrointestinal events. The dorsal vagal complex (DVC) is the major relay site for vagally mediated afferent signals from the GI tract [89] (Fig. 1). Besides close connections to brain nuclei of the central antonomic network like the paraventricular nucleus of the hypothalamus (PVN), which integrate the neurohumoral control of the organism, the DVC also projects to thalamic nuclei, probably thereby modifying nociception, and to parts of the limbic system, like the amygdala, which play a crucial role in emotionality [47, 52, 73]. Further, it has been shown that vagally mediated visceral afferent information modulates the activity of descending bulbospinal pain modulating pathways; e. g. vagally mediated information about aversive conditions like nausea activate the descending pain facilitating system [125, 128]. Thus, perception and emotional quality of gastrointestinal events could be modified by drug action along spinal and vagal afferent pathways.

Pharmacotherapy of altered visceral sensitivity

Efferent and afferent pathways involved in the CNS modulation of GI-function are integrated at the peripheral, spinal and supraspinal level, and neuroanatomical and neurophysiological studies show that alterations at one level of integration affect efferent and afferent activity at other levels of the brain-gut axis [72]. Thus, pharmacotherapy of altered brain-gut interaction could aim to affect one or several of the mechanisms modulating visceral sensitivity.

From various substances which may be effective in the pharmacotherapy of alterations in brain-gut mechanisms by acting at peripheral, spinal, supraspinal or various sites along the CNS-gut axis, most have been tested only in experimental models and proof of effectiveness in therapy of functional gastrointestinal disorders still has to be gained (see Tab. 1 for overview). However, some compounds have already been used in clinical trials.

Compounds modulating visceral sensitivity by acting peripherally

5-HT3 antagonists
It has been suggested that 5-HT receptor antagonists might act as 'visceral analgesics' since serotonin, which can be released by platelets, mast cells and

Table 1: *Substances with modulatory effects on visceral afferent neurotransmission in brain-gut interaction.*

site of drug action	substance	experiment. evidence	clinical evidence
primary sensory neuron ('visceral analgesics')			
(?)	5 HT3 antagonists	animals, humans	(+)
	kappa opioid agonists	animals, humans	(+) (Fedotozine)
	ion channel modulators	animals, humans	−
(?)	somatostatin analogues	animals, humans	+ (Octreotide)
spinal sensory neuron ('spinal analgesics')			
	adrenoreceptor agonists	animals, humans	−
	5-HT1 agonist	animals, humans	−
	opioids (agonists)	animals	−
modulation of spinal neuro-transmission by selective neuropeptides and analogues			
	CCK antagonists	animals	−
	NK-1 antagonists	animals	−
	NK-2 antagonists	animals	−
	somatostatin agonist	animals, humans	? (Octreotide)
	CGRP (no antagonist available)	animals	−
reversion of spinal neuroplastic changes			
	NMDA antagonists	animals	−
supraspinally acting drugs			
	tricyclic antidepressants	animals, humans	++
	serotonin-uptake inhibitors	animals, humans	+
	anxiolytics	animals, humans	+
	anticholinergics	animals	?
	CRF antagonists	animals	?
	CCK-B antagonists	animals	?

ECL cells in the GI-tract, can produce pain and hyperalgesia by action on 5-HT1-3 receptors in various animal models. In addition, 5-HT has been shown to be able to excite spinal and vagal primary sensory neurons [4, 9, 37, 44, 63, 114].

Serotonin can cause a direct excitation of sensory neurons by increasing sodium channel permeability via 5-HT3 receptor activation; this 5-HT effect can be blocked by 5-HT3 antagonists, e.g. by ICS 205.930 [98]. S-HT also indirectly activates sensory neurons via G-protein coupled 5-HT1 and 5-HT2 receptors inducing a decrease in potassium-ion permeability and membrane depolarization. There is some evidence that this may sensitize nociceptors, lowering their threshold to for example pressure stimuli, and may also induce repetitive neuronal firing. These effects seem to be c-AMP-dependent [35, 62, 95].

Therefore, 5-HT3 receptor mediated excitation of sensory neurons might be more important in the mediation of acute pain, whereas 5-HT1 and 5-HT2 receptors seem to play a greater role in peripheral mechanisms of chronic pain. This observation could be important when considering 5 HT receptor antagonists as a therapeutic alternative in the treatment of patients with functional gastrointestinal disorders associated with continual pain.

5-HT3 receptors have been proposed to be localized on spinal and vagal primary sensory neurons, but have also been found on other neuronal structures involved in visceral-afferent neurotransmission. In the spinal cord, 5-HT3 receptors seem to be localized on dorsal horn neurons which give rise to the spinothalamic tract. These neurons are probably the target of descending serotoninergic fibers from raphe nuclei being involved in the descending pain control system. However, the descending serotoninergic fibers might also act via interneurons expressing 5-HT3 receptors. Since serotonin itself unfolds antinociceptive effects in the spinal cord, for example in response to noxious colorectal distension in the rat, it is rather unlikely that the antinociceptive effects of 5-HT3 receptor antagonists are due to action on spinal cord neurons [2, 4, 27, 40, 56, 102].

It has been shown in experimental animal models that serotonin stimulates vagal sensory neurons by 5-HT3 receptors, and 5-HT receptor antagonists diminish pseudoaffective cardiovascular responses to intestinal distension [4, 63]. Also 5-HT3 receptor antagonists affect GI motor activity in animals by acting on vagal afferents [54].

However, 5-HT3 receptors are also localized in the area postrema, where they play a role in emetic responses, and also in higher CNS structures, which are involved in emotional processes [5, 6, 94]. Furthermore, in experimental animals the peripheral administration of 5-HT uptake inhibitors modify CNS-mediated alterations of gastrointestinal function. In patients with non-ulcer dyspepsia the central serotoninergic receptor sensitivity to buspirone is on average significantly greater than in healthy controls [33, 107]. Therefore, and despite the well established effects of serotonin on primary sensory neurons, it is unknown until now if effects of 5-HT3 receptor antagonists on GI sensitivity are exclusively mediated by action on primary sensory neurons or if actions on central nervous system structures are also involved.

In humans, specific 5-HT3 receptor antagonists have been used in experimental settings as well as in small clinical trials. In IBS-patients granisetron reduced rectal sensation (gas, desire or urgency to defecate, discomfort) to distension without changes in motility parameters of the distal colon under basal conditions. However, granisetron showed a dose-dependent reduction in postprandial rectosigmoid motor activity, which was suggested to be the result of a decreased afferent input to the gastrocolonic response by action on mucosal 5-HT3 receptors in the intestinal mucosa [91]. Intravenous or oral (up to 16 mg three times daily) administration of ondansetron, another 5-HT receptor antagonist, prolonged transit in the distal colon without affecting small-intestinal transit times, gastric emptying or mouth-to-caecum transit times in healthy subjects [43, 119–121]. In IBS patients, ondansetron caused a reduction in looseness of stool, mainly in the subgroup of patients with diarrhoea, but had no effects on pain at 4 mg and 16 mg three times daily for 4 weeks [69, 112]. Nevertheless, it has been speculated that the subjective improvement in stool consistency in this study may reflect changes in the perception of defecation since stool frequency and stool weight as well as orocoecal transit time or small-intestinal transit time were not altered by the drug [111, 112]. However, in a recent investigation with a small number of patients studied, ondansetron (16 mg/day) induced firmer stools in IBS patients, decreased the number of episodes of pain although not their severity, but had no significant effects on pain thresholds to rectal distension and rectal sensory thresholds to electrical stimulation [41]. Further, in experimental studies a single dose of ondansetron (0,15 mg/kg i. v.) did not alter gastric or rectal perception to balloon distension in healthy controls and IBS patients [132].

In conclusion, 5-HT3 receptor antagonists are a promising group of new drugs for treatment of functional gastrointestinal disorders, especially for diarrhoea predominant subgroups of IBS. However, results of recent studies suggest that the positive effects in IBS could be simply due to effects of these drugs on GI secretion and motility and independent of antinociceptive action. In this context it is of interest that endogenous serotonin seems to be one of the substances which mediate gastrointestinal responses to stress, and that these effects of 5-HT are mediated by 5-HT3 receptors [75, 76].

Results from animal models and *in vivo* studies also suggest that serotonin antagonists acting on the 5-HT3 receptor might be more beneficial in the treatment of acute pain episodes than in chronic pain, due to differences in the underlying pathophysiological mechanisms. This might have implications for the prospect of this group of substances to be useful in the treatment of recurrent and prolonged periods of abdominal pain, as often seen in functional gastrointestinal disorders like IBS. This also might be a reason for the lack of convincing evidence that 5-HT3 receptor antagonists are beneficial in the treatment of abdominal pain in functional GI disorders. On the other hand, 5-HT3 antagonists might be effective in the treatment of acute pain caused by colonic inflammation, but this question still needs to be further addressed [82].

Kappa-opioid receptor agonists
There is considerable evidence that various exogenous opiates unfold their anti-nociceptive effects by acting on different opioid receptors, which are localized centrally and peripherally. Opiates acting exclusively peripherally would lack sedative and psychotrophic effects and avoid the dependence problem. There-fore, they would be a valuable alternative for the treatment of such functional GI disorders which are associated with abdominal pain [113].

It has been shown that the endogenous kappa-receptor ligand dynorphin, which can be produced in the periphery by immune cells at inflammation, exerts anti-nociceptive action in the periphery in models of inflammatory and neuropathic pain, besides additional effects on sympathetic nerve fibers, at least partly due to direct action on primary afferent nerves [3, 25, 50, 105, 118].

In accordance with the expectation that peripherally acting exogenous kappa opioid receptor agonists should be most beneficial in pain states due to altered primary afferent nerve function, it has been shown that systemic administration of the kappa agonist fedotozine augments autonomic pain reflexes at colonic balloon distension primarily under conditions of peripheral sensitization, for example at acute experimental colitis in animals [59].

Kappa opioid receptors have been proposed to be localized on spinal as well as on vagal primary sensory neurons. In the periphery, kappa opioid receptors are also located in the intestinal mucosa and submucosa [26]. However, kappa opioid receptors have also been found in various CNS structures involved in afferent neurotransmission, especially in brain areas and spinal structures in-volved in the descending pain control system, like periaqueductal grey, the ra-phe nuclei, and the locus coeruleus (LC) [15, 55, 64, 67]. It has been shown that CNS opiate receptors which modulate gastrointestinal motility are also involved in the mediation of opioid analgesic effects [87, 88]; e. g. morphine microinjected into the LC, a brain site which has been shown to be involved in the CNS control of GI secretion and motility, inhibits the response of most dorsal horn cells to noxious stimuli [55, 80, 81]. Further, kappa opioid receptors seem also to be localized on pre-synaptic spinal terminals of sensory C-fibres and other structures of the spinal cord mediating antinociception at spinal levels [7, 31, 123].

However, there is considerable experimental evidence in animals suggesting that at systemic administration kappa receptor agonists like fedotozine and U50488 exert their antinociceptive effects as well as their effects on GI motility by action on peripheral nerve endings of sensory vagal and non-vagal afferent pathways [34, 100, 101].

Interestingly, kappa agonists seem to modify stress induced and CNS mediated alterations of GI motility and cortisol secretion by action on vagal pathways in the periphery [12, 46, 57]. These data emphasize the role of peripheral kappa receptors in the modulation of neurohumoral mechanisms in brain-gut interaction.

The kappa opioid agonist fedotozine has been used in several experimental settings and clinical trials in humans. Under experimental conditions the drug increased sensory threshold volumes to gastric distension in healthy controls and (at 100 mg i. v. versus placebo) the thresholds of first sensation and pain perception to colonic distension in IBS patients without affecting parameters assessing gastrointestinal motor activity. The lack of effect on motility parameters might be due to the fact that dynorphin, the endogenous kappa-receptor ligand, inhibits mainly stimulated intestinal motility [22, 29].

In clinical trials fedotozine at doses of 30−70 mg tid were superior to placebo in relieving the intensity of dyspeptic symptoms like epigastric pain, nausea, postprandial fullness and bloating in functional dyspepsia, and improved the maximal intensity of lower abdominal pain in IBS patients after 6 weeks of treatment [1, 28, 38].

After abdominal surgery, fedotozine reduced pain and digestive symptoms at 50 mg i. v., and also induced an earlier restoration of intestinal transit at 25 mg i. v. [103]. Similar effects regarding the reversal of post-surgery as well as peritonitis-induced ileus have been shown in experimental animals [101]. Therefore, kappa agonists might relieve the intensity of postsurgical discomfort, besides antinociceptive effects, also by an improved restoration of GI motility.

Ion channels modulating drugs
It has been suggested that peripheral sensitization, i. e. increased excitability of primary sensory neurons, might be involved in the pathogenesis of visceral hypersensitivity in functional gastrointestinal disorders. In neuropathic pain, where sensitization of sensory neurons has been shown and conventional analgesic drugs often fail, abnormal sodium-channel action or accumulation of sodium channels in the membrane of primary sensory neurons may be a key element. Also, the effectiveness of agents that reduce membrane excitability, like local anesthetics, anticonvulsants and antiarrhythmics in the treatment of neuropathic pain, most likely reflects that all of these substances are sodium channel blockers [14, 93]. Several groups of sodium channel blocking agents, e. g. anticonvulsants like carbamazepine and antiarrhythmics like mexilitene, have been used as systemic analgesics especially in neuropathic pain [93]. Therefore, one might speculate that sodium channel blockers could be beneficial in the treatment of functional gastrointestinal disorders.

Nociceptive neurons express at least two types of sodium channels. The slow-activating type is selectively expressed in nociceptive afferent neurons [95]. Drugs only acting at this sodium channel will probably have fewer side effects but are not available until now.

In an experimental study mucosal application of the local anesthetic lidocaine 2% failed to affect hypersensitivity to rapid phasic rectal distention in patients with IBS [61, 86]. Studies about the effectiveness of systemic treatment with sodium channel blockers in functional abdominal pain have not been performed until now.

Somatostatin analogues

Somatostatin and its stable analogues octreotide and vaproetide have antinociceptive effects in various animal models and have been shown to induce analgesia in humans after intravenous, epidural or intrathecal administration [20, 65, 78, 108]. This opened the question if somatostatin and its analogues, which are well known to have profound effects on GI motor activity, also affect intestinal-visceral perception [13, 48].

There are indications for possible antinociceptive actions of somatostatin on several sites of the organisms [20, 65, 104]. However, the most convincing evidence for a modulation of nociception by the peptide has been demonstrated for the spinal cord, where somatostatin is released as an antinociceptive mediator in response to neural transmission of painful stimuli. Somatostatin is present in small diameter cells in the dorsal root ganglion and in afferent terminals in the substantia gelatinosa of the spinal cord [11, 51]. In experimental rats, noxious stimuli induce a release of somatostatin in the dorsal horn, where it causes a hyperpolarisation of dorsal horn neurons and a reduction in spontaneous firing [104]. Intrathecal administration of somatostatin induces antinociceptive effects to peripheral stimuli in various pain models [78, 79]. This suggests that somatostatin has an inhibitory role in the dorsal horn, making it the only inhibitory neurotransmitter known to be released by sensory C-fiber endings in the dorsal horn.

It has been shown in healthy controls that subcutaneous application of the long acting somatostatin analogue octreotide (100 μg) reduces sensation of unpleasant or painful rectal distension (probably via inhibition of visceral afferent pathways) without affecting rectal motor activity, local reflexes and cutaneous perception [86]. Perception of thermal or electrical cutaneous stimulation was unaffected by octreotide showing selectivity of the antinociceptive effects for visceral afferents. It has been suggested that the inhibitory effect of octreotide on rectal sensation is due to a direct effect on extrinsic primary afferent neurons with receptive fields in the mucosa, since the somatostatin analogue did not further increase sensory thresholds above the effect of intrarectally administered lidocaine [86]. In contrast, octreotide had no effect on gastric sensitivity but reduced gastric compliance in healthy controls [74, 109]. In diarrhoea-prone patients with irritable bowel syndrome octreotide (100 μg s. c.) reduced perception of rectal distension and also reduced elevated rectal resistance to normal levels [49]. However, in other studies the increase in thresholds for discomfort and pain was not accompanied by effects on rectal compliance and other colorectal motility parameters in IBS-patients and healthy controls [10, 109]. It has been suggested that the effects of octreotide on visceral perception might be mediated by a reduction of spinal afferent transmission since electroencephalographic studies showed diminished evoked spinal and cortical potentials after octreotide [19, 85]. Currently only peptide analogues of somatostatin are available, which do not reach spinal sites when given systemically. Thus, the mechanisms of their effects on GI perception when given systemically remain unclear [106, 126].

Somatostatin analogues show high affinity for opioid receptors and in some studies their analgesic effects were reversible by naloxone. Therefore, it is not clear if these effects in humans are in fact caused by action on a somatostatin receptor.

Despite the fact that somatostatin analogues are expensive and that no oral analogue is available until now, further studies are desirable to determine if somatostatin analogues are beneficial in functional gastrointestinal disorders, especially when associated with abdominal pain.

Compounds modulating visceral sensitivity by acting centrally

Adrenoreceptor agonists

There is strong evidence that noradrenaline (NA) is implicated in opioid- and central stimulation-induced analgesia mediated by descending spinal pathways (Fig. 2). It has been shown that α_2-receptors are the subtype responsible for NA analgesic effects in the spinal cord. The α_2-receptors exist both pre- and postsynaptically, whereby the spinal α_2-receptor sites responsible for antinociception are postsynaptically located (Fig. 3). However, a novel α_2-receptor agonist (S 12813-4) has been shown to reduce the release of substance P from afferent nerve endings by probably acting on a specific presynaptic subtype of the α_2-adrenoreceptors [23, 45].

There are no NA cell bodies in the spinal cord, and major NA fibers descend from the reticular formation and from the locus coeruleus [15, 55, 127]. Since α_2-adrenoreceptor agonists block firing of LC neurons, thereby decreasing the antinociceptive effects of activation of the LC, it seems unlikely that the effects of α_2-adrenoreceptor agonists on nociception are mediated by α_2-adrenoreceptors in the LC [21, 130]. There is some evidence that there is synergistic interaction of NA and serotoninergic sytems in the descending bulbospinal pathways mediating pain inhibition, whereby α_2-adrenoreceptors in raphe nuclei may be involved [127] (Fig. 2).

In a double-blind crossover trial, the alpha 2 agonist lidamidine was found to cause a slight reduction in frequency of defecation but had no significant effect on frequency and severity of abdominal pain or bloating in patients with IBS [92].

Clonidine is an alpha-2-receptor agonist with a mild antinociceptive effect used via systemic or intrathecal administration which potentiates the action of morphine (Fig. 3) [127]. Further, it has been hypothesized that, besides the antinociceptive effects, a stabilization of the responsiveness of brain NA systems like that originating in the locus coeruleus may be a fundamental mechanism of action of clonidine to be effective in the treatment of disorders with a psychosomatic component such as IBS or premenstrual tension [115]. However, in patients with non-cardiac chest pain, effectiveness of clonidine could not be proved [16].

Tricyclic antidepressants (low dose) and serotonin reuptake inhibitors
Low dose tricyclic antidepressants (TCA) are effective in treatment of different types of chronic pain and are often recommended for treatment of chronic pain in functional GI disorders [39, 58]. All antidepressants interfere with monoaminergic sytems in the central nervous system. Tricyclic compounds block the uptake of both NA and serotonin, and also have antihistaminergic, antidopaminergic and anticholinergic effects. TCA unfold antinociceptive effects already at doses too low to affect mood conditions (e. g. trimipramine at 30 mg/day) [58, 83, 84]. Intrathecal administration of TCA potentiates spinally mediated morphine analgesia by NA and 5-HT mechanisms and combined serotonin and catecholamine uptake inhibitors without structural similarity to TCA (e. g. venlafaxine) show similar analgesic effectivity as tricyclic antidepressants. However, selective serotonin (e. g. paroxetine, fluoxetine) and catecholamine uptake inhibitors (e. g. desipramine) have lower analgesic potency [60]. Nevertheless, in an experimental study in humans a significant increase in nociceptive flexion reflex threshold and subjective pain threshold was observed after a 14-day treatment with dothiepin, an antidepressant interacting with serotonin receptors [53]. Further, this effect was modulated during the cold-pressor test, which is known to activate descending inhibitory pain control systems [53]. Further, the onset of the analgesic action of antidepressants is earlier (3 to 10 days) than that of antidepressive action [32]. These observations suggest that antinociceptive effects of these compounds at low doses might be mediated by interference with inhibitory noradrenergic and serotoninergic mechanisms of the descending bulbospinal pain modulating system at spinal sites (Fig. 2).

Tricyclic antidepressants have been shown to be superior to placebo for the management of abdominal pain, nausea, and diarrhoea but not constipation in IBS [83, 84]. Four days administration of the TCA imipramine (100 mg daily) prolongs both orocaecal and whole gut transit time in irritable bowel syndrome patients; the selective 5-HT re-uptake inhibitor paroxetine (30 mg daily) prolongs orocoecal transit without effecting whole gut transit time. These effects on transit precede any effects on mood, supporting the idea that these drugs may have therapeutic actions on gut function in addition to antidepressive effects [42].

In a recent study tricyclic antidepressants (50 mg imipramine nightly) also significantly improved symptoms in patients with non-cardiac chest pain (chest pain and normal coronary angiograms) [16].

Central modulation of visceral afferent neurotransmission by selective analogues, agonists and antagonists of endogenous substances modulating nociception

Starting from the hypothesis that facilitated transmission of visceral afferent information in the dorsal horn might be a key mechanism in the pathophysiology of at least a great proportion of patients with functional GI disorders, as a result of central sensitization or other modulating influences whose activity may be altered in abdominal pain syndromes like IBS, the pharmacological modulation of sensory dorsal horn excitability seems to be an interesting approach. Neuropeptides like CCK, substance P, somatostatin, CGRP and endogenous opioids as well as non-peptide chemical mediators like glutamate, GABA, adenosin and others have been shown to modulate transmission in spinal afferent pathways. Thus, selective analogues, agonists and antagonists acting at the receptors of these substances might be potential new types of drugs in the pharmacotherapy of altered brain-gut interaction (Tab. 1).

Serotonin agonists
In contrast to effects in the periphery where 5-HT can cause pain by excitation of primary sensory neurons, in the spinal cord serotonin seems to have an antinociceptive effect by acting as an inhibitory agonist on dorsal horn neurons [2, 40, 63, 114]. Serotoninergic neurons project from the raphe nucleus to dorsal horn neurons, where they unfold inhibitory action on nociceptive neurotransmission [27, 56, 102] (Fig. 2). However, there is also evidence that this might be an indirect effect of 5-HT by activation of inhibitory GABA interneurons [2]. The pharmacology of spinal 5-HT receptors seems to be complex; preliminary evidence suggests that mainly 5-HT1 receptors mediate the antinociceptive effect of serotonin in the spinal cord [27, 122]. Spinal serotonin receptors are involved in the mediation of stress induced analgesia by bulbospinal pathways [122]. 5-HT, opioids and NA interfere in their antinociceptive action on sensory dorsal horn neurons [60]. Selective 5-HT1A and 5-HT1B agonists have been tested in animal models and shown to reduce acute pain-induced behavioral responses at intrathecal administration [77].

Opioids
Endogenous opioids are main transmitters involved in the descending inhibition of spinal nociceptive pathways, mainly by action on mu- and kappa-receptors. At supraspinal sites of this system mu-receptor binding is found in the periaqueductal grey (PAG) and the nucleus raphe magnus (NRM). Kappa-receptor binding is found in the locus coeruleus (LC), PAG, and NRM (Fig. 2). Local microinjection of opiates into these brain nuclei modulates responses of dorsal horn neurons to noxious stimulation, associated with changes in spinal *c-fos* expression and behavioral responses [15, 55, 64, 125, 128].

Opioid receptors in the spinal cord are the key site of antinociceptive action of bulbospinal pathways of the descending inhibitory pain control system. Opioids have antinociceptive effects in the spinal cord by directly and indirectly modulating dorsal horn neuron excitability. The main effect is indirectly mediated via presynaptic mu- and delta-receptors [7, 31, 67]. Kappa opioid receptors seem also to be localized on pre-synaptic spinal terminals of sensory C-fibres and other spinal neurons mediating transmission of visceral afferent information, and spinal kappa receptors have been shown to mediate opioid-induced antinociception [7, 31, 123]. Opioids seem to increase potassium permeability of the primary sensory neuron, thereby hyperpolarising the nerve terminal. This induces a decreased release of neuropeptides which would have excitatory effects on the dorsal horn neuron, especially of substance P and glutamate [131] (Fig. 3). Therefore, opioids decrease the input to dorsal horn nociceptive neurons, which delays the onset of wind-up (and central sensitization) but does not abolish it [131]. However, in models of neuropathic pain, which is insensitive to opioids, the combination of threshold morphine and NMDA antagonists can restore morphine effectiveness [131]. Therefore, one might speculate about the possibility to approach functional abdominal pain syndromes, which often show similarity to conditions of neuropathic pain, with such treatment in the future.

CCK antagonists
It has been suggested that peripheral CCK may be involved in an enhanced ileo-colonic motor response proposed to be prevalent in patients with IBS; it was therefore speculated that peripherally acting CCK-antagonists might be useful in the therapy of postprandial abdominal pain due to an exaggerated motor response [96]. However, the results of experimental and of small clinical studies were disappointing [8, 96].

CCK in the spinal cord has no direct effect on nociceptive spinal pathways, but unfolds its action by decreasing the efficiency of the endogenous opioid sytem, probably by interference with the mu-opioid receptor. Therefore, CCK has no modulatory effect on nociception under normal conditions, but at increased or decreased activity of antinociceptive spinal opioid mechanisms. Besides other effects, CCK reduces descending- and stress-induced morphine analgesia, inducing hyperalgesia under these conditions [125, 131]. In experimental animals CCK-B antagonists (L-365-260 and C1988) have shown to enhance the analgesic effect of opiates, and may be useful in restoring morphine analgesia at conditions of 'wind up' [110]. However, in the spinal cord of primates the CCK-A receptor dominates and therefore CCK-A antagonists theoretically might be preferable in humans. CCK-antagonists acting selectively on specific spinal sites may enhance the potency of endogenous opioids and provide a useful pharmacological tool for treatment of stress-related abdominal symptoms in the future.

Tachykinins (NK-1 and NK-2 antagonists)
Tachykinins (substance P, neurokinin A (NKA) and neurokinin B (NKB)) play a pivotal role in transmission of nociceptive information in the spinal cord. SP and NKA are released in the spinal cord from sensory C-fiber nerve endings at noxious peripheral stimulation [68, 90]. In acute nociceptive events NKA acting on the NK-2 receptor seems to play the most important role in afferent neurotransmission in the dorsal horn. In pathological pain conditions, e. g. inflammatory hyperalgesia, substance P (SP) acting on the NK-1 receptor of the spinal sensory neuron has been shown to be the most important neurotransmitter. SP induces a long lasting depolarization of the dorsal horn neuron which contributes to a long-lasting facilitation of nociceptive transmission ('wind-up'), which is one important factor contributing to hyperalgesia. Hyperexcitability also increases susceptibility of these neurons to activation by excitatory amino acids like glutamate, which finally causes neuroplastic changes [23, 128, 131] (Fig. 3).

Non-peptide antagonists for NK-1 and NK-2 receptors have been developed in recent years. The selective NK-1 antagonists RP-67580 has been shown to inhibit the development of neuropathic pain in experimental animal models [24]. Neurokinin antagonists seem to be promising compounds for future treatment strategies in functional gastrointestinal disorders associated with chronic pain and discomfort.

Reversion of spinal neuroplastic changes

Excitatory amino acid antagonists (NMDA antagonists)
Central sensitization due to increased excitability of sensory dorsal horn neurons is the result of temporally summated subthreshold synaptic potentials mediated by NMDA and tachykinin receptors, in consequence of increased release of glutamate and substance P from C-fiber nerve endings at for example peripheral inflammation (Fig. 3). This leads to an exponentially increasing cumulative depolarization of the dorsal horn neuron, which is responsible for the wind-up of action potential discharge, and also for *prolonged alterations* in

membrane excitability. This is the basis of heterosynaptic facilitation of nociceptive transmission on the cellular and central sensitization at the physiological level. Other excitatory transmitters released from sensory C-fiber endings might further potentiate this process [131].

There is evidence that the NMDA receptor is responsible for the induction and maintenance of the wind-up phenomenon. Compounds like ketamine are effective NMDA channel blockers and have been shown to be effective in treatment of patients with chronic neuropathic pain. In experimental animals, NMDA antagonists (e. g. MK-801, Memantine, CPP) have been shown not to abolish pain but to block and prevent central sensitization [30, 129]. The combination of low threshold opioid, which decreases the release of substance P and neurokinin A, and NMDA receptor antagonists has been shown to restore morphine effectiveness in neuropathic pain models [18, 129]. Therefore, NMDA antagonists seem to allow a reversion of spinal neuroplastic changes at central sensitization [30, 131]. If the current side effect problems are surmountable, these compounds could be very valuable in the therapy of altered brain-gut interaction.

References

1. Abitol, J. L., N. W. Read, K. D. Bardhan et al.: Fedotozine in functional dyspepsia: Results of a 6 week placebo-controlled multicenter therapeutic trial. Gut 37 (1995) A161.
2. Alhaider, A. A., S. Z. Lei, G. L. Wilcox: Aponal 5-HT$_3$ receptor-mediated antinociception: possible release of GABA. Journal of Neuroscience 11 (1991) 1881–1888.
3. Andreev, N., L. Urban, A. Dray: Opioids suppress spontaneous activity of polymodal nociceptors in raw paw skin induced by ultraviolet irradiation. Neuroscience 58 (1994) 793–798.
4. Andrews, P. L., H. I. M. Davison: Activation of vagal afferent terminals by 5HT is mediated by the 5HT$_3$ receptor in the anaesthetized ferret. J. Physiol. 422 (1990) 982–986.
5. Ashby, C. R., Y. Minabe, E. Edwards et al.: 5-HT$_3$ like receptors in the rat medial prefrontal cortex: an electrophysiological study. Brain Res. 550 (1991) 181–190.
6. Barnes, N. M., B. Costall, R. J. Naylor et al.: Identification of 5-HT$_3$ recognition sites in the ferret area postrema. J. Pharm. Pharmacol. 40 (1988) 17–21.
7. Besse, D., M. C. Lombard, J. M. Zakac et al.: Pre- and postsynaptic distribution of mu, delta and kappa opioid receptors in the superficial layers of the cervical dorsal horn of the rat spinal cord. Brain Res. 521 (1–2) (1990) 15–22.
8. Birmauer, N., H. Flor, W. Lutzenberger et al.: The corticalisation of chronic pain. In: B. Bromm, J. E. Desmedt (Eds.): Pain and the Brain – From Nociception to Cognition, pp. 331–344. Raven Press, New York 1995.
9. Blackshaw, L. A., D. Grundy: 5HT receptor mediated effects on vagal mucosal afferent fibres from the upper gastrointestinal tract of the anaesthetised ferret. J. Physiol. 435 (1996) 64–66.
10. Bradette, M., M. Delvaux, G. Staumont et al.: Octreotide increases thresholds of colonic visceral perception in IBS patients without modifying muscle tone. Dig. Dis. Sci. 39 (1994) 1171–1178.
11. Buck, M., J. H. Walsh, H. I. Yamamura et al.: Neuropeptides in sensory neurons. Life Sci. 30 (1982) 1857–1866.

12. Bueno, L., M. Gue, M.J. Fargeas et al.: Vagally mediated inhibition of acoustic stress-induced cortisol release by orally administered kappa opioid substances in dogs. Endocrinology 124 (1989) 1788−1793.

13. Burroughs, A. K., P. A. McCormick: Somatostatin and octreotide in gastroenterology. Aliment. Pharmacol. Ther. 5 (1991) 331−341.

14. Butterworth, J. F., G. R. Strichartz: Molecular mechanisms of local anesthesia: a review. Anesthesiology 72 (4) (1990) 711−734.

15. Camarata, P. J., T. L. Yaksh: Characterisation of the spinal adrenergic receptors mediating the spinal effects produced by microinjection of morphine into the PAG. Brain Res. 1985 Jun 10; 336 (1) (1985) 133−142.

16. Cannon, R. O., A. A. Quyyumi, R. Mincemoyer et al.: Imipramine in patients with chest pain despite normal coronary angiograms [see comments]. N. Engl. J. Med. 330 (1994) 1411−1417.

17. Cervero, F., J. F. B. Morrison: Visceral sensation. Elsevier, Amsterdam 1986.

18. Chapman, V., A. H. Dickenson: The combination of NMDA antagonisms and morphine produces profound antinociception in the rat dorsal horn. Brain Res. 573 (1992) 321−323.

19. Chey, W. D., A. Beydoun, W. L. Hasler et al.: Octreotide reduces spinal afferent transmission in response to rectal electrical stimulation in diarrhea-predominant irritable bowel patients. Gastroenterology 106 (1994) A478.

20. Chrubasik, J., J. Meynadier, P. Scherpereel et al.: The effect of epidural somatostatin on postoperative pain. Anesth. Analg. 64 (1985) 1085−1088.

21. Clark, F. M., H. K. Proudfit: The projection of locus coeruleus neurons to the spinal cord in the rat determined by anterograde tracing combined with immunocytochemistry. Brain Res. 538 (1991) 231−245.

22. Coffin, B., M. Jian, M. Lemann et al.: Fedotozine increases threshold of discomfort to gastric distension in healthy subjects. Gastroenterology 102 (1992) A437.

23. Collin. E., D. Frechilla, M. Pohl et al.: Differential effects of a novel analgesic, S12813-4, on the spinal release of substance P and calcitonin gene-related peptide-like materials in the rat. Archives of Pharmacology 349 (1994) 387−393.

24. Courteix, C., M. Bardin, C. Chantelauze et al.: A study on the sensitivity of the diabetes induced pain model in rats to a range of analgesics. Pain 57 (1994) 153−160.

25. Czlonkowski, A., C. Stein, A. Herz: Peripheral mechanisms of opioid antinociception in inflammation: involvement of cytokines. Eur. J. Pharmacol. 242 (3) (1993) 229−235.

26. Daniel. E. E., J. E. T. Fox, H. D. Allescher et al.: Peripheral actions of opiates in canine gastrointestinal tract; actions on nerves and muscles. Gastroenterol. Clin. Biol. 11 (1987) 477−495.

27. Danzebrink, R. M., G. F. Gebhart: Evidence that spinal 5-HT1, 5-HT2 and 5-HT3 receptor subtypes modulate responses to noxious colorectal distension in the rat. Brain Res. 538 (1991) 64−75.

28. Dapoigny, M., J. L. Abitol, J. Geneve et al.: Fedotozine in irritable bowel syndrome: Results of a 6 wk placebo-controlled multicenter therapeutic trial. Gut 37 (1995) A159.

29. Delvaux, M., D. Louvel, B. Scherrer et al.: The k-agonist fedotozine increases thresholds of the first sensation and pain perception to colonic distension in patients with irritable bowel syndrome. Gut 37 (1995) A148.

30. Dickenson, A. H.: A cure for wind up: NMDA receptor antagonists as potential analgesics. Trends in Pharmacological Sciences 11 (8): (1990) 307−309.

31. Dickenson, A. H., A. F. Sullivan: Electrophysiological studies on the effects of intrathecal morphine on nociceptive neurones in the rat dorsal horn. Pain (1986) 211−222.

32. Diener, H. C., R. van Schayck, O. Kastrup: Pain and Depression. In: B. Bromm, J. E. Desmedt (Eds.): Pain and the Brain − From Nociception to Cognition, pp. 345−356. Raven Press, New York 1995.

33. Dinan, T. G., A. S. B. Chua, P. W. N. Keeling: Serotonin and physical illness: Focus on non-ulcer dyspepsia. J. Psychopharmacol. 7 (1994) 126−130.

34. Diop, L., P. J. Riviere, X. Pascaud et al.: Peripheral kappa-opioid receptors mediate the antinociceptive effect of fedotozine on the duodenal pain reflex in the rat. Eur. J. Pharmacol. 271 (1994) 65–71.

35. Dray, A.: Tasting the inflammatory soup: role of peripheral neurones. Pain Reviews 1 (1994) 153–171.

36. Drossman, D. A. Psychosocial factors in chronic functional abdominal pain. In: E. A. Mayer, H. E. Raybould (Eds.): Basic and clinical aspects of chronic abdominal pain, 271–280. Elsevier, Amsterdam 1993.

37. Eschalier, A., V. Kayser, G. Guilbaud: Influence of a specific 5-HT3 antagonist on carrageenan-induced hyperalgesia in rats. Pain 36 (1989) 249–255.

38. Fraitag, B., M. Homerin, P. Hecketsweiler: Double blind dose-response multicenter comparison of fedotozine and placebo in treatment of nonulcer dyspepsia. Dig. Dis. Sci. 39 (1994) 1072–1077.

39. Friedman, G.: Treatment of the irritable bowel syndrome. In: G. Friedman (Ed.): Gastroenterology Clinics of North America; The Irritable Bowel Syndrom: Realities and Trends, pp. 325–333. W. B. Saunders Company, Philadelphia 1991.

40. Glaum, S. R., H. K. Proudfit, E. G. Anderson: Reversal of the antinociceptive effects of intrathecally administered serotonin in the rat by a selective 5HT3 receptor antagonist. Neurosci. Lett. 95 (1988) 313–317.

41. Goldberg, P. A., M. A. Kamm, P. Setti-Carraro et al.: Modification of visceral sensitivity and pain in irritable bowel syndrome by 5-HT$_3$ antagonism (ondansetron). Digestion (1996) in press.

42. Gorard, D. A., G. W. Libby, M. J. Farthing: Effect of a tricyclic antidepressant on small intestinal motility in health and diarrhea-predominant irritable bowel syndrome. Dig. Dis. Sci. 40 (1995) 86–95.

43. Gore, S., I. T. Gilmore, C. G. Haigh et al.: Colonic transit in man is slowed by ondansetron (GR38032F) a selective 5-hydroxytryptamine receptor (type 3) antagonist. Aliment. Pharmacol. Therap. 4 (1990) 139–144.

44. Grubb, B. D., D. S. McQueen, A. Iggo et al.: A study of 5-HT-receptors associated with afferent nerves located in normal and inflamed rat ankle joints. Agents Actions 25 (1988) 216–218.

45. Gue, M., J. Fioramonti, J. L. Junien et al.: Orally administered kappa but not mu opiate agonists enhance gastric emptying of a solid canned food meal in dogs. J. Pharm. Pharmacol. 40 (1988) 873–875.

46. Gue, M., C. Honde, X. Pascaud et al.: CNS blockade of acoustic stress induced gastric motor inhibition by kappa opiate agonists in dogs. Am. J. Physiol. 254 (1989) G802–G807.

47. Hammond, D. L., R. Presley, K. R. Gogas et al.: Morphine or U-50,488 suppresses fos protein-like immunoreactivity in the spinal cord and nucleus tractus solitarii evoked by a noxious visceral stimulus in the rat. Journal of Comparative Neurology 315 (1992) 244–253.

48. Haruma, K., J. A. Wiste, M. Camilleri: Effect of octreotide on gastrointestinal pressure profiles in health and in functional and organic gastrointestinal disorders. Gut 35 (1994) 1064–1069.

49. Hasler, W. L., H. C. Soudah, C. Owyang: Somatostatin analog inhibits afferent response to rectal distension in diarrhea-predominant irritable bowel patients. J. Pharmacol. Exp. Ther. 268 (1994) 1206–1212.

50. Hassan, A. H., R. Pzewlocki, A. Herz et al.: Dynorphin, a preferential ligand for kappa-opioid receptors, is present in nerve fibers and immune cells within inflamed tissue in the rat. Neurosci. Lett. 140 (1992) 85–88.

51. Ho, R. H., M. Berelowitz: Somatostatin 28(1-14) immunoreactivity in primary afferent neurons of the rat spinal cord. Neurosci. Lett 46 (1984) 161–166.

52. Holstege, G.: Some anatomical observations on the projections from hypothalamus to brainstem and spinal cord: an HRP and autoradiographic tracing study in the cat. J. Comp. Neurol. 260 (1987) 98−126.

53. Inoue, M.: Pharmaceutical treatment of irritable bowel syndrome. Nippon Rinsho 50 (1992) 2746−2751.

54. Itoh, Z., A. Mizumoto, Y. Iwanaga et al.: Involvement of 5-hydroxytryptamine 3 receptors in regulation of interdigestive gastric contractions by motilin in the dog. Gastroenterology 100 (1991) 901−908.

55. Jones, S. L., G. F. Gebhart: Inhibition of spinal nociceptive transmission from the midbrain, pons and medulla in the rat. Brain Res. 460 (1988) 281−296.

56. Jones, S. L., A. R. Light: Serotonergic medullary raphespinal projection to the lumbar spinal cord in the rat: a retrograde immunohistochemical study. Journal of Comparative Neurology 322 (1992) 599−610.

57. Junien, J. L., M. Gue, X. Pascaud et al.: Central and peripheral opioid inhibitory pathways on stress induced gastric motor alteration in fasted dogs: a pharmacological approach. In: E. Bueno, S. Collins, J. L. Junien (Eds.): Stress and Digestive Motility, pp. 187−195. John Libby, London, Paris 1996.

58. Krishnan, K. R., R. D. France: Antidepressants in chronic pain syndromes. American Family Physician 39 (1989) 233−237.

59. Langlois, A., L. Diop, P. J. Riviere et al.: Effect of fedotozine on the cardiovascular pain reflex induced by distension of the irritated colon in the anesthetized rat. European. J. Pharmacol. 27 (1994) 245−251.

60. Larsen, J. J., J. Arnt: Spinal 5-HT or noradrenaline uptake potentiates supraspinal morphine antinociception in rats. Acta Pharmacol. Toxicol. 54 (1984) 72−75.

61. Lembo, T., J. Munakata, H. Mertz et al.: Evidence for the hypersensitivity of lumbar splanchnic afferents in irritable bowel syndrome. Gastroenterology 107 (1994) 1686−1696.

62. Levine, J. D., H. L. Fields, A. I. Basbaum: Peptides and the primary afferent nociceptor. Journal of Neuroscience 13 (1993) 2273−2286.

63. Lew, W. Y. M., J. C. Longhurst: Substance P, 5HT and bradykinin stimulated abdominal visceral afferents. Am. J. Physiol. 250 (1986) 464−473.

64. Llewelyn, M. B., J. Azami, M. H. Roberts: Brain stem mechanisms of antinociception. Effects of electrical stimulation and injection of morphine into the nucleus raphe magnus. Neuropharmacology 25 (1986) 727−735.

65. Madrazo, I., R. E. Franco-Bourland, V. M. Leon-Maza et al.: Intraventricular somatostatin-14, arginine vasopressin, and oxytocin: analgesic effect in a patient with intractable cancer pain. Appl. Neurophysiol. 50 (1987) 427−431.

66. Malagelada, J. R.: Altered visceral sensation in functional dyspepsia and related syndromes. In: E. A. Mayer, H. E. Raybould (Eds.): Basic and clinical aspects of chronic abdominal pain, pp. 55−59. Elsevier, Amsterdam 1993.

67. Mansour, A., C. A. Fox, H. Akil et al.: Opioid-receptor mRNA expression in the rat CNS: anatomical and functional implications. Trends Neurosci. 18 (1995) 22−29.

68. Massari, V. J., Y. Tizabi, C. H. Park et al.: Distribution and origin of bombesin, substance P and somatostatin in cat spinal cord. Peptides 4 (1983) 673−681.

69. Maxton, D. G., C. G. Haigh, P. J. Whorwell: Clinical trial of ondansetron, a selective 5-HT$_3$ antagonist in irritable bowel syndrome (IBS). Gastroenterology 100 (1991) A468.

70. Mayer, E. A.: The sensitive and reactive gut. European Journal of Gastroenterology & Hepatology 6 (1994) 470−477.

71. Mayer, E. A., G. F. Gebhart: Functional bowel disorders and the visceral hyperalgesia hypothesis: In: E. A. Mayer, H. E. Raybould (Eds.): Basic and clinical aspects of chronic abdominal pain, pp. 3−28. Elsevier, Amsterdam 1993.

72. Mayer, E. A., H. E. Raybould: Role of visceral afferent mechanisms in functional bowel disorders. Gastroenterology 99 (1990) 1688−1704.

73. McCann, M. J., R. C. Rogers: Central modulation of the vagovagal reflex: influence on gastric function. In: Y. Tache, D. L. Wingate (Eds.): Brain-Gut Interactions, pp. 57−69. CRC Press, Boca Raton 1991.

74. Mertz, H., V. Plourde, B. Sytnik et al.: Effect of a somatostatin analogue on gastric sensory perception and compliance. Dig. Dis. Sci. 37 (1996) A23.

75. Miyata, K., H. Ito, M. Yamano et al.: Comparison of the effects of trimebutine and YM114 (KAE-393), a novel 5-HR$_3$ receptor antagonist, on stress-induced defecation. European. J. Pharmacol. 250 (1993) 303−310.

76. Miyata, K., T. Kamato, H. Nishida et al.: Role of serotonin$_3$ receptor in stress-induced defecation. J. Pharma. Exp. Ther. 261 (1992) 297−307.

77. Mjellem, N., A. Lund, P. K. Eide et al.: The role of 5-HT1A and 5-HT1B receptors in spinal nociceptive transmission and in the modulation of NMDA induced behavior. Neuroreport 3 (1992) 1061−1064.

78. Mollenholt, P., C. Post, I. Paulsson et al.: Intrathecal and epidural somatostatin in rats: can antinociception, motor effects, and neurotoxicity be separated? Pain 43 (1990) 363−370.

79. Mollenholt, P., C. Post, N. Rawal et al.: Antinociceptive and 'neurotoxic' actions of somatostatin in rat spinal cord after intrethecal administration. Pain 32 (1988) 95−105.

80 Mönnikes, H., B. G. Schmidt, J. Tebbe et al.: Microinfusion of corticotropin releasing factor into the locus coeruleus/subcoeruleus nuclei stimulates colonic motor function in rats. Brain Res. 644 (1994) 101−108.

81. Mönnikes, H., J. Tebbe, C. Bauer et al.: Microinfusion of corticotropin-releasing factor into the locus coeruleus/subcoeruleus nuclei inhibits gastric acid secretion via spinal pathways in the rat. Brain Res. (1996) in press.

82. Morteau, O., V. Julia, C. Eeckhout, et al.: Influence of 5-HT$_3$ receptor antagonists in visceromotor and nociceptive responses to rectal distension before and during experimental colitis in rats. Fundam. Clin. Pharmacol. 8 (1994) 553−562.

83. Myren, J., B. Lovland, S. E. Larssen et al.: A double-blind study of the effect of trimipramine in patients with the irritable bowel syndrome. Scand. J. Gastroenterol. 19 (1984) 835−843.

84. Myren, J., B. Lovland, S. E. Larssen et al.: Psychopharmacologic drugs in the treatment of the irritable bowel syndrome. A double blind study of the effect of trimipramine. Ann. Gastroenterol. Hepatol. Paris 20 (1984) 117−123.

85. Owyang, C.: Octreotide in gastrointestinal motility disorders. Gut 35 (1994) S11−4.

86. Plourde, V., T. Lembo, Z. Shui et al.: Effects of the somatostatin analogue octreotide on rectal afferent nerves in humans. Am. J. Physiol. 265 (1993) G742−51.

87. Porreca, F., J. J. Galligan, T. F. Burks: Central opioid receptor involvement in gastrointestinal motility. Trends Pharmacol. Sci. 7 (1986) 104−107.

88. Porreca, F., H. I. Mosberg, R. Hurst et al.: Roles of mu, delta and kappa opioid receptors in spinal and supraspinal mediation of gastrointestinal transit effects and hot-plate analgesia in the mouse. J. Pharmacol. Exp. Ther. 230 (1984) 341−348.

89. Powley, T. L., H.-R. Berthoud, J. C. Prechtl et al.: Fibers of the vagus nerve regulating gastrointestinal function. In: Y. Tache, D. L. Wingate (Eds.): Brain-Gut Interactions, pp. 73−82. CRC Press, Boca Raton 1991.

90. Pretel, S., Piekut, D. T.: Enkephalin, substance P, and serotonin axonal input to c-fos-like immunoreactive neurons of the rat spinal cord. Peptides 12 (1991) 1243−1250.

91. Prior, A., N. W. Read: Reduction of rectal sensitivity and postprandial motility by granisetron, a 5HT$_3$ receptor antagonist, in patients with irritable bowel syndrome (IBS). Aliment. Pharmacol. Therap. 7 (1993) 175−180.

92. Prior, A., K. M. Wilson, P. J. Whorwell: Double-blind study of an alpha 2 agonist in the treatment of irritable bowel syndrome. Aliment. Pharmacol. Ther. 2 (1988) 535−539.

93. Ragsdale, D. S., T. Scheuer, W. A. Catterall: Frequency and voltage-dependent inhibition of type IIA Na$^+$ channels, expressed in a mammalian cell line by local anesthetic, antiarrhythmic, and anticonvulsant drugs. Molecular Pharmacology 40 (5) (1991) 756−765.

94. Raiteri, M., G. Maura, P. Paudice: Different 5-HT Receptors Modulate Glutamate Release in Cerebellum (5-HT1 and 5-HT2) and Cholecystokinin Release in Nucleus Accumbens (5-HT3) − Possible Relevance to Cerebellar Ataxias and to Anxiety. Serotonin Receptor Subtypes. Pharmacological Significa 12 (1992) 1105−1110.

95. Rang, H. P., S. J. Bevan, A. Dray: Nociceptive peripheral neurones: cellular properties. In: P. D. Wall, R. Melzack (Eds.): Textbook of Pain, pp. 57−78. Churchill Livingstone, Edinburgh 1994.

96. Read, N. W.: The rational use of CCK antagonists in irritable bowel syndrome. In: G. Adler, C. Beglinger (Eds.): Cholecystokinin Antagonists in Gastroenterology, pp. 214−219. Springer-Verlag, Berlin−Heidelberg 1991.

97. Read, N. W.: Visceral afferent innervation and functional bowel disease: evidence for dyssensation and altered reflex function. In: E. A. Mayer, H. E. Raybould (Eds.): Basic and clinical aspects of chronic abdominal pain, pp. 87−96. Elsevier, Amsterdam 1993.

98. Richardson, B. P., G. Engel, P. Donatsch et al.: Identification of serotonin M-receptor-subtypes and their specific blockade by a new class of drugs. Nature 316 (1985) 126−131.

99. Richter, J. E., M. D. Laurence, A. Bradley: The irritable esophagus. In: E. A. Mayer, H. E. Raybould (Eds.): Basic and clinical aspects of chronic abdominal pain, pp. 45−54. Elsevier, Amsterdam 1993.

100. Riviere, P. J., X. Pascaud, E. Chevalier et al.: Fedotozine reversal of peritoneal-irritation-induced ileus in rats: possible peripheral action on sensory afferents. J. Pharma. Exp. Ther. 270 (1994) 846−850.

101. Riviere, P. J., X. Pascaud, E. Chevalier et al.: Fedotozine reverses ileus induced by surgery of peritonitis: action at peripheral kappa opiod receptors. Gastroenterology 104 (1993) 724−731.

102. Rivot, J. P., C. Y. Chiang, J. M. Besson: Increase of serotonin metabolism within the dorsal horn of the spinal cord during raphe magnus stimulation, as revealed by in vivo electrochemical detection. Brain Res. 238 (1995) 117−126.

103. Salet, G. A.M., J. M. M. Heyligers, J. M. Lautenschutz et al.: Effect of fedotozine on digestive symptoms following abdominal surgery. Gut 37 (1995) A48.

104. Sandkühler, J., Q. G. Fu, C. Helmchen: Spinal serotonin superfusion in vivo affects activity of the cat nociceptive dorsal horn neurons: comparison with spinal morphine. Neuroscience 34 (1990) 565−576.

105. Schäfer, M., L. Carter, C. Stein: Interleukin 1 beta and corticotropin-releasing factor inhibit pain by releasing opioids from immune cells in inflamed tissue. Proc. Natl. Acad. Sci. USA 91 (1994) 4219−4223.

106. Schmidt, K., P. H. Althoff, A. G. Harris et al.: Analgesic effect of the somatostatin analogue octreotide in two acromegalic patients: a double-blind study with long term follow up. Pain 53 (2) (1993) 223−227.

107. Schockley, R. A., K. J. LePard, R. L. Stephens Jr.: Fluoxetine pretreatment potentiates intracisternal TRH analogue-stimulated gastric acid secretion in rats. Regul. Pept. 38 (1992) 121−128.

108. Sicuteri, F., P. Geppetti, S. Marabini et al.: Pain relief by somatostatin in attacks of cluster headache. Pain 18 (1984) 359−365.

109. Soudah. H. C., W. L. Hasler, C. Owyang: Differential effects of the somatostatin analog on perception of visceral distension in the rectum versus the stomach. Gastroenterology 102 (1992) A518.

110. Stanfa, L., A. H. Dickenson, X. Xu et al.: Cholecystokinin and morphine analgesia: variations on a theme. Trends in Pharmacological Sciences 15 (1994) 65−66.

111. Steadman, C. J., N. J. Talley, S. F. Phillips et al.: Trial of a selective serotonin type 3 (5HT3) receptor antagonist, ondansetron (GR 3802F) in diarrhoea predominant irritable bowel syndrome (IBS). Gastroenterology 98 (1990) A394.

112. Steadman, C. J., N. J. Talley, S. F. Phillips et al.: Selective 5-hydroxytryptamine type 3 receptor antagonism with ondansetron as treatment for diarrhoea-predominant irritable bowel syndrome: A pilot study. Mayo Clinic Proceedings 67 (1992) 732−738.

113. Stein, C.: Peripheral mechanisms of opioid analgesia. Anesth. Analg. (1993) 967−973.

114. Sufka, K. J., F. M. Schomburg, J. Giordano: Receptor mediation of 5-HT-induced inflammation and nociception in the rat. Pharmacol. Biochem. Behav. 41 (1991) 53−56.

115. Svensson, T. H.: Clonidine treatment in vegetative dysfunction − experimental rationales. Acta Obstet. Gynecol. Scand. Suppl. 132 (1985) 23−28.

116. Taché, Y.: Central control of gastrointestinal transit and motility by brain-gut peptides. In: W. J. Snape (Ed.): Pathogenesis of Functional Bowel Disease, pp. 55−76. Plenum Press, New York 1989.

117. Taché, Y., H. Mönnikes: CRF in the central nervous system mediate stress-induced stimulation of colonic motor function: relevance to the pathophysiology of IBS. In: E. A. Mayer, H. E. Raybould (Eds.): Basic and clinical aspects of chronic abdominal pain, pp. 141−151. Elsevier, Amsterdam 1993.

118. Taiwo, Y. Q., J. D. Levine: Kappa- and delta-opioids block sympathetically dependent hyperalgesia. J. Neurosci. 11 (1991) 928−932.

119. Talley, N. J., S. F. Phillips, A. Haddad et al.: Effect of selective 5HT$_3$ antagonist (GR 38032F) on small intestinal transit and release of gastrointestinal peptides. Dig. Dis. Sci. 34 (1989) 1511−1515.

120. Talley, N. J., S. F. Phillips, A. Haddad et al.: GR 38032F (ondansetron), a selective 5-HT$_3$ receptor antagonist, slows colonic transit in healthy man. Dig. Dis. Sci. 35 (1990) 477−480.

121. Talley, N. J., S. F. Phillips. L. J. Miller et al.: A specific 5HT$_3$ antagonist delays colonic transit and inhibits postprandial neurotensin (NT) release. Gastroenterology 95 (1988) 891.

122. Tokuyama, S., M. Takahashi, H. Kaneto: Involvement of serotonergic receptor subtypes in the production of antinociception by psychological stress in mice. Jpn. J. Pharmacol. 61 (1993) 237−242.

123. Watkins, L. R., E. P. Wiertelak, S. F. Maier: Kappa opiate receptors mediate tail-shock induced antinociception at spinal levels. Brain Res. 582 (1992) 1−9.

124. Whitehead, W. E.: Psychophysiology of irritable bowel syndrome. In: E. A. Mayer, H. E. Raybould (Eds.): Basic and clinical aspects of chronic abdominal pain, pp. 239−247. Elsevier, Amsterdam 1993.

125. Willis, W. D.: Anatomy and physiology of descending control of nociceptive responses of dorsal horn neurons: comprehensive review. In: H. L. Fields, H. L. Besson (Eds.): Pain Modulation. Progress in Brain Research, pp. 1−29. Elsevier, New York 1988.

126. Wolfe, F., M. A. Cathey: Somatostatin therapy in patients with severe fibromyalgia: a preliminary report. Pain 55 (1990).

127. Yaksh, T. L.: Pharmacology of spinal adrenergic system which modulates spinal nociceptive processing. Pharmacology, Biochemistry & Behavior 22 (1985) 845−858.

128. Yaksh, T. L., A. B. Malmberg: Central pharmacology of nociceptive transmission. In: P. D. Wall, R. Melzack (Eds.): Textbook of Pain, pp. 165−200. Churchill-Livingstone, Edinburgh 1993.

129. Yamamoto, T., T. L. Yaksh: Studies on the spinal interaction of morphine and the NMDA antagonist MK-801 on the hyperesthesia observed in a rat model of sciatic mononeuropathy. Neurosci. Lett. 135 (1992) 67−70.

130. Yeomans, D. C., F. M. Clark, J. A. Paice et al.: Antinociception induced by electrical stimulation of spinally projecting noradrenergic neurons in the A7 catecholamine cell group of the rat. Pain 48 (1992) 449−461.

131. Zieglgänsberger, W., T. R. Tölle, A. Zimprich et al.: Endorphins, pain relief, and euphoria. In: B. D. Bromm, J. E. Desmedt (Eds.): Pain and the Brain — From Nociception to Cognition, pp. 439–458. Raven Press, New York 1995.
132. Zighelboim, J., N. J. Talley, S. F. Phillips et al.: Visceral perception in irritable bowel syndrome. Rectal and gastric responses to distension and serotonin type 3 antagonism. Dig. Dis. Sci. 40 (1995) 819–827.

Behavioral treatment of altered brain-gut mechanisms

G. A. Fava

Since the early fifties, there has been a steady growth in psychotherapy research. Use of control groups, standardized assessments, follow-up evaluations, blind raters has built the research evidence necessary to verify the effectiveness of psychotherapeutic approaches in a number of psychiatric and medical disorders [3]. In many controlled studies, no significant differences between psychotherapeutic modalities emerged. This suggested the presence of some common and non-specific therapeutic ingredients that even very different psychotherapeutic techniques may share. Such ingredients include attention to the patient, disclosure of psychological distress and feelings, high arousal, interpretation (and thus rationalization) of symptoms, and the rituals associated with the psychotherapeutic setting [7]. Psychotherapy research has shown that the benefits of psychotherapy are maximal when a specific technique is used in the setting of well-specified psychiatric disorders. For instance, behavioral therapies were found to be most effective in phobic and anxiety disorders, whereas cognitive therapies had a higher impact on depressive disorders [3]. At times, different psychotherapeutic approaches are combined (e. g., cognitive-behavioral treatment). The heading cognitive-behavioral has characterized the most effective approaches in psychiatric disorders [3]. The cognitive hypothesis proposes that emotions of any kind arise from a person's idiosyncratic interpretation of the meaning of situations and events [10]. Such emotions may result in physical sensations and symptoms and/or in misinterpretation of health-related information. Cognitive therapy is aimed at changing beliefs about the consequences of the problem and at suggesting alternative interpretations. Behavioral therapies are aimed at modifying maladaptive behavior (e. g. avoidance in phobias) and include techniques such as exposure in vivo, relaxation and biofeedback.

Several psychotherapeutic approaches have been proposed to alleviate psychological distress and improve physical symptoms in irritable bowel syndrome (IBS). Such approaches have included cognitive-behavior therapy, relaxation training, hypnosis, and brief dynamic psychotherapy (the forming of an intense relationship with the patient, linking symptoms to feelings, and then understanding the relationship of symptoms to problems or emotional difficulties in the patient's life). At times, a combination of these treatment modalities has been attempted. These studies have been reviewed in detail elsewhere [2, 9]. The majority of the controlled investigations showed the superiority of psychological treatments associated with conventional medical treatment compared to medical therapy alone. No significant differences between treatment modalities emerged, suggesting a strong impact of non-specific ingredients of psychotherapy.

These studies, however, have limited impact on clinical practice, unless they are filtered by a sequential approach.

Should all patients with irritable bowel syndrome be referred for psychotherapy?

The answer is obviously not. A physician already encounters considerable resistance in referring a patient with functional gastrointestinal symptoms to a psychiatrist or psychologist. Psychotherapy is a time consuming process that requires considerable motivation, that can be attained only by selected patients. Further, the majority of patients with IBS (up to 83%) respond to conventional medical treatment in conjunction with explanation and reasssurance [9]. In one of the most important psychotherapy trials in IBS, Guthrie et al. [8], included only patients with continuous symptoms for at least one year, who attended a gastrointestinal clinic for at least 6 months and who were unresponsive to conventional medical treatment. These criteria provide a reasonable gastroenterologic background for further exploring the psychological dimension in IBS patients. Obviously, such criteria should be supplemented by customary clinical judgement (e. g., marked depressive features).

Psychological assessment of patients

In the controlled studies available, irritable bowel syndrome patients were treated as if psychological mechanisms were homogeneous in the patients. Research evidence just shows the contrary: patients are very heterogeneous as to psychopathology and psychometric dimensions [2, 9]. Often referral to a psychiatrist becomes a source of frustration for the gastroenterologist. This is also because current diagnostic criteria used in clinical psychiatry such as DSM-IV [1], fail to provide a satisfactory description of the psychosomatic syndromes and problems (4, 6]. For this reason, new diagnostic criteria for psychosomatic patients have been developed [5]. Table 1 outlines the diagnostic criteria for functional somatic symptoms secondary to a psychiatric disorder. In these cases, treatment of the primary psychiatric disorder (whether pharmacological or psychological or both) according to well defined guidelines is likely to entail disappearance or considerable decrease of bowel symptoms. Other cases (Table 2) would present clinical characteristics that are likely to respond to psychotherapy instead of drug treatment [7]. Another example may involve the persistent

Table 1: *Diagnostic criteria for functional somatic symptoms secondary to a psychiatric disorder (A through D are required).*

A. Symptoms of autonomic arousal (e. g., palpitations, sweating, tremor, flushing) or functional medical disorder (e. g., irritable bowel syndrome, fibromyalgia, neurocirculatory asthenia), causing distress, or repeated medical care, or resulting in impaired quality of life.

B. Appropriate medical evaluation uncovers no organic pathology to account for the physical complaints.

C. A psychiatric disorder (which includes the involved somatic symptoms within its manifestations) preceded the onset of functional somatic symptoms (e. g., panic disorder and cardiac symptoms).

D. Even though health anxiety may occur, the patient does not meet the criteria for hypochondriasis or disease phobia.

From Fava et al. [5], by permission.

Table 2: *Diagnostic criteria for demoralization (A through D are required).*

A. A feeling state characterized by the patient's consciousness of having failed to meet his or her own expectations (or those of others) or being unable to cope with some pressing problems. The patient experiences feelings of helplessness, or hopelessness, or giving up.

B. The feeling state should be prolonged and generalized (at least one month duration).

C. The feeling closely antedated the manifestations of a medical disorder or exacerbated its symptoms.

D. Demoralization is not secondary to a psychiatric disorder (such as major depression or panic disorder).

From Fava et al. [5], by permission.

Table 3: *Diagnostic criteria for persistent somatization (A through C are required).*

A. Functional medical disorder (e. g., fibromyalgia, fatigue, esophageal motility disorders, non ulcer dyspepsia, irritable bowel syndrome, neurocirculatory asthenia, urethral syndrome), whose duration exceeds 6 months, causing distress, or repeated medical care, or resulting in impaired quality of life.

B. Additional symptoms of autonomic arousal (involving also other organ systems) and exaggerated side effects from medical therapy are present, indicating low sensation or pain thresholds and high suggestibility.

C. Somatic symptoms do not occur in the course of a mood, anxiety or organic mental disorder.

From Fava et al. [5], by permission.

somatizers (Table 3). Kellner [9] suggested that it may be advantageous to conceptualize a somatizing patient as someone in whom psychophysiological symptoms have clustered. These patients are more likely to respond to explanation,

Table 4: *Diagnostic criteria for health anxiety (A through C are required).*

A. Generic worry about illness, concern about pain and bodily preoccupations (tendency to amplify somatic sensations) of less than 6 months duration.
B. Worries and fears readily respond to appropriate medical reassurance, even though new worries may ensue after some time.
C. Worries and fears are not secondary to mood or anxiety disorders.

From Fava et al. [5], by permission.

Table 5: *Diagnostic criteria for conversion symptoms (A through D are required).*

A. One or more symptoms or deficits affecting voluntary motor or sensory function, characterized by lack of anatomical or physiological plausibility, and/or absence of expected physical signs or laboratory findings, and/or inconsistent clinical characteristics. If symptoms of autonomic arousal or functional medical disorder are present, conversion symptoms should be prominent, causing distress, or repeated medical care, or resulting in impaired quality of life.
B. At least 2 of the following features are present:
   (1) ambivalence in symptom reporting (e. g. the patient appears relaxed or unconcerned as he describes distressing symptoms)
   (2) hystrionic personality features (colorful and dramatic expression, language and appearance; demanding dependency; high suggestibility; rapid mood changes)
   (3) precipitation of symptoms by psychological stress, the association of which the patient is unaware
   (4) history of similar physical symptoms experienced by the patient, or observed in someone else, or wished on someone else.
C. Appropriate medical evaluation unconvers no organic pathology to account for the physical complaints.
D. Somatic symptoms do not occur in the course of a mood, anxiety or organic mental disorder.

From Fava et al. [5], by permission.

reassurance, and support by the treating physician than to complex and time consuming psychotherapeutic techniques [4]. Similar considerations apply to health anxiety (Table 4) − and conversion symptoms (Table 5).

Referral for psychotherapy

It is conceivable, even though yet to be tested in controlled studies, that patients with IBS who are properly screened and selected may offer a better response to brief psychotherapy than unselected patients. Diagnostic developments in psychosomatic diagnosis may thus pave the way for more targeted psychotherapeutic efforts in altered brain-gut mechanisms. Controlled studies may then determine whether a specific technique (e. g., cognitive-behavioral therapy) is more likely to yield successful results than others. Until more research evidence is at hand, gastroenterologists should not dismiss the considerable therapeutic potential of psychotherapy in the setting of irritable bowel syndrome.

References

1. American Psychiatric Association: Diagnostic and statistical manual of mental disorders (DSM-IV), APA, Washington, DC 1994.
2. Drossman, D. A., F. H. Creed, G. A.Fava et al.: Psychosocial aspects of the functional gastrointestinal disorders. Gastroenterology Int. 8 (1995) 47–90.
3. Fava, G. A.: Psychotherapy research: clinical trials versus clinical reality. Psychother. Psychosom. 46 (1986) 6–12.
4. Fava, G. A.: The concept of psychosomatic disorder. Psychother. Psychosom. 58 (1992) 1–12.
5. Fava, G. A., H. J. Freyberger, P. Bech et al.: Diagnostic criteria for use in psychosomatic research. Psychother. Psychosom. 63 (1995) 1–8.
6. Fava, G. A., H. Freyberger (Eds.): New developments in psychosomatic medicine. International Universities Press, Madison, CT 1996.
7. Frank, J. D., J. B. Frank: Persuasion and healing. The Johns Hopkins University Press, Baltimore 1991.
8. Guthrie, E., F. Creed, T. Dawson et al.: A controlled trial of psychological treatment for the irritable bowel syndrome. Gastroenterology 100 (1991) 450–457.
9. Kellner, R.: Psychosomatic syndromes and somatic symptoms. American Psychiatric Press, Washington 1991.
10. Salkovskis, P.: The cognitive-behavioral approach. In: F. Creed, R. Mayou, A. Hopkins (Eds.): Medical symptoms not explained by organic disease, pp. 70–84. Royal College of Psychiatrists and Royal College of Physicians, London 1992.

The barostat: a tool to evaluate visceral sensitivity

M. Delvaux

Introduction

Functional digestive disorders (FDD), of which irritable bowel syndrome (IBS) is the most frequent condition, are very often the reason for consultation in Gastroenterology. Clinically, FDD are essentially characterized by an association of various disturbances with pain, the location of which depends on the organ thought to be involved. IBS has been recently defined by the Rome criteria as an association of abdominal pain with changes in stool habits and/or abdominal bloating [49]. The pathophysiology of pain in FDD and IBS has been poorly studied for the lack of a standard methodology for its investigation and this little knowledge of the role of visceral afferents in comparison to that so far acquired on somatic afferent nerve pathways [10].

In the two last decades some studies have shown that the thresholds for perception of visceral pain are lower in IBS patients than in controls during the test of rectal distension [44, 30]. In patients with non cardiac chest pain (NCCP), a hypersensitivity of the oesophagus has been observed after mechanical distension [26] or intraluminal acid infusion [27]. More recently, the availability of electromechanical barostats for the study of digestive tone and visceral perception has led to an increasing knowledge about the pathophysiological role of the altered visceral perception in patients with FDD. These alterations could result from abnormalities of pain perception at the level of visceral afferent nerve pathways and/or of the central nervous system (CNS) [11, 45]. Pharmacological studies in animals have shown that many neurotransmitters are involved in the regulation of visceral afferent function [5, 39]. Moreover, some results indicate that visceral perception may be pharmacologically modulated in healthy humans [25] as well as in patients with IBS [13].

Initially the barostat was designed by Malagelada and Azpiroz to evaluate the tone of a hollow organ [6]. To maintain the pressure constant in a bag placed in the organ, the barostat inflates or deflates the bag. The movements of air are thought to reflect changes in tone of the organ. However, the barostat has since been used by many investigators as a distending device to evaluate visceral sensitivity. Luminal distension is one of the most common methods to elicit visceral sensations. Although a barostat is not needed to perform distension studies, it has made those easier to design and has allowed to obtain more complete results.

We would like to review in this chapter the technical characteristics of the barostat that are important for distension studies, the protocols of such studies, the methods to elicit subject's response and the factors able to influence their results. In a second part, we will provide a quick overview of the studies performed with a barostat and showing that patients with FDD may have altered visceral sensitivity, with some comments regarding the possibility to use drugs to modify visceral perception and we will finally discuss the impact of barostat studies on the clinical approach to FDD.

Technical characteristics of the barostat

The barostat is made of a pumping device controlled by a computer which maintains constant the pressure in the bag connected to the inflation line (Fig. 1). To achieve this, the barostat aspirates or inflates air in the bag and the changes in bag volume reflect changes in tone of the gut. The pumping device may either be a bellows or a syringe [24]. Both have advantages and disadvantages. It is beyond the scope of this chapter to discuss those in detail. However, we must point out that some calculations must be performed by the system to compensate artifacts in pressure and volume measurements. A careful calibra-

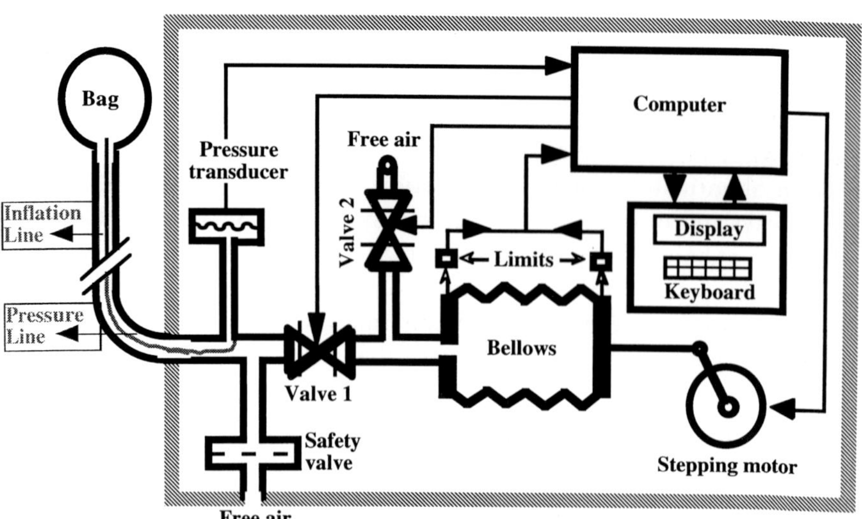

Fig. 1: *Scheme of a barostat using a bellows as pumping device and showing the air circuit within the barostat. It is important to note that the probe attached to the barostat must ideally have distinct lines for inflation of air within the bag and measurement of the intrabag pressure. A safety valve triggered by a mechanical button allows the investigator to deflate very rapidly the bag in case of emergency.*

tion of the system is also mandatory. Some technical issues have recently been addressed by a group of experts in the field, regarding the use of a barostat for distension studies [52].

The advantages of using a barostat as distending device are multiple. The size of the bellows or the syringe may be adapted to the organ to distend and thus it is possible to obtain very fast inflation of the bag which provokes a rapid stretch of the gut wall. Because of the computer driven inflation system, the barostat allows one to perform various types of distending protocol (see later, "Methods") and to inflate the bag several times in a reproducible way. Speed of inflation, duration of the inflation, pressure or volume limits are electronically controlled and thus reproducible repetitions of distensions are ensured. The main advantage of the barostat is that it measures precisely both the volume and the pressure when a distension is performed. Whenever the fixed parameter defining the distension step is the pressure (*isobaric distensions*) or the volume (*isovolumic distensions*), the other parameter is measured at the same time. This is important for the studies about compliance of the gut wall to distension (see later, "Evaluation of compliance").

An important point is the question whether a balloon or a bag should be used for barostat studies. This question has not been definitively answered so far [29]. The latex balloons made from condoms have been widely used in the past [4, 54, 33]. These balloons have frequently an ovoid or cylindrical form and are characterized by a rapid increase in internal pressure for small volume changes that reflect their elastic properties (Fig. 2). Then, when the pressure increases above the elastance threshold, they become plastic and may accommodate large volumes with little increase in pressure [50]. By contrast, polyethylene bags display an infinite compliance at low pressure until the volume of air within the bag is equal to the volume of the bag itself. Thereafter, any further increase in volume will induce a rapid increase in internal pressure [11, 47, 9]. In distension studies, the bag or the balloon should not interfere with the measurements of volume (or pressure when thresholds are defined by the volume) needed to reach a given pressure level in order not to modify the pressure-volume relationship (compliance). For these reasons, we would recommend to use a bag instead of a balloon. The sole advantage of a latex balloon is that it is more compact and thus easier to pass through the mouth or anus but, finely folded, bags pass through both routes.

An additional characteristic of the bag is that it must be oversized, relatively to the organ to be distended. The capacity volume of the bag must be greater than the larger volume of air to be injected. Indicative sizes are given in Table 1 for bags designed to distend the various segments of the gut. Indeed, at volumes larger than 90% of its maximal capacity, the bag will interfere with pressure and volume measurements. Moreover, it is emphasized that the diameter of the

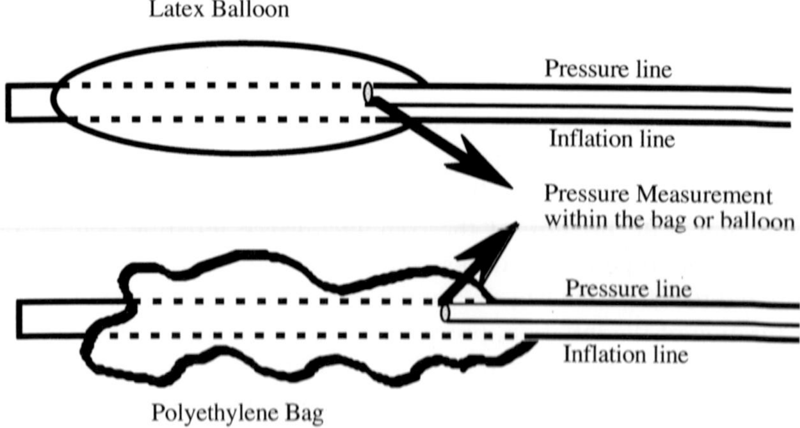

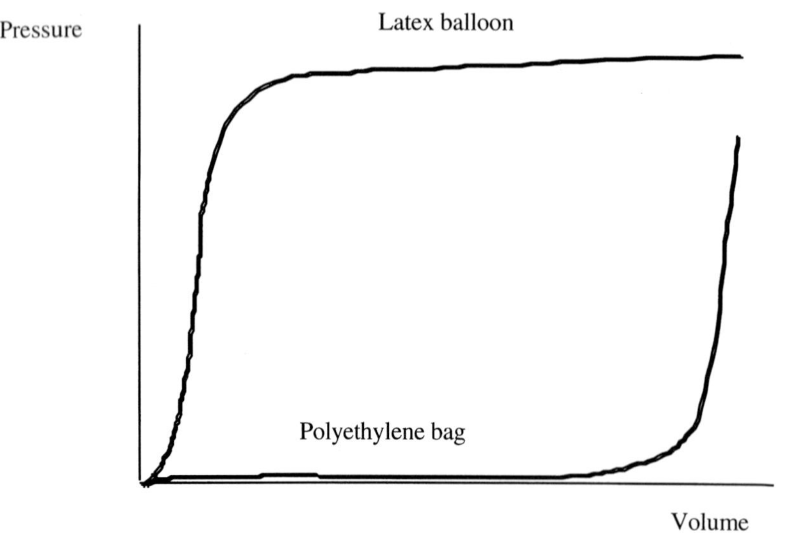

Fig. 2: *Schematic representation of a polyethylene bag and a latex balloon that can be used for distension studies. Note the separation between the pressure and the inflation lines. Shape and size of the bag or balloon has to be fixed depending on the organ studied (cfr Table 1). The chart shows theoretical compliance curves of the polyethylene bag and latex balloon when they are inflated in air. The polyethylene bag is infinitely compliant until the volume of air inflated is up to 90% of the maximal capacity of the bag. On the contrary, latex balloons are poorly compliant and the pressure increases rapidly within them.*

bag must be larger than the maximal diameter of the gut segment being tested. The form of the bag should also be adapted to the organ. For studies in reservoir organs like the stomach [7, 46], the rectum [9] or the bladder, it is advisable

Table 1: *Examples of bag design for barostat studies in the various parts of the gut.*

Organ	Shape	Length	Diameter	Capacity
Esophagus	Cylindrical	5 cm	6 cm	
Stomach	Spherical	n. r.		tone: 700 ml distension = 1,100 ml
Small intestine	Cylindrical	10 cm	18 cm	
Colon	Cylindrical	10 cm	15 cm	700 ml
Rectum	Spherical	n. r.		500 ml

to use bags that, when inflated, conform to a spherical shape. For tubular regions of the gastrointestinal tract, such as the esophagus, small intestine [8] or colon [11] (except rectum), cylindrical bags with a fixed length should be used, i. e., the bag should be attached to the probe at both ends in order to avoid any appreciable change in length during inflation.

The distension protocols

The distension protocol may considerably affect the results of visceral perception studies. The pressure or volume defining a sensory threshold and subsequently the concept of hyperreactivity or hypersensitivity to distension will be influenced by the method of distension.

Isobaric or isovolumic distensions

When the barostat is used to perform luminal distension of a digestive segment, the first parameter to be predetermined is whether the level of distension will be defined according to the pressure level reached in the bag (isobaric distensions) or to the volume of air present in the bag (isovolumic distensions). Some problems may arise with volume-scaled stimuli. Volume is not linearly related to balloon diameter or pressure because (i) air is inflated into a bag of approximately cylindrical shape in most cases, (ii) air is compressible, (iii) small variations in bag shape and dimensions may affect the measurements and dimensions of the bag and thus affect the pressure—volume relationship and (iv) finally the volume is to some extent influenced by the anatomy of the subject. Therefore the measure of balloon or bag pressure is more reproducible among laboratories and among subjects because the pressure scale compensates for the different factors possibly influencing the volume of the bag: bag shape, gut wall compliance, contractile activity and subject's anatomy. It is thus recommended to define sensory thresholds by the distending pressure. Some authors have recently proposed to consider the wall tension induced by the distending bag, which is defined as $T = 2Pr$ where P is the pressure and r, the radius of the distending bag [37]. This calculation does not bring significant additional information and is based on the "in vitro" or theoretical calculation of the radius of the distending bag which may not fully reflect the actual shape of the bag within the tested segment of the gut.

Cumulative versus phasic distension stimuli

Various distension protocols have been proposed. They are mainly based on the use of 2 different types of stimulus: the continuous, progressive and cumulative distension (*ramp distension*) and the rapid and time-limited distension inducing an abrupt stretch of the gut wall (*phasic distension*). Using these different protocols (Fig. 3), some authors have reported variations in subject's responses elicited by luminal distension. Comparing ramp distension to phasic distension, Mayer and coworkers found that hypersensitivity to rectal distension characterizing the patients with IBS was only triggered by phasic distension [33]. In another study reporting results obtained with 2 types of distensions (rapid phasic distension and cumulative stepwise distension), the pain threshold elicited by rapid phasic distension was significantly lower than the one elicited by stepwise distension [11]. This observation may suggest that different afferent nerve pathways are triggered by the various types of distension but a role for distinct mechanoreceptors or for multisensitive nociceptors within the gut wall has not been ruled out so far [28].

Although ramp or phasic distension may be used in distension studies depending on the question to be addressed, it it important to know that some sensory tests protocols (e.g. double random staircase or signal detection) can only be done with phasic distensions. As a general recommendation, when phasic stimuli are used, the duration of distension steps has to be at least 60 seconds and the interval between steps, also equal to or higher than 60 seconds. In case of phasic distensions, the subject's sensations will not be recorded immediately after the onset of the pressure in the balloon since the time required for wall adaptation may be 3 to 5 seconds and that reflex contractions may occur during 10 to 20 seconds after onset of inflation [7, 53].

Other factors influencing the measurements of sensory thresholds

Sensory thresholds are higher for rapid inflation than for slow inflation rates [48] and the differences between irritable bowel patients and healthy controls are greater for rapid distension than for slow distension [33]. Rates up to 40 ml/sec are able to efficiently compensate for changes in balloon pressure associated with coughing or other movement artifacts. Whatever rate of inflation is

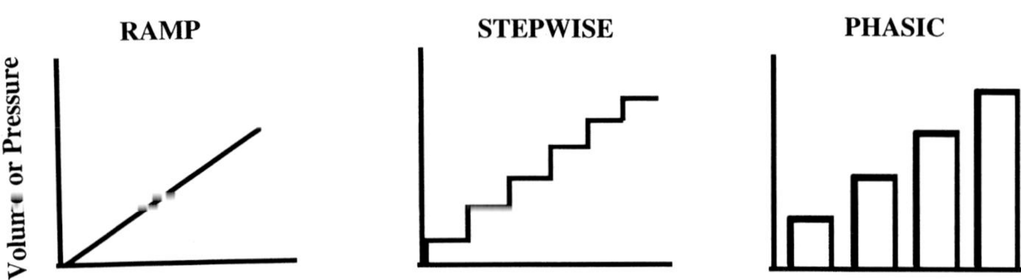

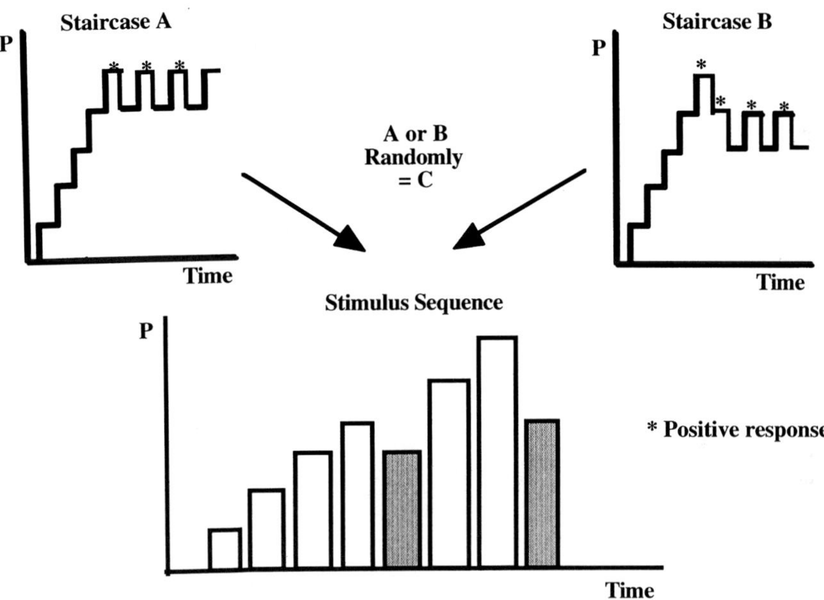

Fig. 3: *Schematic representation of the most common distension protocols. Advantages and disadvantages of these protocols are discussed in Table 2.*

chosen, it should be constant for all distension steps in one experiment. This will have the effect that distensions at high pressure levels require longer to reach the target pressure (or volume) but this is preferable to inflating at different rates in order to predetermine the duration of inflation.

Air compressibility in the system also influences the results of pressure and volume measurements. Adapted calculations and corrections should be performed to obtain a true assessment of pressure-volume relationship.

Distension protocols

The response of the subject to distension of the gut may be influenced by his past experience and psychological factors such as the fear of pain, which are collectively called response bias. Therefore, some distending protocols were designed to eliminate this bias (Fig. 3).

Ascending limit protocols are based on the progressive increase in intensity of the distending stimulus, using either ramp, stepwise or phasic distension, until the subject reports pain or another sensation of interest (Fig. 3). The assumption underlying the "ascending limit method" is that pain is qualitatively different from other sensations produced by distension and that there is a discrete threshold at which pain is first experienced. This method is believed to be maximally sensitive to psychological biases, especially the fear or pain, because stimuli are predictable to the subject. In addition, the patient learning history may influence where on the continuum of stimulus intensity he/she reports pain. Therefore the thresholds recorded using this method seem less reliable and it should not be recommended. However, in our opinion, the "ascending limit method" has nevertheless some advantages including its simplicity, the smaller number of presentations of the stimulus and it has been recently proven reproducible in careful double-blind controlled studies [18, 20].

Various protocols have then been designed to circumvene the problem of response bias. They are based on the presentation of multiple stimuli to the subject, using a random order or jumping randomly from one technique of tracking the response of the subject to another one. This latter method is called the "double random staircase". One may even make the sequence of stimuli unpredictable to the investigator when the computer program determines this sequence, based on the response of the subject, without any intervention of the investigator. We must emphasize that independently of the protocol used, the trial must start with an "ascending limit method" phase to detect the pressure (or volume) threshold at which the subject will report pain or discomfort. This is mandatory to detect the pain threshold and avoid inflation of the bag at pressures higher than this threshold during the second part of the trial. Then, multiple stimuli are presented around this threshold pressure in order to assess the reliability of the subject's response. Finally, the threshold pressure is defined as the mean intensity of the thresholds eliciting the sensation of interest.

Signal detection uses two stimuli of rather similar intensity so that most of the subjects cannot distinguish between them without making mistakes. The stimuli are presented a large number of times in a random order (up to 200 in some studies on somatic perception). One counts the number of times the stimuli have qualified as painful or non-painful [51, 14]. One practical problem with these protocols is that it is difficult to predetermine the distension pressure to

Table 2: *Advantages and disadvantages of the various distension protocols.*

Method	Definition	Advantages	Disadvantages
Ascending method of limits	Each distension larger than last until subject reports pain.	Simple. Few trials.	Vulnerable to psychological bias. Stimuli are predictable. Only one judgment depicts thresholds.
Random sequence	Random series. Subject rates each distension.	Less psychological bias. Sequence is unpredictable. Relatively few trials.	Impossible to use because some distensions would be too painful. Must use pseudo-random sequence, approximating ascending limit method.
Tracking technique	After each pain report, next distension is randomly same or lower. After each report of no pain, next distension is randomly same or higher.	Sequence is unpredictable. Threshold is based on multiple judgments.	Requires large number of distension (up to 45 trials).
Double random staircase	In staircase A, distension decreases after every pain report and increases after report of no pain. Staircase B works in the same way. Computer randomly alternates A and B.	Sequence is unpredictable. Threshold is based on multiple judgments.	Requires large number of distensions (up to 30 trials), but fewer than tracking.

be used during the test. If the same distending pressure is used for all the subjects, some will report only non painful sensations while some others will report only painful ones. Therefore, a search for pain threshold by an "ascending limit protocol" is needed beforehand.

One could summarize the problem of choice of a distending protocol with the following statements:
— Multiple distensions at each pressure or volume step yield more reliable estimates of sensory thresholds. However practical considerations may limit the number of trials which can be presented.

– For measuring the threshold for urgency, discomfort or pain, the ascending method of limits is frequently used but is more vulnerable to psychological influence on sensory reports.

Advantages and disadvantages of the various distension protocols are summarized in Table 2.

Methods of eliciting the subject's response

The perception of pain is dependent on the past experience of the subject, his cultural environment and various psychological factors. Objective measurements like pressure or volumes in case of distending studies reflect the intensity of the stimulus used to trigger a painful sensation. However, these objective measurements do not evaluate the sensations felt by the subject which are a sum of the factors influencing the perception of pain and the specific consequences of the painful stimulus applied during the study.

Various methods have been proposed to record pain sensations in humans. The most simple one is the presentation of a single question to the patient: "Do you have pain or not?". This question induces a binary answer "Yes or No" without quoting the intensity of painful sensations. Associated with a distension protocol using ascending method of limits, it is simple to use and has proven reproducible for some authors [18, 20]. However this method is limited and less sensitive since it does not explore intensity and allows only to detect threshold stimuli.

Therefore, it is recommended to use rating scales which allow the subject to report the intensity of the sensation. Usually verbal rating scales (ordinal scales) or visual analog scales are used (Table 3). The subject must be asked to rate on

Table 3: *Example of visual and verbal rating scales.*

A. Verbal rating scales of pain and unpleasantness

Pain		Unpleasantness	
0	None	0	None
1	Weak	1	Mild
2	Mild	2	Discomforting
3	Moderate	3	Distressing
4	Strong	4	Horrible
5	Intense	5	Excruciating

B. Visual analog scale for pain

No pain	Worst ever

←——————————————————————→

2 separate scales the intensity of pain and the unpleasantness of sensations. Examples of scales are available from the literature [22, 36].

Azpiroz and Malagelada developed a unique approach to assessing the sensations which occur in response to distension of the gastrointestinal tract [1]. They provide the subject with several 7 point numeric scales, defining the various sensations that can be triggered by distension and ask the subject for quoting each sensation at each distension step. Then, they express the intensity of sensations induced by distension at a given level of pressure by the mean of the intensity descriptors reported by the subjects of one group and compare it to the mean of sensations reported by the subjects of another group.

Evaluation of compliance

Compliance is the capacity of a hollow organ to adapt to distension. It is defined as the ratio dV/dP which characterizes the derived function of the pressure-volume curve and is expressed in ml.mmHg^{-1}, when isobaric distensions are performed (Fig. 4). To evaluate compliance, one needs to measure the volume of the distending bag at each pressure step, build the pressure-volume curve and calculate the slope of this curve, which represents the compliance.

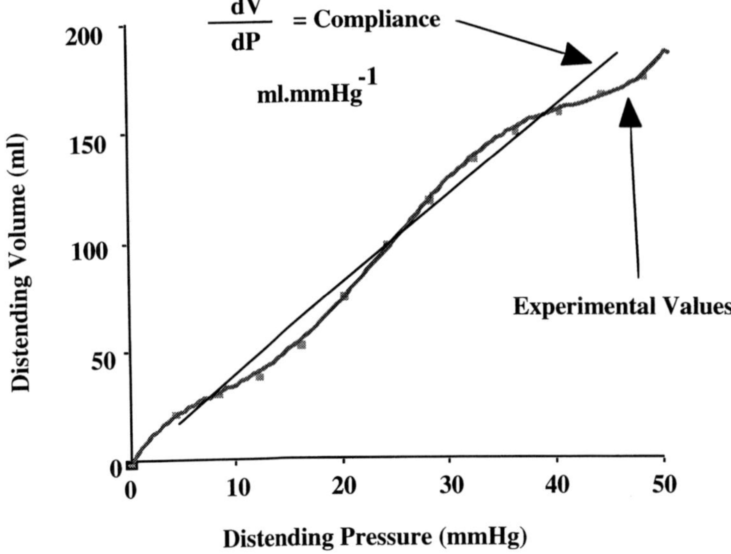

Fig. 4: *Theoretical pressure-volume curve observed when the colon is distended by a polyethylene bag. The first derived function of the curve dV/dP is a straight line. The compliance corresponds to the slope of this line and is expressed in ml.mmHg^{-1}.*

The shape of the pressure-volume relationship may be considerably different, depending on the studied organ. It is usually linear in the range of the intermediate pressure steps but may show inflection points at lower or higher pressure steps [37].

Compliance is influenced by many factors including the tone of the organ, the contractile activity, the surrounding anatomy. It may also be influenced by the elastic properties of the distending device (barostat + probe and bag). We have seen that polyethylene bags and latex balloons behave quite differently when inflated in air (paragraph 1). Latex balloons are poorly compliant and influence dramatically the compliance measurements, so that when latex balloons are used, the compliance of the system must be carefully evaluated in air before performing distension studies and then subtracted from the compliance measured during distension sessions. On the contrary, polyethylene bags are extremely compliant if they are oversized as compared to the range of volumes to be used during the distension studies, so that the maximal distending volume never exceeds 80% of the maximal capacity of the bag.

Evaluation of compliance is important when one compares the sensitivity of an organ in different experimental conditions, e. g. in fasted versus fed state, or on placebo or a drug which is thought to modify sensory thresholds. Changes in compliance may then explain variations of volumes observed during isobaric distensions [42]. Changes in compliance may also interfere with results of studies comparing thresholds detected by isovolumic distensions under various conditions. The slopes of pressure-volume curves need to be carefully compared in such cases to rule out changes in compliance before concluding that the sensory thresholds are modified.

On the other hand, the absence of changes in compliance while pressure thresholds are significantly different between various experimental conditions or between various groups of subjects indicate that these changes are related to modifications of sensory pathways and not to changes in elastic properties of the wall of the organ.

The barostat to explore visceral sensitivity in patients with functional bowel disorders

Irritable bowel syndrome

Hypersensitivity of the gut to distension was suggested twenty years ago by Ritchie, who showed that during rectal distension IBS patients experienced pain at lower distending volumes than controls [44]. In another study, pain thresholds elicited by rectal distension were much lower in patients with functional diarrhea than in constipated patients, suggesting an influence of colonic transit on visceral perception [41]. Colonic hypersensitivity has also been observed in patients with constipation-prone IBS [11, 54] and the lowered pain threshold observed in these patients could be normalized by octreotide up to the distending pressure required to induce pain in controls [13].

Like in the colon, visceral hypersensitivity has been observed when distending the jejunum in IBS patients as compared to controls [1]. It has been recently shown by Whorwell's group that in IBS patients, hypersensitivity to distension was a diffuse disorder involving the oesophagus, the various segments of the small intestine, the colon and the rectum [21]. The pathophysiology of visceral hypersensitivity in patients with IBS remains controversial. Some authors have claimed that it could be related to a default in relaxation of the colonic wall resulting in an increase in parietal tension when a contraction occurs and in a subsequent stimulation of parietal mechanoreceptors. However, Whitehead has simultaneously recorded colonic phasic activity by manometry and distended the colon by a balloon and has shown that abdominal pain was induced by distension in the absence of any alteration of colonic motility [54]. This observation was confirmed by studies performed with the barostat which concluded that colonic compliance, i.e. the elastic properties of the colon, was not different in IBS patients and in controls [11, 50]. These results suggest that the primary disorder responsible for the visceral hypersensitivity in patients with functional bowel disorders could be located on visceral afferents. However the exact level of this abnormality has not yet been defined. The daily clinical experience suggests that some psychological factors may influence abdominal symptoms in IBS patients. Some authors have suggested that psychological factors could account for hyperalgesia observed in patients [31]. However, there are some experimental data supporting the involvement of peripheral afferents in the pathophysiology of visceral hypersensitivity in IBS. As already said, octreotide restores sensory thresholds to colonic distension in IBS patients without modifying colonic compliance [25, 13] and decreases the intensity of cortical and spinal evoked potentials [45]. Comparison between electrical stimulation of jejunal afferents and mechanical distension of the jejunum to induce an intestino-intestinal reflex in IBS patients and healthy volunteers has shown that only thresholds of pain perception triggered by mechanical distension were lower in IBS than in controls while perception of electrical stimulation was rather similar in both groups [2]. This observation suggests that the primary disorder could be located at the level of parietal mechanoreceptors themselves.

However, many questions remain open: the relationship between the intensity of abdominal symptoms and the measure of lowered thresholds to mechanical distension has been suggested [37] but is not firmly established. The influence of various parameters like age, sex, anxiety of the patients, stress or tone of the digestive wall has not been evaluated so far. One important issue that needs to be addressed in view of the clinical implications of distension tests with a barostat is the question whether these tests may be regarded as a diagnostic tool to fairly discriminate between IBS patients and normals or non-IBS patients. The cumulative frequency curves of positive responses for a given pressure show some overlap between patients and controls [11] (Fig. 5). Large multicenter trials will be needed to answer these questions.

Other functional digestive disorders

Distension studies have also shown an hypersensitivity of patients with other functional digestive disorders. Very few studies have been performed with the barostat in the oesophagus. Oesophageal hypersensitivity has initially been demonstrated by Castell and Richter [15, 43]. However the mechanical environment of the oesophagus is quite different from that of the abdominal viscera since it is placed in a rigid enclosure (the chest). Contrary to IBS, oesophageal balloon distension has been recognized as a diagnostic tool for the investigation of patients with non cardiac chest pain of suspected oesophageal origin [26].

In patients with functional dyspepsia, it has also been shown that a painful sensation was triggered by lower distending pressures than in controls [32, 12]. Implications are rather similar to those of recto-colonic studies in IBS patients and deal with the specificity of the sensory thresholds, the conditions affecting the results of such studies and the clinical use of these tests.

Pharmacological modulation of sensory thresholds

The possibility of performing distension studies with a good reproducibility of sensory thresholds has led some investigators to evaluate the effect of drugs on visceral sensitivity. Somatostatin has been studied in many trials which have shown that it was able to increase sensory thresholds during rectal [25, 40] and colonic [13] distension. Moreover, somatostatin decreases the intensity of evoked potentials triggered by electrical stimulation of the rectal wall [45]. This observation suggests that somatostatin could act directly on peripheral afferent pathways.

The second class of compounds which has been evaluated over the last 4 years is the group of 5HT-3 antagonists. The 5HT-3 receptors are one of the best known examples of receptors involved in the activation of peripheral afferents. They play an important role in somatic afferents [35] and possibly in digestive afferents too [38, 39]. Indeed, Moss and coworkers have observed that in rat, granisetron decreases the intensity of the cardiovascular response to duodenal distension [39]. In the same way, 5HT-3 receptors are involved in visceral reflexes triggered by recto-colonic distension in animals with a chemically-in-

A. First sensation Threshold

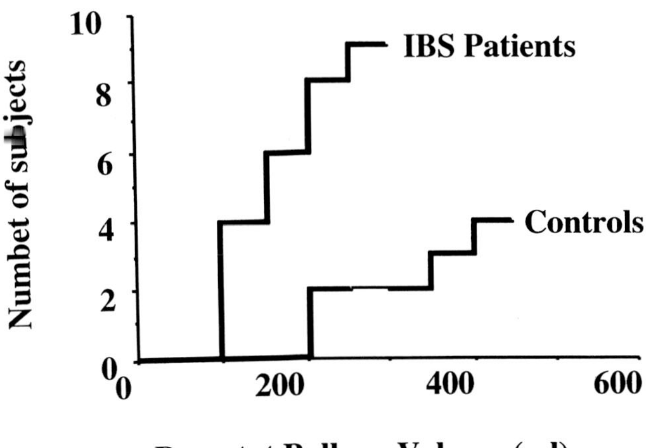

B. Pain Threshold

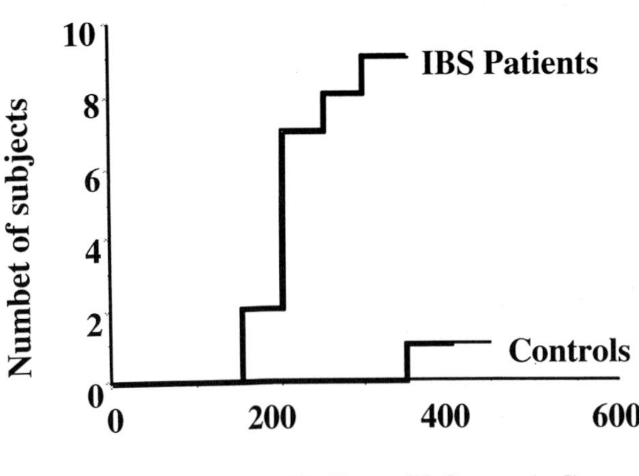

Fig. 5: *Cumulative number of patients with IBS and controls giving a positive response for a given step of distension of the left colon. Distensions were phasic intermittent isovolumic distensions by steps of 40 ml maintained for 5 minutes. One sees that, for the first sensation threshold, an overlap exists between IBS and controls. The pain threshold was not reached by most of the controls in this study using a limited range of distending volumes (up to 600 ml).*

duced experimental colitis [38]. On the contrary, in humans 5HT-3 antagonists did not influence the response to gastro-duodenal distension nor to transcutaneous electrical stimulation [16]. By contrast, the role of 5HT-3 receptor antagonists has been demonstrated in drug-induced emesis [4]. Finally, in man, granisetron increases the thresholds of visceral perception induced by rectal distension in IBS patients [42] and some studies are currently being performed with new drugs of this family in IBS patients. However, in the study by Prior and Read, which was performed on patients with functional diarrhea, granisetron also modified the compliance of the rectum.

Recently, we have also shown that fedotozine, which acts peripherally as an agonist of K-opiate receptors, was able to inhibit hypersensitivity of IBS patients to colonic distension [20]. Fedotozine has also been shown to improve the abdominal symptoms of patients with IBS [17]. Moreover, in animals, fedotozine was shown to affect viscero-visceral reflexes, indicating that it could act on afferent pathways [23]. On the other hand, fedotozine does not alter the compliance of the colonic wall.

Among the other drugs which are acting on sensory thresholds, we have shown that oxytocin is acting on sensory thresholds in a cut-off manner, independent of the dose [34]. Recently, we have obtained experimental evidence that this effect of oxytocin is not mediated through a release of enkephalins since it is not inhibited by naloxone [34]. The beta-3 agonist SR58611A also increases sensory thresholds to rectal distension in healthy volunteers but it does only affect the pain threshold [19]. These drugs do not modify the rectal or colonic compliance.

Conclusion

The barostat has been widely used over the last 5 years to explore the sensitivity of the gut to luminal distension. The results of these studies have brought new insights in the pathophysiology of functional bowel disorders and have demonstrated the importance of visceral perception disturbances in these patients. The knowledge has also been increased about visceral afferents and their implication in perception disorders.

Drug trials based on the evaluation of sensory thresholds become now published and will in future provide an interesting approach to test the potential therapeutic effect of drugs designed to treat functional bowel disorders. However the distension tests lack at the moment specificity to discriminate between functional patients and normals or patients with organic diseases. Therefore, the results of drug trials based on the evaluation of effects on sensory thresholds must presently be considered as indicative but not predictive of the clinical action of the drug. Multicenter trials will answer these questions in the future.

Finally, we would like to stress the dramatic influence of the technical conditions of distension studies on their results. As stated here above, we need some standardisation of the experimental procedures, in order to enable comparisons between different studies. At least, the reports of these studies should include a clear description of methods and procedures and provide technical specifications of distending devices, probes and bags or balloons. The Working Party Report that will be published soon by a group of investigators with expertise in the use of barostat [52] is intended to provide the users of barostat with recommendations to accurately address these technical issues.

References

1. Accarino, A. M., F. Azpiroz, J. R. Malagelada: Symptomatic responses to stimulation of sensory pathways in the jejunum. Am. J. Physiol. 263 (1992) G673−G677.
2. Accarino, A. M., F. Azpiroz, J. R. Malagelada: Selective dysfunction of the mechanosensitive intestinal afferents in Irritable Bowel Syndrome. Gastroenterology 108 (1995) 636−643.
3. Akervall, S., S. Fasth, S. Nordgren et al.: Rectal reservoir and sensory function studied by graded isobaric distention in normal man. Gut 30 (1989) 496−502.
4. Andrews, P. L. R., W. G. Rapeport, G. J. Sanger: Neuropharmacology of emesis induced by anticancer therapy. Trends in Pharmacol. Sci. 9 (1988) 334−341.
5. Arletti, R., A. Benelli, A. Bertolini: Influence of oxytocin on nociception and morphine antinociception. Neuropeptides 24 (1993) 125−129.
6. Aspiroz, F., J. R. Malagelada: Physiological variations in canine gastric tone measured by an electronic barostat. Am. J. Physiol. 248 (1985) G229−G237.
7. Azpiroz, F., J. R. Malagelada: Gastric tone measured by an electronical barostat in health and postsurgical gastroparesis. Gastroenterology 92 (1987) 934−943.
8. Azpiroz, F., J. R. Malagelada: Isobaric intestinal distention in humans: sensorial relay and reflex gastric relaxation. Am. J. Physiol. 258 (1990) G202−G207.
9. Bell, A. M., J. H. Pemberton, R. B. Hanson et al.: Variations in muscle tone of the human rectum: recordings with an electromechanical barostat. Am. J. Physiol. 260 (1991) G17−G25.
10. Besson, J. M.: La douleur: aspects physiopharmacologiques. Biologie. Comptes rendus (C. R. Soc. Biol.) 186 (1992) 26−36.
11. Bradette, M., M. Delvaux, G. Staumont et al.: Evaluation of colonic sensory thresholds in IBS patients using a barostat: definition of optimal conditions and comparison with healthy subjects. Dig. Dis. Sci. 39 (1994) 449−457.
12. Bradette, M., P. Pare, P. Douville et al.: Visceral perception in health and functional dyspepsia. Crossover study of gastric distension with placebo and domperidone. Dig. Dis. Sci. 36 (1991) 52−58.
13. Bradette, M., G. Staumont, M. Delvaux et al.: Somatostatin analogue increases thresholds of discomfort and pain perception to colonic distension in irritable bowel syndrome patients. Dig. Dis. Sci. 39 (1994) 1171−1178.
14. Bradley, L. A., I. C. Scarinci, J. E. Richter: Pain threshold levels and coping strategies among patients who have chest pain and normal coronary arteries. Med. Clin. North. Am. 75 (1991) 1189−1202.

15. Castell, D. O.: Esophageal chest pain. Am. J. Gastroenterol. 79 (1984) 969−976.

16. Coffin, B., F. Aspiroz, J. R. Malagelada: Mécanismes des réponses sensorielles à des stimulations viscérales et somatiques. Gastroenterol. Clin. Biol. 15 (1991) A28 (abstract).

17. Dapoigny, M., J. L. Abitbol, G. Méric et al.: Fedotozine in Irritable Bowel Syndrome: Results of a 6 week placebo-controlled multicenter therapeutic trial. Gastroenterology 108 (1995) A588 (abstract).

18. Delvaux, M., D. Louvel, E. Lagier et al.: Reproducibility of sensory thresholds triggered by rectal distension in healthy volunteers. Gastroenterology 108 (1995) A590 (abstract).

19. Delvaux, M., D. Louvel, P. Peronnet et al.: Effect of SR58611A, an agonist at the adrenergic beta-3 receptor on rectal sensory thresholds in healthy volunteers. Gastroenterology 108 (1995) A589 (abstract).

20. Delvaux, M., D. Louvel, B. Scherrer et al.: : The k-agonist fedotozine increases thresholds of first sensation and pain perception to colonic distension in patients with irritable bowel syndrome. Gastroenterology 108 (1995) A590 (abstract).

21. Francis, C. Y., L. A. Houghton, P. J. Whorwell et al.: Enhanced sensitivity of the whole gut in patients with irritable bowel syndrome. Gastroenterology 108 (1995) A601 (abstract).

22. Gracely, R. H., P. McGrath, R. Dubner: Ratio scales of sensory and affective verbal pain descriptors. Pain 5 (1978) 5−18.

23. Gué, M., J. L. Junien, L. Buéno: The kappa-agonist fedotozine modulates colonic distension-induced inhibition of gastric motility and emptying in dogs. Gastroenterology 107 (1994) 1327−1334.

24. Hachet, T., M. Caussette: A multifunction programmable computerized barostat. Gastroenterol. Clin. Biol. 17 (1993) 347−351.

25. Hasler, W., H. Soudah, C. Owyang: A somatostatine analogue inhibits afferent pathways mediating perception of rectal distension. Gastroenterology 104 (1993) 1390−1397.

26. Humeau, B., D. Cloarec, J. Simon et al.: Douleurs pseudo-angineuses d'origine œsophagienne. Résultats de l'exploration fonctionnelle et intérêt du test de distension mécanique par ballonnet. Gastroenterol. Clin. Biol. 14 (1990) 334−341.

27. Janssens, J., G. Vantrappen, G. Ghillebert: 24 hours recording of esophageal pressure and pH in patients with noncardiac chest pain. Gastroenterology 90 (1986) 1978−1984.

28. Jaenig, W., M. Koltzenburg: On the function of spinal primary afferent fibers supplying colon and urinary bladder. J. Autonom. Nerv. Syst. 30 (1990) 589−596.

29. Khan, M. I., C. Feinle, N. W. Read: Investigating gastric and sensory response to distention: comparative studies using flaccid bags and latex balloons. 2nd United European Gastroenterology Meeting (1993) A: 175.

30. Kullman, G., J. F. Fielding: Rectal distensibility in the irritable bowel syndrome. Ir. Med. J. 74 (1981) 140−142.

31. Latimer, P., D. Campbell, M. Latimer et al.: Irritable bowel syndrome: a test of the colonic hyperalgesia hypothesis. J. Behav. Med. 2 (1979) 285−295.

32. Lémann, M., J. P. Dederding, B. Flourié et al.: Abnormal perception of visceral pain in response to gastric distension in chronic idiopathic dyspepsia. The irritable stomach syndrome. Dig. Dis. Sci. 36 (1991) 1249−1254.

33. Lembo, T., J. Munakata, H. Mertz et al.: Evidence for the hypersensitivity of lumbar splanchnic afferents in irritable bowel syndrome. Gastroenterology 107 (1994) 1686−1696.

34. Louvel, D., M. Delvaux, J. Fioramonti et al.: Effect of various doses of oxytocin on sensory thresholds in patients with irritable bowel syndrome. Gut (1996) in press.

35. Meller, S. T., S. J. Lewis, M. J. Brody et al.: The peripheral nociceptive actions of intravenous administered 5-HT in the rat requires dual activation of both 5-HT2 and 5-HT3 receptor subtypes. Brain Res. 561 (1992) 61−68.

36. Melzak, R.: The McGill Pain Questionnaire: major properties and scoring methods. Pain 1 (1975) 277−299.

37. Mertz, H., B. Naliboff, J. Munakata et al.: Altered rectal perception is a biological marker of patients with irritable bowel syndrome. Gastroenterology 109 (1995) 40−52.
38. Morteau, O., C. Eeckhout, L. Buéno: Effect of 5-HT3 antagonists (granisetron and KC9946) on viscerosensitive response to colorectal distension before and during experimental colitis in awake rats. Fundam. Clin. Pharmacol. 8 (1994) 553−562.
39. Moss, H., G. J. Sanger: Antagonism by BRL43694 of pseudoaffective reflexes evoked by duodenal distension. Br. J. Pharmacol. 92 (1987) 531P.
40. Plourde, V., T. Lembo, Z. Shui et al.: Effects of the somatostatin analog, octreotide on rectal afferent nerves in humans. Am. J. Physiol. 265 (1993) G742−G745.
41. Prior, A., D. G. Maxton, P. J. Whorwell: Anorectal manometry in irritable bowel syndrome: differences between diarrhoea and constipation predominant subjects. Gut 31 (1990) 458−462.
42. Prior, A., N. W. Read: Reduction of rectal sensitivity and postprandial motility by granisetron, a 5-HT3 receptor antagonist, in patients with irritable bowel syndrome. Gut 31 (1990) A1174 (abstract).
43. Richter, J. E., C. F. Barish, D. O. Castell: Abnormal sensory perception in patients with esophageal chest pain. Gastroenterology 91 (1986) 845−852.
44. Ritchie, J.: Pain from distension of the pelvic colon by inflating a balloon in the irritable colon syndrome. Gut 14 (1973) 125−132.
45. Roberts, D., W. D. Chey, W. Hasler et al.: Somatostatin analog reduces perception of rectal distension by specific inhibition of spinal afferent pathways. Gastroenterology 104 (1993) A571 (abstract).
46. Ropert, A., S. Bruley de Varannes, Y. Bizais et al.: Simultaneous assessment of liquid emptying and proximal gastric tone in humans. Gastroenterology 105 (1993) 667−674.
47. Steadman, C. J., S. F. Phillips, M. Camilleri et al.: Variation of muscle tone in the human colon. Gastroenterology 101 (1991) 373−381.
48. Sun, W. M., N. W. Read, A. Prior et al.: The sensory and motor responses to rectal distension vary according to the rate and pattern of balloon inflation. Gastroenterology 99 (1990) 1008−1013.
49. Thompson, W. G., F. Creed, D. A. Drossman et al.: Functional bowel disorders and chronic functional pain. Gastroenterol. Int. 5 (1992) 75−91.
50. Toma, T. D., J. Zighelboim, S. F. Phillips et al.: Methods for studying intestinal sensitivity and compliance: In vitro studies of balloons and a barostat. Neurogastroenterol. Mot. (1995) in press.
51. Whitehead, W. E., M. D. Crowell, A. Davidoff et al.: Is sexual abuse associated with lower thresholds for pain due to balloon distention of the rectum? Gastroenterology 106 (1993) A588 (abstract).
52. Whitehead, W. E., M. Delvaux: Standardization of procedures for testing smooth muscle tone and sensory thresholds in the gastrointestinal tract. Dig. Dis. Sci. (1996) in press.
53. Whitehead, W. E., B. T. Engel, M. M. Schuster: Irritable bowel syndrome. Physiological and psychological differences between diarrhea-predominant and constipation-predominant patients. Dig. Dis. Sci. 25 (1980) 404−413.
54. Whitehead, W. E., B. Holtkotter, P. Enck et al.: Tolerance for recto-sigmoid distention in irritable bowel syndrome. Gastroenterology 98 (1990) 1187−1192.

Stimulation techniques of the gastrointestinal tract: evaluation of the responses and factors which determine the responses

F. Azpiroz

Physiological stimuli in the gastrointestinal tract induce specific reflexes to accomplish the digestive function. Normally, the whole process evolves unperceived, and only in some circumstances do patients develop symptoms. Studies on visceral sensitivity in healthy subjects require perceptible probing stimuli, and over the years distension of the gut has been the most common stimulus used for this purpose.

Distension of the gastrointestinal tract

Basically there are two methods to produce distension of the gut: fixed-volume distension and fixed-pressure distension. Fixed-volume distension can be produced with a method as simple as an inflatable balloon. A fixed volume of air is inflated into the balloon, and the intraballoon pressure during the distension is monitored with a pressure transducer via the connecting tube. High-compliance latex balloons made with condoms have relatively low intrinsic pressures, and compliance can be calculated with a reasonably small error [2, 5]. Flaccid balloons with a negligible intrinsic pressure require no corrections and may be preferable [14]. Alternatively, distension of the gut can be produced by fixed pressure increments by using a barostat, in which a feedback mechanism maintains a constant pressure within an air-filled balloon [4, 6].

For most purposes both fixed-pressure and fixed-volume distensions are equivalent, provided proper intraluminal probes are used. It has been suggested that pressure thresholds are more reliable and reproducible measures of pain than volume thresholds. However, we have consistently found the same variability using fixed-pressure and fixed-volume distensions of the stomach and the small intestine [6, 14]. However, these methods do not give identical results. For instance, the relaxed stomach tolerates large volumes because intragastric pressure remains small, but a relatively low distending pressure level set by the barostat may produce a painful elongation of the gastric wall [14].

Responses to distension

Perception of gut distension can be both quantitatively and qualitatively measured using specific questionnaires, similar to those used to evaluate somatic sensitivity [8]. With such methods it has been shown that the symptomatic response to distension is rather uniform from the stomach down to the mid small bowel [1, 5, 6, 16]. Most subjects perceive the distensions as a diffuse pressure sensation felt in the epigastrium and the paraumbilical region. A relatively small proportion of distensions in the stomach and proximal duodenum induce nausea, which is rarely induced by jejunal distension. In contrast, jejunal distensions are frequently perceived as colicky or as a stinging sensation. The intensity of perception is stimulus related, but the same type of sensations are induced by low distensions near the threshold for perception and by distensions at threshold for discomfort. Furthermore, the sensitivity along the gastrointestinal tract seems quite uniform, although standardization of distending stimuli in different segments of the gut is problematic. These observations indicate a low discriminative value of gastrointestinal sensitivity, and emphasize the difficulty that exists in ascribing these kinds of symptoms (also described by patients with abdominal complaints) to a specific segment of the gut. The distending levels that induce perception and discomfort may vary considerably in different studies depending on several factors, such as body position for gastric studies, the length of the segment stimulated in the intestine, and the corrections applied. A point of caution in interpreting old studies is the extremely high distending pressures usually reported.

Gut stimuli that induce perception may also induce reflex responses. These types of reflex responses have been well characterized in experimental animals, because they have been used as an indirect index of nociception. However, responses in healthy humans differ from those in acute experiments in anesthetized animals, mainly because the magnitude of the stimuli applied in conscious subjects is much smaller. For instance, in testing gastrointestinal stimuli up to the threshold for discomfort, we have never detected consistent cardiovascular responses, a pseudoaffective reflex commonly used in animal experiments.

Any method used to measure gastrointestinal activity could potentially be applied to measure reflex responses to gut stimuli. Manometry and electromyography are well-established methods to measure phasic motor activity of the gut in humans. However, since phasic activity is intermittent, it may be difficult to assess responses to brief stimuli, more so taking into account that most reflexes induced by distension are inhibitory [3, 16]. The electronic barostat, previously described to produce fixed-pressure distension of the gut, can also function to measure changes in gut tone. For this purpose, the barostat is set at a low and constant pressure level and measures isobaric volume changes; under these conditions a volume expansion reflects a relaxation, and vice versa [4, 6, 16].

Using the barostat it has been shown that intestinal distension induces a gastric relaxation by a vagal enterogastric reflex. However, the specific responses depend on the region stimulated. Distension of the small intestine also induces intestinal reflexes. In contrast to the uniformity of perception, the reflex responses to gut distension are quite heterogeneous. In recent years new techniques have been developed, such as cerebral evoked potentials, positron emission tomography (PET) and single-photon emission computed tomography (SPECT) that image the topography of nervous circuits activated by visceral stimuli. However, in some cases it cannot be ascertained whether the responses are recorded precisely at perception pathways or at other afferents. It is important to emphasize that perception and reflex responses are dissociable and hence, both responses may be independently altered in some conditions [6, 9, 16].

Other techniques of gastrointestinal stimulation

Testing somatic sensitivity involves a variety of stimuli, each activating a specific pathway. For instance, A-beta low-threshold mechanoreceptors, which produce a faint tactile sensation at levels near the detection threshold, can be assessed by cotton wisps. At detection, electrical stimulation activates the same pathways, by directly stimulating afferent axons independently of the receptors [11, 15]. Likewise, nonpainful thermal stimuli provide important information in somatosensory testing. Thinly myelineated A-delta-fibers mediate the sensation of cool, and C-fibers mediate warmth detection. Hence, warmth and cool detection can be used to evaluate these specific pathways [11].

Transmucosal electrical nerve stimulation

In analogy to transcutaneous electrical nerve stimulation, transmucosal electrical nerve stimulation can be used as an alternative test of visceral sensitivity. Electrical stimuli can be applied via intraluminal electrodes [1, 3]. The conductive surfaces of a bipolar electrode are mounted at opposite rims of a suction hole on a tube. When the tube is positioned in the intestine, suction should be applied through the lumen of the tube to ensure firm contact of the electrodes with the gut wall. Transmucosal electrical nerve stimulation is then produced by a constant current stimulator.

Transmucosal electrical nerve stimulation of the small intestine induces intensity-related perception. Interestingly, most sensations elicited by electrical stimuli correspond to clinical-type abdominal symptoms such as abdominal pressure, fullness, colicky or stinging sensation, similar to those elicited by distension. Only about one-third of electrical stimuli induce paraesthesia or somatic flutter-like sensation [1]. Conceivably, these sensations originate by stimulation of surrounding somatic structures across the intestinal wall. There is no relation between the intensity of electrical stimulation and the type of sensation elicited;

that is, similar sensations are produced by weak, barely perceptible stimuli and by strong uncomfortable stimuli. Transmucosal nerve stimulation does not modify the intrinsic basal myoelectrical rhythm in the intestine [1]. Furthermore, electrical stimulation induces neither local activation nor reflex inhibition of intestinal motor activity, suggesting that it activates afferent pathways distinct from those activated by distension [3].

Transmucosal electrical nerve stimulation may depolarize all afferents within the gut wall. Whereas distending stimuli activate sensory pathways and induce perception by specific stimulation of mechanoreceptors on the gut wall, transmucosal electrical nerve stimulation induces similar perception by nonspecific stimulation of afferent pathways, that is, without relaying on any specific receptor.

Thermal stimulation

Thermal stimulation of the gut can be produced via intraluminal water-filled tubular bags positioned either in the stomach, duodenum, or jejunum [18]. The temperature within the bag is continuously monitored by an intrabag telethermometer, and the desired temperature is achieved by recirculating water at adjusted temperatures through thermally insulated connecting tubes. Temperature changes are achieved fairly rapidly, so that brief stimuli can be tested. The stomach and the intestine exhibit similar stimulus-related thermal sensitivity. About half of the thermal stimuli applied in the stomach (warm and cold alike) are perceived as abdominal pressure, fullness, or nausea; the rest of the stimuli induce warm or cold sensation. In contrast, only 10% of intestinal stimuli induce clinical type symptoms. Gastric stimuli, but not intestinal stimuli, induce changes in gastric tone. Warm stimuli in the stomach induce a gastric relaxation, whereas cold stimuli induce a gastric contraction [18]. The responses have a brief latency and revert shortly after discontinuation of the stimulus. Both with warm and cold stimuli the magnitude of the gastric responses is stimulus-related. Thermal sensitivity of the gastrointestinal tract in humans remains poorly explored, and the specific type of afferents activated by warm and cold stimuli has not been characterized. Nevertheless, thermal stimuli could be potentially applicable in conjunction with mechanical and electrical stimuli for the evaluation of gastrointestinal sensory dysfunctions.

Factors which determine the responses

Both perception and visceral reflexes induced by gut stimuli are modulated by a variety of mechanisms at different levels of the brain-gut axis. In the assessment of visceral sensitivity it is very important to control for these factors which may modify the responses. Moreover, altered sensitivity in some clinical conditions could conceivably be due to dysfunction of these modulatory mechanisms, a possibility that still remains to be explored.

Interaction of stimuli

Perception of gut stimuli in humans depends on the temporo-spatial relationship of different stimuli in the gut. That is, the responses to a given stimulus may be modified by either simultaneous or previous stimulation.

The effects of previous stimulation on the responses to intestinal distension are rather complex; the effects may be facilitatory or inhibitory depending on the intensity of the previous stimulus and the elapsed time interval from the exposure. Mild distension produces a brief period of local desensitization, and reduces both perception and the reflex relaxation induced by a second stimulus applied 10 seconds later at the same site [17]. However it has been shown that intense, painful distensions may sensitize the sigmoid colon in humans [13]. On the other hand, the lack of built-up effects during the stimulation is remarkable; perception of prolonged intestinal distension remains stable at least throughout a 90-minute period [17].

Perception of simultaneous stimuli is additive, so that the gut responds by a phenomenon of spatial summation. For instance, two distensions that are well tolerated alone may produce discomfort when applied simultaneously [17]. Spatial summation can also be elicited by the interaction of different types of stimuli. It has been shown that low-intensity transmucosal electrical nerve stimulation increases the sensitivity of the intestine to distension applied at an adjacent site, and these effects are not due to changes in muscular activity and compliance of the intestinal wall.

Interestingly, the same type of electrical stimulation applied in the somatic area has opposite effects. Indeed, application of transcutaneous electrical nerve stimulation on the hand reduces the discomfort produced by gastric and by duodenal distensions [10]. This form of viscerosensory modulation by somatic stimulation is exerted without alteration of basal gut tone or visceral reflexes. It has been also shown that noxious cutaneous stimuli in rats inhibit the activity in spinal somatosensory neurons evoked by colorectal distension [13]. It seems that acupuncture operates by the same type of antinociceptive mechanisms as those activated by other forms of somatic stimulation, and hence, may have similar effects.

Sympathetic and cortical modulation

The sympathetic nervous system regulates gastrointestinal secretory-motor function by a series of reflex arcs, but also participates in the modulation of sensory responses to gut stimuli. Several models of experimental stress increase sympathetic activity and modify gastrointestinal responses. However, these methods of sympathetic activation involve cognitive processes or unpleasant somatic sensations, and both factors per se may modify visceral perception [2, 10]. Normally, change in body position from supine to orthostatism induces a sympathetic reflex that increases vascular resistance and prevents a fall in blood pressure. This phenomenon has served as the basis to develop a form of non-hypotensive, nontachycardiac lower body negative pressure, which is a clean and elegant method to produce sympathetic activation without involving pain, stress, or changes in basal physiological activity that could interfere with other responses. Using this technique, it has been shown that the sympathetic nervous system exerts modulatory control of visceral but not somatic sensitivity. Increased sympathetic activity significantly heightened perception of intestinal stimuli, but did not modify perception of somatic stimuli [12]. Furthermore, sympathetic activation magnified the relaxatory responses of the gut to both vagal enterogastric and sympathetic intestinointestinal reflexes.

The precise mechanisms by which the sympathetic nervous system modulates visceral perception and reflexes are still unknown, but animal studies have shown that viscerosensory neurons in the spinal cord are controlled by descending excitatory pathways of supraspinal origin [7].

In addition to the modulatory mechanisms stratified at different levels of the brain-gut axis, the cortex exerts the final control of visceral perception. In a series of very carefully designed experiments, we showed that anticipatory knowledge increases perception of intestinal distension as compared to mental distraction [2]. Furthermore, anticipatory knowledge increases the area of referred sensation, and the stimuli are perceived over a wider abdominal region. Mental activity does not modify intestinal compliance or the reflex response to distension. Hence, cognitive processes selectively regulate sensitivity to gut stimuli, while visceral reflexes operate independently.

Conclusion

Proper assessment of visceral sensitivity should involve different stimuli to activate specific afferent pathways, appropriate methodologies to evaluate perception and reflex responses, and a careful control of the factors involved in the modulation of the responses.

References

1. Accarino. A. M., F. Azpiroz, J.-R. Malagelada: Symptomatic responses to stimulation of sensory pathways in the jejunum. Am. J. Physiol. 263 (1992) G673–G677.

2. Accarino, A. M., F. Azpiroz, J.-R. Malagelada: Focusing attention at the gut: effects on viscero-visceral reflexes and perception. Gastroenterology 104 (1993) A468.

3. Accarino, A. M., F. Azpiroz, J.-R. Malagelada: Selective dysfunction of mechanosensitive intestinal afferents in the irritable bowel syndrome. Gastroenterology 108 (1995) 636−643.

4. Azpiroz, F., J.-R. Malagelada: Gastric tone measured by an electronic barostat in health and postsurgical gastroparesis. Gastroenterology 92 (1987) 934−943.

5. Azpiroz, F., J.-R. Malagelada: Perception and reflex relaxation of the stomach in response to gut distention. Gastroenterology 98 (1990) 1193−1198.

6. Azpiroz, F., J.-R. Malagelada: Isobaric intestinal distension in humans: sensorial relay and reflex gastric relaxation. Am. J. Physiol. 258 (1990) G202−G207.

7. Cerveró, F.: Visceral pain: what's in the gut and what's in the brain. In: Y. Taché, D. Wingate (Eds.): Brain-gut interactions, pp. 339−346. CRC Press, Boca Raton FL 1991.

8. Chapman, C. R., K. L. Casey, R. Dubner et al.: Pain measurements: an overview. Pain 22 (1985) 1−31.

9. Coffin, B., F. Azpiroz, F. Guarner et al.: Selective gastric hypersensitivity and reflex hyporeactivity in functional dyspepsia. Gastroenterology 107 (1994) 1345−1351.

10. Coffin, B., F. Azpiroz, J.-R. Malagelada: Somatic stimulation reduces perception of gut distension. Gastroenterology 107 (1994) 1636−1642.

11. Gracely, R. H.: Studies of pain in normal man. In: P. D. Wall, R. Melzack (Eds.): Textbook of Pain, 3rd ed, pp. 315−336. Churchill Livingstone, Edinburgh 1994.

12. Iovino, P., F. Azpiroz, E. Domingo et al.: The sympathetic nervous system modulates perception and reflex responses to gut distension in humans. Gastroenterology 108 (1995) 680−686.

13. Mayer, E. A., G. F. Gebhart: Basic and clinical aspects of visceral hyperalgesia. Gastroenterology 107 (1994) 271−293.

14. Notivol, R., B. Coffin, F. Azpiroz et al.: Gastric tone determines the sensitivity of the stomach to distension. Gastroenterology 108 (1995) 330−336.

15. Price, D. D., S. Long, C. Huitt et al.: Sensory testing of pathophysiological mechanisms of pain in patients with reflex sympathetic dystrophy. Pain 49 (1992) 163−173.

16. Rouillon, J. M., F. Azpiroz, J.-R. Malagelada: Sensorial and intestino-intestinal reflex pathways in the human jejunum. Gastroenterology 101 (1991) 1606−1612.

17. Serra, J., F. Azpiroz, J.-R. Malagelada: Perception and reflex responses to intestinal distension are modified by simultaneous or previous stimulation. Gastroenterology, 109 (1995) 1742−1749.

18. Villanova, N., F. Azpiroz, J.-R. Malagelada: Gut thermosensitivity in humans: sensorial and motor responses. Gastroenterology 100 (1991) A505.

Vesico-urethral sensitivity: clinical implications

F. Pesce

Introduction

Bladder and urethral sensory innervation plays an important role in the micturition mechanism, and both the storing and the voiding phase may be significantly affected by an impaired sensory output from the lower urinary tract. Unfortunately, we still have a limited knowledge of all the sensory pathways, and we are unable to effectively treat most lower urinary tract sensory disorders.

Neuroanatomy

In the bladder wall there are three types of sensory endings: mechanoceptors (small myelinated A-delta fibers), thermoreceptors, and pain receptors (unmyelinated C fibers). These receptors are most likely to be free, unmodified nerve endings: the more complex receptors (Ruffini's, Meisner's, Kruse's bodies) are not involved. Afferent impulses from the bladder, urethra and the perineal floor travel through the hypogastric, pelvic, and pudendal nerves in the pelvis and enter the spinal cord via the posterior roots at the sacral and distal thoracic levels. The posterior root ganglia of S2−S4 contain the cell bodies for all of these sensory nerves of the pelvis and these, in turn, project to the dorsal root entry zone (Substantia gelatinosa Rolandi) [2]. Within the spinal cord, both proprioceptive and exteroceptive information from the bladder ascends the spinothalamic tracts (lateral funiculi) to the pontine micturition centre, while proprioception from the urethra passes through the dorsal columns [9]. Pain sensations project to the thalamus [9] through two pathways [8]. Neurons from the substantia gelatinosa cross the mid-line in the anterior white commissure and ascend in the lateral spinothalamic tract to the thalamic nuclei and to the cortex. This pathway is concerned with sharper and better localised pain. A second pathway diverges from this lateral tract, primarily in the brain stem, to disperse in the periaqueductal grey matter of the reticular formation (hypothalamus and limbic lobes). This tract deals with dull, less localised and more disabling pain. These paleospinothalamic tracts have a significant input to the limbic structures of the brain. Many of the patients with pelvic pain have a significant emotional component [13].

Whereas the autonomic sensory information travelling in the pelvic nerve is a crucial part of the sacral reflex arc, the somatic afferent information travelling in the pudendal nerve is not essential for the micturition cycle. The former is of clinical relevance, since bladder hyperactivity can be abolished in various clinical conditions by instilling lignocaine or capsaicin in the bladder, or by sectioning the posterior sacral roots (sacral rhizotomy).

Classification

Many clinical conditions can affect the vesico-urethral sensation, which may be either reduced or enhanced. The principal causes of depressed sensation are spinal cord diseases and diabetes mellitus. In cases of significant diabetic neuropathy, the functional bladder capacity is usually increased, the detrusor contractility is impaired and a post-voiding residual may be present.

On the other hand, an increased sensation may be the result of several processes, such as bacterial urethro-cystitis, interstitial cystitis, urethral syndrome, prostatodynia, chronic pelvic pain syndrome, etc. (Table 1). All of these conditions are characterised by a diminished sensory threshold, a reduced functional bladder capacity, with varying degrees of urinary frequency and, at times, pain in the suprapubic, urethral and perineal areas.

Table 1: *Hypersensitive conditions of lower urinary tract and pelvis.*

Urethritis
Cystitis
Prostatitis
Urethral syndrome
Interstitial cystitis
Prostatodynia
Chronic pelvic pain

Diagnosis

The most common means of assessing bladder proprioception is to record the first bladder filling sensation threshold during cystometry. This is a somewhat imprecise and subjective method, and the information gathered is rarely consistent and reproducible. It may vary according to several parameters, such as the filling medium, its temperature, and the infusion rate. The total bladder capacity can also influence this threshold, as in case of a very large bladder, the sensory threshold may be delayed even in the presence of intact sensory innerva-

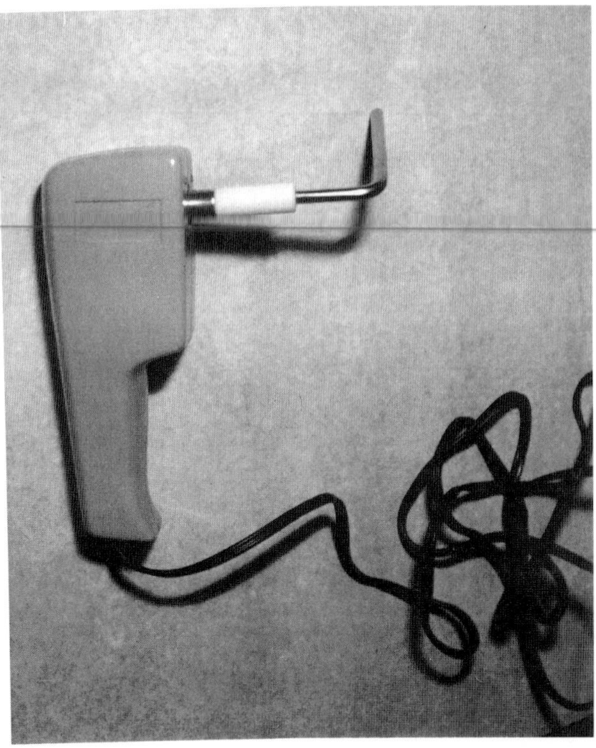

Fig. 1: *Modified Biothesiometer. The button-like vibrating tactor has been replaced with a smooth and thin probe which easily fits the female urethra. The probe is metallic and detachable and can be adequately sterilised.*

tion. Cystometry is useful, however, in evaluating bladder sensation by other means. An increase in intravesical pressure should always be recognised by the patients, especially if a phasic detrusor contraction occurs. In case of detrusor hyperreflexia, many patients feel no sensation during the uninhibited detrusor contractions. A markedly reduced bladder capacity unrelated to uninhibited contractions is referred to as "sensory urgency" and denotes a hypersensitive condition of the bladder and/or urethra. A more sensitive, but more complicated way of assessing bladder sensation is the mucosal electrosensitivity technique [4, 12, 10]. By this method it is possible to determine the sensory threshold of bladder and urethra to electrical stimuli of increasing intensity. A catheter mounted electrode is employed to deliver square wave pulses from a constant current stimulator. In the normative study published by Opsomer and co-workers [10] the median value in males and females was 10.7 and 8.5 mA respectively. Among symptomatic patients, they found higher values in patients with stranguria and in diabetics. Overall, they found the method reproducible and useful in the objective assessment of sensory output from the lower urinary tract.

Distal urethral proprioceptive sensation has also been assessed by means of biothesiometry [11]. By this method it is possible to assess the urethral vibratory sensitivity threshold (UVST) using a modified biothesiometry unit (Fig. 1). The smooth vibrating tip of the unit is inserted in the (female) distal urethra and the vibratory excursion (amplitude) is gradually increased until the subject perceives it (vibratory threshold). The relative value in volts is then read on a scale of the control unit. Attention must be paid not to use any anaesthetic jelly which could alter the normal sensation. Several measurements are taken to achieve reproducible results. In order to test the patient's alertness and reliability, it is also advisable in some occasions to ask if he or she can feel the vibration without effectively giving any stimulus. The mean normal values are considerably higher in older subjects. The test is simple and inexpensive and can be easily performed in the urologist's or gynaecologist's office.

Therapy

Unfortunately, there is no specific therapy for decreased or absent sensation in the lower urinary tract. In the presence of residual urine, intermittent catheterisation is the best choice to empty the bladder while avoiding urinary tract infections.

Therapy of hypersensitive conditions is aimed at removing possible causes, such as urinary infections. Much more unpredictable are the therapeutical results in case of the chronic pelvic pain syndrome. This condition is usually sustained by increased muscle contractility and muscle spasm in the perineal floor (anal sphincter, urethral sphincter, bulbo-cavernosous muscles, levator ani etc.). The pain, usually intolerable, is localised in the perineum, vulva, scrotum or in the suprapubic area and is almost invariably associated with voiding disturbances in terms of frequency, dysuria, hesitancy, intermittent voiding. An increased number of daily bowel movements is also quite common. Sometimes behaviour therapy (counselling and biofeedback) can achieve some relief. The goal of such therapy is to restore patient's awareness and correct concepts of pelvic muscle relaxation. Unfortunately only the less severe cases are likely to respond to the therapy. Nevertheless, this kind of physical therapy is otherwise innocuous and it is usually worth trying it as a first-line treatment.

Other non-surgical-non-medical kinds of management are the external electrical stimulation (transcutaneous, transvaginal, transanal) and acupuncture. In the latter method the needles are placed in the skin area above the medial malleolus

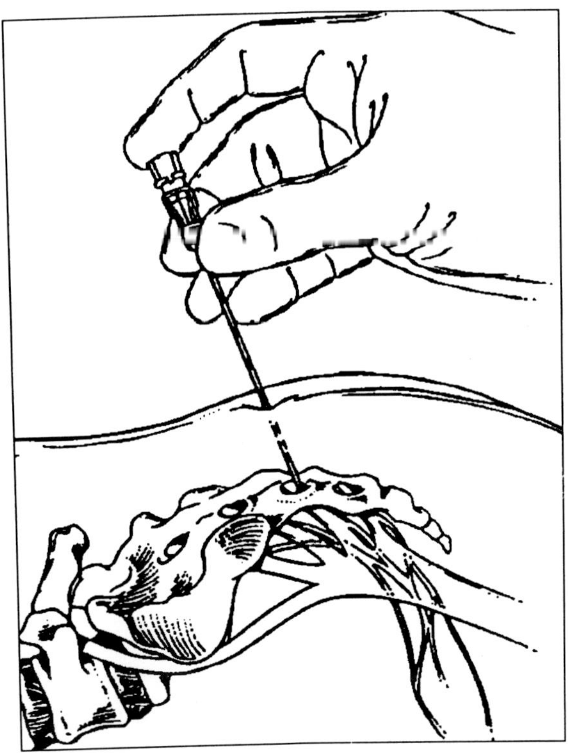

Fig. 2: *Schematic representation of the Peripheral Nerve Evaluation Test (PNE). The stimulating needle approaches the root in the third sacral foramen and the muscular responses are observed. A temporary lead is passed through the needle and is secured in situ for a 4–7 days stimulation period.*

and behind tibia [7]. The general belief is that for both methods the results are short-lasting.

Very good results can be obtained with tricyclic antidepressant agents, especially if the patient can tolerate the anticholinergic type of side-effects, thus allowing a reasonable therapeutical dose. Probably the most commonly used drug is amitriptyline, taken at bed-time with a starting dose of 25 mg, slowly increased every week by 25 mg increments until the effecive dosage is reached, usually 75 mg. Sometimes it is necessary to reach 150 mg or a higher dosage. The results are likely to become manifest in 2 to 4 weeks.

Should the described conservative therapies fail, there still is the possibility of managing this syndrome by means of an implanted neurostimulator continuously delivering electrical stimuli to the third sacral root monolaterally [14]. This technique, referred to as Neuromodulation, is believed to beneficially act on the pelvic pain by lowering the perceived intensity of the pain by exciting

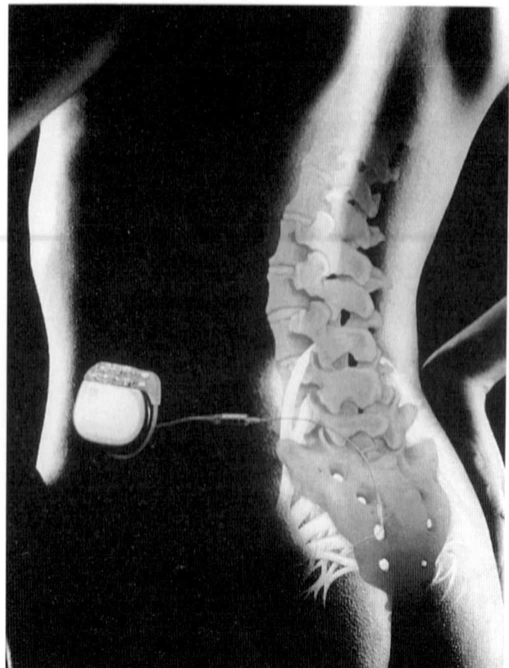

Fig. 3: *Schematic representation of the implanted stimulation kit: a programmable battery-powered pulse generator (ITREL® II 7424) and a permanent electrode fixed in the right third sacral foramen (courtesy of Medtronic Inc. Minneapolis, Minn).*

antinociceptive fibers and masking the pain through the sensation of the electrical stimulation. Before resorting to the permanent implant, a temporary electrode is percutaneously positioned in the third sacral foramen and is connected with an external pulse generator for a test period of 4–7 days (Fig. 2). If there is a significant symptomatic improvement the patient becomes a candidate for the surgical implant (see scheme in Fig. 3).

Besides treating the hypersensitive conditions affecting the lower urinary tract and the pelvis, it is also possible to successfully manage neurogenic overactive bladder conditions (detrusor hyperreflexia) by altering the bladder sensation. This can be obtained chemically, by bladder instillation of capsaicin [3], or surgically, by sectioning the posterior sacral roots [6, 5, 1]. In both instances the underlying rationale is the interruption of the sacral reflex arc, which eventually results in an areflexic bladder. Such therapeutical options are indicated in case of urinary incontinence intractable by more conventional and conservative methods (oral or intravesical anticholinergic therapy and intermittent catheterisation).

References

1. Brindley, G. S.: The first 500 patients with sacral anterior root stimulator implants: general description. Paraplegia 32 (1994) 795–805.
2. Cervero, F., A. Iggo: The substantia gelatinosa of the spinal cord — critical review. Brain 103 (1980) 717–772.
3. Fowler, C. J., R. O. Beck, S. Gerrard et al.: Intravesical capsaicin for treatment of detrusor hyperreflexia. J. Neurol. Neurosurg. Psychiatry 57 (1994) 169–172.
4. Frimodt-Moller, C.: A new method for quantitative evaluation of bladder sensibility. Scand. J. Urol. Nephrol. 6 (suppl. 15) (1972) 135–142.
5. McGuire, E. J.: The effects of sacral denervation on bladder and urethral function. Surgery, Gynecology & Obstetrics 144 (1977) 343–346.
6. Meirowsky, A. M.: Studies on the sacral arc in paraplegia. Differential sacral neurotomy: an operative method. J. Neurosurg. 7 (1950) 39–43.
7. Mendelson, G.: Acupuncture analgesia. I. review of clinical studies. Aust. N.Z. J. Med. 7 (1977) 642–648.
8. Milne, R. J., R. D. Foreman, G. J. Giesler et al.: Convergence of cutaneous and pelvic visceral nociceptive inputs onto primate spinothalamic neurones. Pain 2 (1981) 163–183.
9. Nathan, P. W., M. C. Smith: The centripetal pathway from the bladder and urethra within the spinal cord. J. Neurol. Neurosurg. Psychiatry 14 (1951) 262–280.
10. Opsomer, R. J., T. C. Gerstemberg, P. Klarskov et al.: The electrical sensitivity threshold in the bladder and urethra. Presented at the XIIIth meeting of the International Continence Society (1983).
11. Pesce, F., M. Cervigni, M. Panei et al.: Assessment of urethral sensation by means by vibratory threshold: a normative study. Presented at the 22nd meeting of the International Continence Society (1992).
12. Powell, B. J.: The role of urethral sensation in clinical urology. Urology 52 (1980) 539–541.
13. Schmidt, R. A.: Chronic pelvic pain. AUA Meeting Instructional Course, Washington, D.C. (1992).
14. Thon, W. F., L. S. Baskin, U. Jonas et al.: Neuromodulation of voiding dysfunction and pelvic pain. World J. Urol. 9 (1991) 138–141.

Assessment of digestive sensitivity by a reflexologic technique

R. Jian, D. Bouhassira, B. Coffin, J. C. Willer

*"If a patient be subject to two pains arising in different parts of
the body simultaneously, the stronger blunts the other"*
(*Hippocrates*)

In the last few years, gut hypersensitivity has become a major component of
the pathophysiology of functional disorders and might play a role in inflammatory or other kinds of organic diseases [18]. Consequently, methods that allow
objective and quantitative evaluation of digestive sensations, that can identify
the afferent neural pathways and receptors implicated in each circumstance
to be studied, and that permit exploration of the inhibitory and facilitating
mechanisms that control visceral sensations are required for physiologic, clinical and therapeutic purposes.

Two methods are mainly used to assess digestive sensitivity in humans [16, 1].
The first consists of subjective reporting of the sensation elicited by visceral
stimulation (usually an intraluminal distention). Although very useful, this
method is greatly affected by emotional and cognitive factors, and ignores the
unconscious afferent activity that represents most of the signals arising from
the gut. The second method of assessing digestive sensitivity consists of studying
the changes in phasic or tonic motility patterns in response to gut stimuli. It is
not specific for digestive sensitivity, since these changes may be not only affected
by afferent pathways and/or nervous centers, but also by efferent pathways.

Several new techniques provide more specific and objective approaches to gut
sensitivity than the above methods. Sensory evoked potentials objectively assess
the function of the nerve tracts from the digestive viscera to the central nervous
system [19]. However, this method needs iterative gut stimulations and the site
at which the recorded potentials are generated and its clinical significance are
still controversial. Techniques of biologic imaging of the brain such as positron
or single photon emission tomography [21] are promising but they are expensive and not easily available. We report here the theoretical basis and some
practical applications of a reflexologic technique developed by the group of
Willer and Le Bars for the study of somatic nociception [24, 27, 4]. This technique is based on the recording of a polysynaptic nociceptive cutaneomuscular
flexion reflex described by Hugon [11], and called the RIII reflex because it
involves type III (Aδ) afferent fibers.

Basic concepts

Principle and test procedure

The RIII reflex is a nociceptive flexion reflex of a flexor muscle (usually the biceps femoris) elicited by ipsilateral nociceptive somatic stimulation (usually electrical stimulation of the sural nerve). Even though the recording of this reflex requires adequate muscular relaxation, the feasibility and tolerance of the technique is good, at least in normal volunteers.

The experimental set-up most often used in humans is schematized in Fig. 1. The RIII reflex is elicited and recorded by an entirely computerized system (Physio Labo System, Notocord Systems, Igny, France). The sural nerve is electrically stimulated at a frequency of 0.17 Hz (10 stimulations per minute) through a pair of surface electrodes placed 2 cm apart on the degreased skin overlying the nerve within its retromalleolar path. Each electrical stimulation consists of a train of five constant current pulses of 1 ms duration. Electromyographic responses are recorded from the ipsilateral biceps femoris muscle via a pair of surface electrodes placed 2 cm apart on the degreased skin over the muscle. The RIII reflex response is identified as a multiphasic signal appearing between 90 and 180 ms after each stimulation. After amplification, each reflex response is digitized, full-wave rectified and integrated. The integrated surface is used to quantify the RIII response. The reflex threshold is first determined

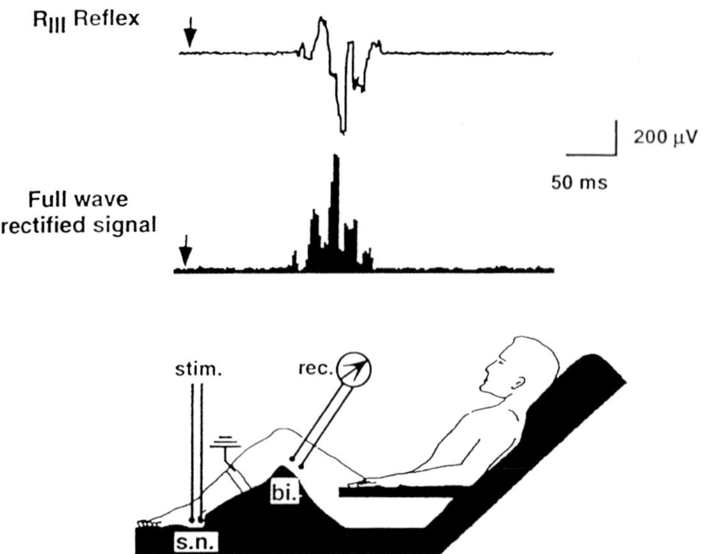

Fig. 1: *Experimental setup for recording the RIII reflex. s. n.: sural nerve, bi.: biceps femoris, stim.: electrical stimulation, rec. electromyographic recording.*

and the intensity of the electrical stimulation of the sural nerve is then adjusted to 20% above the threshold and kept constant for the rest of the experiments. The amplitude of the RIII reflexes in response to each stimulation is usually expressed as a percentage of the mean value obtained during a control period.

Significance of the RIII reflex response

The RIII reflex response is closely related to the concomitant sensation of pain evoked by electrical stimulation. For instance, the reflex threshold is closely related to the pain threshold around a similar value of 10 mA. This value is reliably reproducible in the same subject from one session to the other, as well as in different subjects with minimal inter-individual variations [26]. This close relation was confirmed in dose-response studies performed with morphine [25], and in other clinical experiments involving patients affected either by a pathologic lack of pain sensations or complaining of pain of various origins [26].

Therefore, the RIII reflex response can be considered as a specific and objective physiological correlate of the pain sensation elicited by stimulation of the sural nerve.

Counter-irritation

The application of heterotopic somatic painful conditioning stimuli powerfully and specifically depresses the RIII reflex response and the concurrent sensation of pain, to a degree which is directly and linearly related to the intensity of the conditioning stimuli [27, 29]. This depressive effect is not associated with changes in autonomic functions and is not the result of emotional or stressful reactions [28]. Nor is it due to the postsynaptic inhibition of the motoneurons involved in the spinal flexion reflexes [27]. It corresponds to a decrease in the activity of spinal horn nociceptive neurons [5]. It is noteworthy that in patients with thalamic analgesia, the application of nociceptive stimulation to the anesthetized hand still inhibits the RIII reflex [6]. Therefore, the perception of pain is not involved in RIII reflex inhibition.

On the basis of analogous animal studies, Le Bars and Willer [5, 6, 7, 14] proposed that the depression of the RIII reflex response by painful conditioning stimuli is due to the stimulation of the diffuse noxious inhibitory controls (DNIC). These controls are triggered when two noxious stimuli are applied to distinct areas of the body, thus inducing a competitive effect. Therefore, DNIC are the neuronal substrate of counter-irritation processes, i. e. the masking of pain by a heterotopic painful focus. They are triggered exclusively by heterotopic nociceptive stimuli. They specifically affect the convergent neurons of the spinal dorsal horn [7], which have a key role in the transmission of nociceptive signals. DNIC are anatomically sustained by a loop involving supraspinal structures, and involve opioid peptides and serotonin as neuromediators [14].

In summary, the inhibition of the RIII reflex by heterotopic stimuli can be used for the objective evaluation of the afferent signals triggered by a somatic pain; it does not directly involve sensory experience of pain, and thus limits the influence of emotional and cognitive factors on the evaluation of sensitivity in humans; it is related to the inhibitory process that controls nociceptive signals.

Applications of the RIII reflex technique to the assessment of digestive sensitivity

Effect of gastric distention on the RIII reflex response

Although the inhibition of nociceptive reflexes by visceral stimulation has been evidenced in animals [5, 9, 20], the RIII reflex technique was not applied to the study of visceral sensitivity in man until recently [2]. We have shown that isovolumic gastric distentions inhibit the RIII reflex response in the same way as painful heterotopic somatic conditioning stimuli (Fig. 2). At distention levels of 200 ml and 400 ml, which induced a little or no epigastric discomfort, no significant change in the reflex response was observed, whereas the 600 ml,

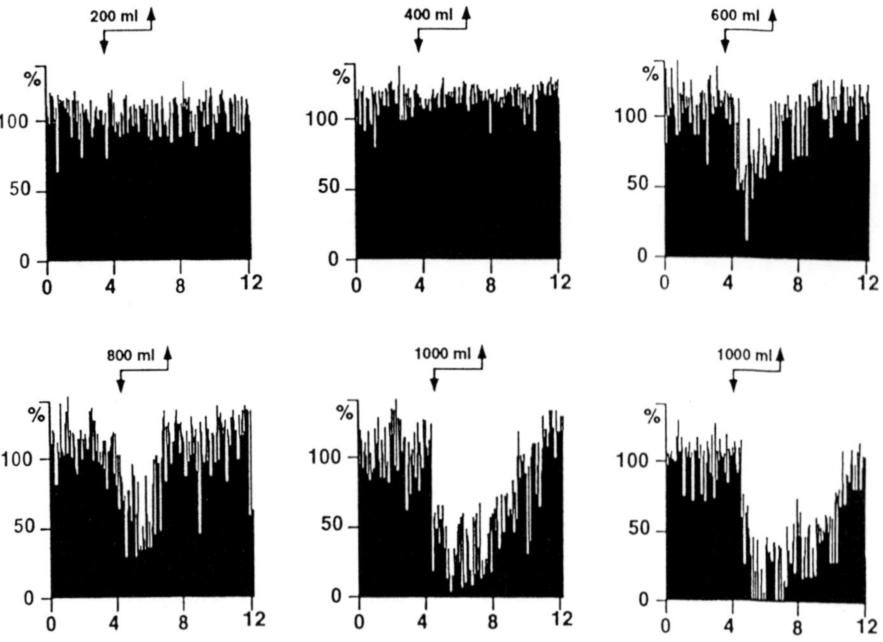

Fig. 2: *Individual examples showing the effects of graded gastric distentions on the RIII reflex response. Each bar represents a single reflex response expressed as a percentage of control (predistension recording) values.*

800 ml, and 1000 ml distention levels inhibited this response by 25, 35 and 55% respectively. The amplitude of the inhibition correlated significantly with both the level of distention and the intensity of visceral perception. The reproducibility of this technique was evidenced by the very similar inhibitions induced by the two 1000 ml distentions performed at an interval of more than two weeks. The only difference between the gastric and somatic conditioning stimuli is that significant inhibition of the RIII reflex was observed with gastric distention levels that did not elicit painful sensations, whereas only painful somatic stimuli inhibited the RIII reflex. The inhibitions observed with nonpainful gastric distention were weaker than those observed with painful distention, and were not followed by post-stimulus effects like those observed for several minutes after painful distentions. Such weaker inhibitions, without postconditioning effects, are still present in spinalized animals [5, 20], which suggests they are sustained by segmental or propriospinal mechanisms. It can therefore be proposed that the inhibitions induced by nonpainful stimuli are only organized spinally and do not involve DNIC.

We conclude from these experiments that RIII reflex inhibition by visceral stimulation permits the objective and quantitative evaluation of visceral sensitivity in humans, and more especially the study of the inhibitory controls of visceral pain.

Effect of fedotozine on RIII reflex inhibition

To further assess the advantages of the above technique, a pharmacological study was performed with a similar experimental design to that just described. The effect of the kappa agonist fedotozine was tested in gastric sensitivity [3]. This drug has been shown to decrease gut sensitivity without affecting somatic sensitivity in several animal models and in humans [8, 13]. Ten healthy subjects, included in a double-blind cross-over study, were given fedotozine (30 mg tid) and a placebo in randomized order for one week. Experiments were performed before each seven-day therapeutic sequence (pre-treatment experiments) and at the end of each sequence. The results of this study are shown in Fig. 3. In pre-treatment experiments, gastric distention, performed at a nociceptive level of 1000 ml for 3 minutes, induced a marked and sustained inhibition of the RIII reflex response. The degree of this inhibition was identical in the two basal experiments, and was not significantly modified by placebo. Fedotozine reduced RIII reflex inhibition, but compared to placebo, this reduction was only significant during the first minute of distention. We conclude that fedotozine reduces gastric nociception by acting on afferent visceral pathways, and that its antinociceptive effect is mainly exerted during the first minute of distention, i. e. during the induction of nociception. It is possible that fedotozine either selectively inhibits a subset of receptors triggered by rapid intermittent distention [12] or

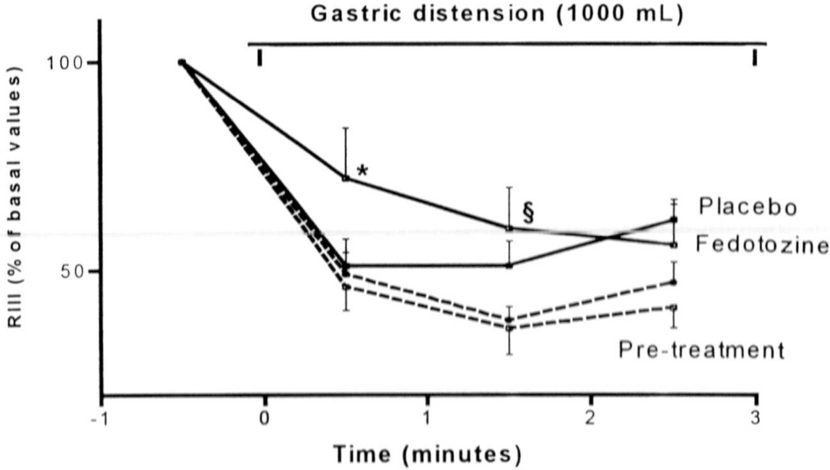

Fig. 3: *Effect of fedotozine on the inhibition of the RIII reflex response induced by gastric distention. Experiments were performed before (pretreatment) and at the end of a 7-day period of treatment by fedotozine and placebo. *: p < 0.05 vs. all other experiments; §: p < 0.05 vs. basal experiments.*

that, under the present experimental conditions, its effect was not strong enough to achieve sustained inhibition of gastric nociception.

However that may be, these results confirm that the RIII technique is of interest for the objective and accurate assessment of the pharmacological action of drugs on visceral sensitivity.

Assessment of rectal afferent visceral pathways

In several recent studies, the possibility was investigated that different sets of mechanoreceptors are involved in signaling rectal sensation by using perception questionnaires together with different modalities of rectal distention and pharmacological manipulation [17, 22, 23]. It was concluded that slow ramp distention preferentially activates mucosal receptors by friction of the mucosa, whereas rapid phasic distention preferentially activates muscular and perhaps serosal receptors. On the basis of these studies, it was also suggested that both types of rectal stimulation primarily activate sacral parasympathetic afferents [22]. The stimulation of nonmucosal receptors can also activate throracolumbar splanchnic (sympathetic) afferents, a neural pathway that seems to be implicated in the hypersensitivity of patients with irritable bowel syndrome [17]. To supply further neurophysiological evidence in support of this hypothesis, we applied the RIII technique to the study of rectal sensitivity. We began by using the same experimental set-up as that used for the stomach to elicit and record the RIII reflex. Four different levels of rapid phasic rectal distention (10, 20, 30

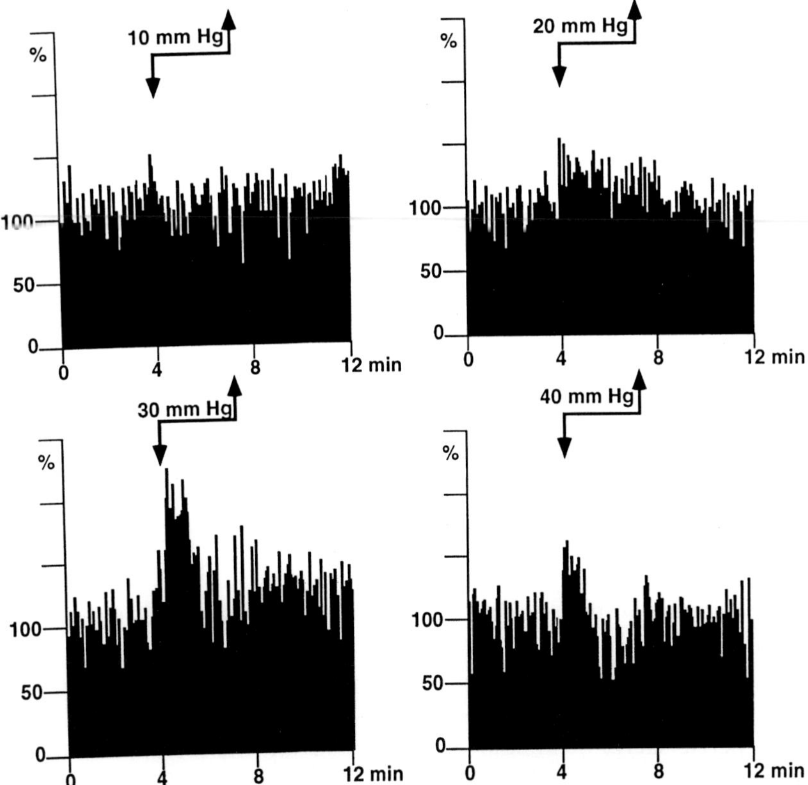

Fig. 4: *Individual example of facilitation of the RIIII reflex response by rapid phasic rectal disten-tions (inflation and deflation rates: 180 ml/min; plateau: 10, 20, 30 and 40 mmHg for 3 minutes). Each bar represents a single reflex response expressed as a percentage of control (pre-distention recording) values.*

and 40 mmHg) were performed in randomized order. Each distention (inflation and deflation rates: 180 ml/min) was maintained constant for three minutes. Surprisingly, rapid phasic distention significantly increased the amplitude of the reflex response (Fig. 4). However, during the higher distention level (40 mmHg), a biphasic response was observed, in which facilitation of the reflex was fol-lowed by its inhibition. Continuous slow ramp rectal distention was also per-formed (inflation rate: 40 ml/min; maximal distending volume: 600 ml). This distention inhibited the RIII reflex (Fig. 5) to a degree which correlated with the intensity of the sensation elicited by the distention ($r = 0.88$; $p < 0.05$). In another series of experiments, the RIII reflex was elicited and recorded in a dermatome clearly different from the rectal viscerotome. The reflex was elicited from the cubital nerve instead of the sural nerve and recorded on the brachial biceps instead of the biceps femoris. In this case, rapid phasic rectal distentions

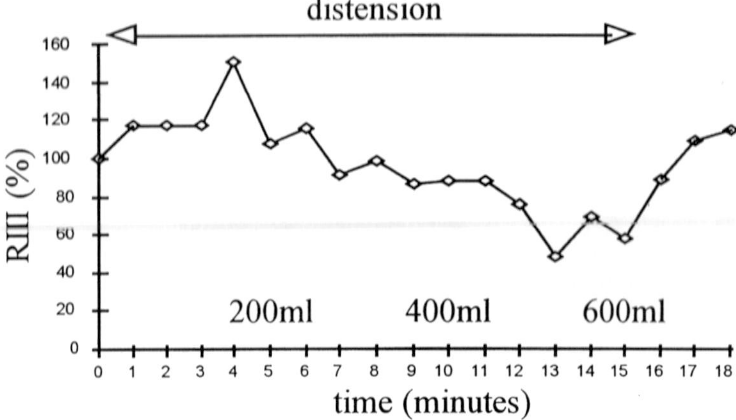

Fig. 5: *Individual example of inhibition of the RIIII reflex response during continuous slow ramp rectal distention performed at 40 ml/minute from 0 to 600 ml. Each point represents the reflex response expressed as a percentage of control (pre-distension recording) values.*

inhibited the RIII reflex response. On the basis of the spinal and supraspinal processing of afferent inputs [15, 10], we postulate that the facilitation of the reflex induced by rapid phasic distentions when the RIII is stimulated and recorded from the leg may be explained by convergence into the same spinal cord segment (upper pelvic sacral or lumbar) of afferents from the rectum and from the somatic territory involved in the RIII reflex. The inhibition of the reflex by slow ramp distention could be due to the fact that this type of distention involves afferents which are not concerned by the above convergence process and therefore, the RIII reflex can be inhibited by DNIC. The convergence process obviously does not concern experiments in which RIII is stimulated and recorded from the arm, which explains why inhibition was observed under these conditions.

The results of the studies described above provide at least one piece of objective evidence that two populations of receptors with specific afferent pathways are present in the rectum.

In conclusion, the reflexologic technique based on the inhibition of the RIII reflex in response to digestive sensory stimulations seems promising for the objective evaluation of visceral sensitivity, the identification of the receptors and afferent pathways it involves, and the exploration of the facilitating and inhibitory mechanisms controlling viscerosensitivity. Studies of patients with disturbed digestive sensitivity are now needed to confirm the clinical relevance of this technique.

References

1. Azpiroz, F.: Sensitivity of the stomach and small bowel: human research and clinical relevance. In: G. F. Gebhart (Ed.): Visceral pain. Progress in pain research and management. Vol. 5, pp. 391−428. IASP Press, Seattle 1995.
2. Bouhassira, D., R. Chollet, B. Coffin et al.: Inhibition of a somatic nociceptive reflex by gastric distension in humans. Gastroenterology 107 (1994) 985−992.
3. Bouhassira, D., B. Coffin, R. Chollet et al.: Effect of fedotozine on gastric nociception assessed by a reflexologic technique. Gastroenterology 108 (1995) A576.
4. Bouhassira, D., L. Villaneuva, Z. Bing et al.: Involvement of subnucleus reticularis dorsalis in diffuse noxious inhibitory controls in the rat. Brain Res. 595 (1992) 353−357.
5. Cadden, S. W., L. Villanueva, D. Chitour et al.: Depression of activities of dorsal horn convergent neurones by propriospinal mechanisms triggered by noxious inputs; comparison with diffuse noxious inhibitory controls (DNIC). Brain Res. 275 (1983) 1−11.
6. De Broucker, T., P. Cesaro, J. C. Willer et al.: Diffuse noxious inhibitory controls (DNIC) in man: involvement of the spinoreticular tract. Brain 113 (1990) 1223−1234.
7. Dickenson, A. H., D. Le Bars, J. M. Besson: Endogenous opiates and nociception: a possible functional role in both pain inhibition and detection as revealed by intrathecal naloxone. Neurosci. Lett. 24 (1981) 161.
8. Diop, L., P. Rivière, X. Pascaud et al.: Peripheral kappa opioid receptors mediate the antinociceptive effect of fedotozine on the duodenal pain reflex in rat. Eur. J. Pharmacol. 271 (1994) 65−71.
9. Falinower, S., J. C. Pascaud, J. C. Willer et al.: A new model to investigate visceral pain in anaesthetized rat. Gastroenterology 104 (1993) A505.
10. Foreman, R. D.: Spinal and supraspinal processing of nociceptive inputs from the urinary bladder and somatic receptive fields. In: E. A. Mayer, H. E. Raybould (Eds.): Basic and clinical aspects of chronic abdominal pain. Pain research and clinical management, Vol. 9, pp. 113−124. Elsevier, Amsterdam 1993.
11. Hugon, M.: Exteroceptive reflexes to stimulation of the sural nerve in normal man. In: J. E. Desmedt (Ed.): New Developments in Electromyography and clinical Neurophysiology, Vol. 3, pp. 713−729. Karger, Basel 1973.
12. Khan, M. I., N. W. Read, D. Grundy: Effect of varying the rate of and pattern of gastric distension on its sensory perception and motor activity. Am. J. Physiol. 264 (1993) G824−G827.
13. Langlois, A., L. Diop, P. Rivière et al.: Effect of fedotozine on the cardiovascular pain reflex induced by distension of the irritated colon in the anaesthetized rat. Eur. J. Pharmacol. 271 (1994) 245−251.
14. Le Bars, C., D. Chitour, E. Kraus et al.: The effect of systemic morphine upon diffuse noxious inhibitory controls (DNIC) in the rat. Evidence for a lifting of certain descending inhibitory controls of dorsal horn convergent neurones. Brain Res. 215 (1981) 257−274.
15. Le Bars, D., H. Dickenson, J. M. Besson et al.: Aspects of sensory processing through convergent neurons. In: T. L. Yaksh (Ed.): Spinal afferent processing, pp. 467−504. Plenum Publishing Corporation, New York 1986.
16. Lémann, M., B. Coffin, R. Chollet et al.: Sensibilité viscérale digestive. Méthodes d'étude chez l'homme et implications physiopathologiques. Gastroenterol. Clin. Biol. 19 (1995) 270−281.
17. Lembo, T., J. Munakata, H. Mertz et al.: Evidence for the hypersensitivity of lumbar splanchnic afferents in irritable bowel syndrome. Gastroenterology 107 (1994) 1686−1696.
18. Mayer, E. A., G. F. Gebhart: Functional bowel disorders and the visceral hyperalgesia hypothesis. In: E. A. Mayer, H. E. Raybould (Eds.): Basic and clinical aspects of chronic abdominal pain. Pain research and clinical management, Vol. 9, pp. 3−28. Elsevier, Amsterdam 1993.

19 Meunier, P., L. Collet, R. Duclos et al.: Endorectal cerebral evoked potentials in humans. Int. J. Neurosci. 37 (1987) 193−196.

20. Ness, T. J., F. G. Gebhart: Interactions between visceral and cutaneous nociception in the rat. II. Noxious visceral stimuli inhibit cutaneous nociceptive neurones and reflexes. J. Neurophysiol. 66 (1991) 29−39.

21. Phelps, M. E.: PET: biological imaging of the brain. In: E. A. Mayer, H. E. Raybould (Eds.): Basic and clinical aspects of chronic abdominal pain. Pain research and clinical management, Vol. 9, pp. 293−310. Elsevier, Amsterdam 1993.

22. Plourde, V., T. Lembo, Z. Shui et al.: Effects of the somatostatin analogue octreotide on rectal afferent nerves in humans. Am. J. Physiol. 265 (1993) G742−G751.

23. Sun, M. W., N. W. Read, A. Prior et al.: Sensory and motor responses to rectal distension vary according to rate and pattern of balloon inflation. Gastroenterology 99 (1990) 1008−1015.

24. Willer, J. C.: Comparative study of perceived pain and nociceptive flexion reflex in man. Pain 3 (1977) 69−80.

25. Willer, J. C.: Studies of pain. Effects of morphine on a spinal nociceptive flexion reflex and related pain sensation in man. Brain Res. 331 (1985) 105−114.

26. Willer, J. C.: Exploration clinique de la nociception par des techniques de réflexologie. Neurophysiol. Clin. 20 (1990) 335−356.

27. Willer, J. C., T. De Broucker, D. Le Bars: Encoding of nociceptive thermal stimuli by diffuse noxious inhibitory controls in humans. J. Neurophysiol. 62 (1989) 1028−1038.

28. Willer, J. C., D. Le Bars, T. De Broucker: Diffuse noxious controls in man: involvement of an opioidergik link. Eur. J. Pharmacol. 182 (1990) 347−355.

29. Willer, J. C., A. Roby, D. Le Bars: Psychophysical and electrophysiological approaches to the pain relieving effect of heterotopic nociceptive stimuli. Brain 107 (1984) 1095−1112.

Gastrointestinal manifestations
of movement disorders

C. D. Marsden

Introduction

The field of Movement Disorders comprises two main categories, the akinetic-rigid syndrome of parkinsonism, and abnormal involuntary movements or dyskinesias. There are many causes of parkinsonism, including classical Parkinson's disease, the Parkinsonism-plus syndromes (such as Multiple System Atrophy, Progressive Supranuclear Palsy, and Corticobasal Degeneration), drug-induced parkinsonism, and parkinsonism in the setting of diffuse cerebral disorders such as in the dementias and cerebrovascular disease. The major categories of dyskinesias include Tremors, Choreas, Tics, Myoclonus, Dystonias, and Paroxysmal Dyskinesias.

Surprisingly little attention has been given to gastrointestinal dysfunction in movement disorders, despite the fact that difficulties in salivation, swallowing, gastric emptying, colonic and rectal function occur frequently and cause severe disability in parkinsonian syndromes. Table 1 gives a survey of gastrointestinal symptoms in 98 cases of Parkinson's disease, compared to 50 matched controls [5]. Excess salivation and drooling, difficulty in swallowing, constipation, and defecatory problems (straining and incomplete emptying) are common.

In fact, some of these disorders are even more evident and disabling in other movement disorders such as the Parkinsonism-plus syndromes and generalised symptomatic dystonias. In particular, drooling and dysphagia, associated with a striatal pseudobulbar palsy, are a major cause of handicap in these illnesses.

Table 1: *Gastrointestinal symptoms in Parkinson's disease (Edwards et al. [5]).*

	PD	Controls
Excess salivation	70	6
Dysphagia	52	6
Nausea	24	8
Constipation	29	10
Straining	66	28

98 cases (79 on dopaminergic drugs, 29 on anticholinergics), 50 matched controls. Percentages are shown.

In contrast to the Parkinsonian syndromes and severe dystonic conditions, gastrointestinal disorders are not a feature of most other dyskinesias. Patients with tremor or tics do not complain of gastrointestinal symptoms. Nor do patients with the many different forms of myoclonic syndromes. Accordingly, I will here review the main gastrointestinal problems seen in parkinsonism and severe dystonia.

The reasons for drooling, dysphagia, alterations in gastric emptying, and in defaecation in Parkinson's disease are complex (see [6] for review). Rigidity and slowness of movement affects bulbar and pelvic striated muscles. Autonomic function is impaired in some patients, and is an integral part of Multiple System Atrophy. Autonomic disturbances may compromise gastrointestinal function, as well as causing problems with sweating, blood pressure control, the bladder and achieving erections. Pathological changes in the myenteric and submucosal plexuses also occur in Parkinson's disease [13].

Drooling

About three quarters of patients with Parkinson's disease experience a feeling of increased saliva in the mouth and drooling and wetting of the pillow during sleep [4, 5]. The extent of these problems is related to the severity of the disease. Eventually, some patients require the constant use of a tissue or handkerchief to mop up saliva dripping from the mouth. Drooling in Parkinson's disease is thought to be due to decreased frequency of swallowing, and difficulty in the oropharyngeal process of swallowing, rather than to excess production of saliva [4]. Bateson et al. [1] found that the output of saliva was the same in those with drooling compared to those with a dry mouth; both groups produced less saliva than controls. Such drooling of saliva is an even greater problem in those with Parkinsonism-plus syndromes and severe dystonic disorders. In these conditions there is even greater striatal pseudobulbar dysfunction than in Parkinson's disease.

The management of excessive salivation and drooling can be exceedingly difficult. Obviously anything that can improve swallowing will help. Radiation of the salivary glands has been employed, but in our experience has not proved satisfactory. Anticholinergic drugs to dry up saliva rarely produce much benefit in those with severe difficulty. Surgical diversion of salivary ducts also has been attempted.

Dysphagia

The complex process of swallowing is frequently affected in those with Parkinson's disease, and particularly in those with a severe striatal pseudobulbar palsy due to the Parkinsonism-plus syndromes and severe dystonic disorders. Difficulties in chewing and then in moving the bolus of food with the tongue towards the pharynx commonly interfere with the oral phase of swallowing. Likewise, there are difficulties with propelling the bolus from the back of the mouth into the pharynx, and in transferring the bolus through the upper oesophageal sphincter into the oesophagus itself. However, there is no single characteristic videographic abnormality of swallowing in Parkinson's disease [2].

The major cause of swallowing difficulties in Parkinson's disease appears to relate to dysfunction of the striated muscles involved in the earlier stages of the process. Autonomic dysfunction may contribute to abnormalities of the oesophageal phase of swallowing. This may be due to degeneration of the dorsal motor nucleus of the vagus [3], Lewy body degeneration of the myenteric plexus [11], and even peripheral dopamine depletion.

Gastric emptying

Abnormalities of gastric emptying play two important roles in Parkinson's disease. First, they may cause symptoms of postprandial fullness, nausea and even vomiting. Second, they may delay or prevent the therapeutic effects of levodopa treatment for Parkinson's disease. Levodopa is absorbed from the upper small bowel, so that anything that delays gastric emptying will affect its therapeutic response.

Patients with Parkinson's disease who have developed the long-term complications of fluctuations and dyskinesias become critically dependent upon an adequate plasma levodopa level for therapeutic benefit. Below the critical level, patients are immobile and "off"; above the critical level they rapidly switch "on" to become mobile but with dyskinesias. Delay in gastric emptying may cause failure of adequate levodopa absorption such that patients experience a long interval between drug intake and switching "on", or even fail to turn "on" at all. Drugs that enhance gastric emptying may therefore improve the response to levodopa treatment in such cases.

Constipation and defecatory dysfunction

Constipation, excessive straining and incomplete emptying of stool are common and distressing problems in Parkinson's disease. At the extreme, megacolon and even sigmoid volvulus may occur.

Colonic transit time is significantly prolonged in Parkinson's disease [7]. In addition, there are anorectal abnormalities causing "outlet" dysfunction, which can be demonstrated on defecatory imaging studies [7].

Mathers et al. [9, 10] have described paradoxical puborectalis contraction during straining in Parkinson's disease, along with anismus, suggesting disordered control of the muscles of the pelvic floor. This can be reversed by administration of a dopamine agonist such as apomorphine.

The defects in striated muscle control characteristic of Parkinson's disease may be responsible for some of the outlet dysfunction causing straining and faecal retention. However, the presence of Lewy bodies in colonic enteric ganglion cells [8] is an added factor. In addition, Singaram et al. [12] have described abnormalities of dopaminergic innervation of colonic tissue in patients with Parkinson's disease.

Gastrointestinal influences on movement disorders

While most of the information available concerns the impact of movement disorders on gastrointestinal function as discussed above, the reverse occasionally is of importance.

Sandifer's syndrome is a rare but fascinating condition in which children with oesophageal reflux develop head posturing or even more frankly dystonic movement after eating. Thus they may present to the neurologist with a paroxysmal movement disorder, but one that is clearly related to food intake. How oesophageal reflex provokes such abnormal movements is not clear, although it is assumed that they represent compensatory attempts to gain relief from the effects of reflux oesophagitis. Treatment of the oesophageal reflux, which often requires surgery, can abolish the condition.

A similar mechanism occasionally is responsible for exacerbations of a movement disorder, commonly athetoid cerebral palsy, at the time of feeding.

References

1. Bateson, M. C., F. B. Gibberd, R. S. E. Wilson: Salivary symptoms in Parkinson's disease. Arch. Neurol. 29 (1973) 274–275.
2. Bushmann, M., S. M. Dobmeyer, L. Leeker et al.: Swallowing abnormalities and their response to treatment in Parkinson's disease. Neurology 39 (1989) 1309–1314.
3. Eadie, M. J.: The pathology of certain medullary nuclei in parkinsonism. Brain Res. 86 (1963) 781–792.
4. Eadie, M. J., J. H. Tyrer: Alimentary disorders in parkinsonism. Aust. Ann. Med. 14 (1965) 13–22.
5. Edwards, L. L., R. F. Pfeiffer, E. M. M. Quigley et al.: Gastrointestinal symptoms in Parkinson's disease. Mov. Dis. 6 (1991) 151–156.
6. Edwards, L. L., M. M. Quigley, R. F. Pfeiffer: Gastrointestinal dysfunction in Parkinson's disease: Frequency and pathophysiology. Neurology 42 (1992) 726–732.

7. Edwards, L. L., E. M. M. Quigley, R. K. Harned et al.: Characterization of swallowing and defecation in Parkinson's disease. Am. J. Gastroenterol. 89 (1994) 15–25.

8. Kupsky, W. J., M. M. Grimes, J. Sweeting et al.: Parkinson's disease and megacolon: Concentric hyaline inclusions (Lewy bodies) in enteric ganglion cells. Neurology 37 (1987) 1253–1255.

9. Mathers, S. E., P. A. Kempster, M. Swash et al.: Constipation and paradoxical puborectalis contraction in anismus and Parkinson's disease: a dystonic phenomenon. J. Neurol. Neurosurg. Psychiat. 51 (1988) 1503–1507.

10. Mathers, S. E., Kempster, P. A., Law, P. J., Frankel, J. P., Bartram, C. I., Lees, A. J., Stern, G. M., Swash, M. Anal sphincter dysfunction in Parkinson's disease. Arch. Neurol. 46 (1989) 1061–1064.

11. Qualman, S. J., Haupt, H. M., Yang, P., Hamilton, S. R. Esophageal Lewy bodies associated with ganglion cell loss in achalasia. Gastroenterology 87 (1984) 848–856.

12. Singaram, C., W. Ashraf, E. A. Gaumnitz et al.: Dopaminergic defect of enteric nervous system in Parkinson's disease patients with chronic constipation. Lancet 346 (1995) 861–864.

13. Wakabayashi, K., H. Takahashi, E. Takeda et al.: Parkinson's disease: the presence of Lewy bodies in Auerbach's and Meissner's plexuses. Acta Neuropathol. 76 (1988) 217–221.

Epidemiology and pathophysiology of gastrointestinal manifestations in Parkinson's disease

E. M. M. Quigley

Gastrointestinal symptoms are common among patients with a variety of movement disorders, but have been best characterized in Parkinson's disease. Thus, while dysphagia, and especially difficulty with the oropharyngeal phase of swallowing may occur in any movement disorder which involves the tongue or pharyngeal musculature, the prevalence of symptoms among these patient populations has not been established and little is known of other aspects of gastrointestinal function. In contrast, recent studies have delineated the prevalence of various gastrointestinal symptoms among patients with Parkinson's disease and have noted, in particular, a high frequency of disordered salivation, dysphagia, constipation and defecatory dysfunction [25]. Furthermore, a pathophysiological basis for some, at least, of these symptoms has been established, and relationships between the central nervous and gastrointestinal manifestations of this disorder are currently under investigation. This review will concentrate, therefore, on gastrointestinal manifestations in Parkinson's disease.

Gastrointestinal symptoms in Parkinson's disease

Gastrointestinal features were recognized by Sir James Parkinson in his original monograph published in 1817 [41]. Indeed, he described, in some detail, the cardinal gastrointestinal features of this disorder; namely, disordered swallowing: "food is with difficulty retained in the mouth until masticated; and then as difficultly swallowed ... the saliva fails of being directed to the back part of the fauces, and hence it is continually draining from the mouth"; constipation: "the bowels which all along had been torpid, now in most cases, demand stimulating medicines of very considerable power" and difficult defecation: "the expulsion of the feces from the rectum sometimes requiring mechanical aid". However, the true frequency of gastrointestinal symptoms in Parkinson's disease remains unclear. While some, recent studies have provided some information on the frequency of various gastrointestinal symptoms among those Parkinson's disease patients who attend a movement disorders clinic [13, 22−24, 27, 38] − it remains to be established whether or not this is a true reflection of their prevalence among those many patients with symptoms of Parkinson's disease in the community [9].

These limitations notwithstanding, available surveys have, in general, confirmed the high prevalence of gastrointestinal symptoms among PD patients and have also clarified which symptoms are most closely related to PD. Thus, when Parkinson's disease patients were compared with age-matched controls, disordered salivation, dysphagia, nausea, constipation and defecatory dysfunction were the gastrointestinal symptoms which were truly more common. In one study, in 98 patients with Parkinson's disease, abnormal salivation, dysphagia, nausea, constipation and defecatory dysfunction were present in 70.2, 52.1, 24.4, 28.7 and 65.9% of Parkinson's disease patients, respectively [24]. Thus, either abnormal salivation, dysphagia or defecatory dysfunction were present in over 50% of these patients. In this same study, the contribution of various constitutional and behavioral factors to the prevalence of gastrointestinal symptoms was also evaluated. Of the various parameters studied, only Parkinson's disease activity and duration of Parkinson's disease correlated with gastrointestinal symptoms — patient age, gender, level of activity, dietary fiber intake and anti-Parkinsonian therapy did not [24]. These findings appear to support Parkinson's original hypothesis, namely, that gastrointestinal symptoms are a component of the disease process itself.

Dysphagia

Dysphagia is common among patients with Parkinson's disease, and usually presents as a sensation of food sticking or "holding up" at the back of the throat, most commonly at the level of the thyroid cartilage [31].

Dysfunction in the oral and pharyngeal phases of swallowing is the major abnormality in patients with Parkinson's disease and disordered swallowing. Bushmann and colleagues described a number of abnormalities which included abnormal lingual control, lingual festination, stasis in the anterior and lateral sulci, vallecular stasis, repetitive and involuntary reflux from the vallecular and pyriform sinuses into the oral cavity and aspiration [13]. In a recent study, Ali and colleagues performed simultaneous video radiography and pharyngeal manometry in 19 patients with Parkinson's disease [1]. While demonstrating that some alterations in oral function may be non-specific, they noted that lingual tremor appeared to be unique to Parkinson's disease, and to directly correlate with the presence of dysphagia. They confirmed that pharyngeal dysfunction was strongly associated with Parkinson's disease, and that coating of the pharyngeal wall, post-swallow vallecular pooling, pyriform sinus pooling, and abnormal pharyngeal wall motion were significantly more common among Parkinson's disease patients than controls. Indeed, impaired pharyngeal bolus transport appeared to be the major determinant of dysphagia; pharyngeal contraction pressures were, on average, lower in patients.

The relevance of cricopharyngeal dysfunction to dysphagia among PD patients has been the subject of considerable debate, some contending that cricopharyngeal achalasia is a major abnormality [40], while others failed to describe the occurrence of cricopharyngeal achalasia among their patients [15, 23, 42]. Several clinical studies have, indeed, described an association between Zenker's diverticulum, cricopharyngeal bars and PD [1, 14, 37] and we recently reported successful relief of dysphagia following cricopharyngeal myotomy in a small group of Parkinson's disease patients with evidence of cricopharyngeal dysfunction [11].

Recent studies on the pathogenesis of cricopharyngeal dysfunction in non-PD patients have suggested that while opening of the upper esophageal sphincter is initiated by relaxation of the cricopharyngeus, the major contribution to opening is provided by the physical distraction of the sphincter, which results in anterior movement and elevation of the hyoid [30]. Full distention of the sphincter is modulated by intrabolus pressures, which are, in turn, generated primarily by the piston-like action of the tongue, rather than pharyngeal peristalsis. Based on these physiological studies and on clinical observations, it is now felt that impaired opening, and not sustained spasm, delayed relaxation or premature contraction is the primary abnormality in the upper sphincter in patients with idiopathic cricopharyngeal bars, Zenker's diverticulum and dysphagia [20]. It is thought that impaired opening is, in turn, related to fibrosis of the cricopharyngeus. Ali and colleagues have now clarified the role of UES dysfunction in the pathogenesis of symptoms in Parkinson's disease [1]. Thus, resting sphincter pressure did not differ between Parkinson's disease patients or controls. Incomplete relaxation was, however, prevalent, upper esophageal sphincter pressure, on average, reduced and, accordingly, the hypopharyngeal intrabolus pressures increased during trans-sphincter flow.

Three factors, perhaps interrelated, appear fundamental, therefore, to the pathogenesis of oropharyngeal dysphagia in PD: lingual tremor (or festination), pharyngeal peristaltic dysfunction and impaired opening of the upper esophageal sphincter.

It is important to remember that drooling and difficulty with saliva are manifestations of disordered swallowing and not of a primary abnormality in salivary flow [22]. Indeed, available evidence indicates that problems with saliva in Parkinson's disease are not due to salivary hypersecretion, but rather to impaired transfer of saliva to the pharynx. When directly studied, salivary output proved similar in both Parkinsonian patients with drooling and those who complained of a dry mouth. Indeed, both groups produced less saliva than controls [8]. Given the location of the swallowing dysfunction, it is not surprising that up to 30% of patients with Parkinson's disease describe associated respiratory symptoms (coughing, choking, nocturnal dyspnea).

While acknowledging the primacy of oral and pharyngeal dysfunction in dysphagia in PD, it is important, from a clinical point of view, to bear in mind that patients with Parkinson's disease may falsely localize dysphagia. In one review of patients with Parkinson's disease presenting with dysphagia, while all localized dysphagia to the oropharynx, a significant proportion were found, on detailed investigation, to exhibit major pathology in the esophageal body or in the lower esophagus [14]. Several, in particular, had advanced reflux disease and esophagitis − effective anti-reflux measures led to significant improvement in dysphagia.

Clinical experience, as well as symptom surveys, associated dysphagia with advanced PD; more detailed investigations suggest that the relationship between oropharyngeal dysfunction and PD activity may be less precise [10, 48]. Thus, Ali and colleagues found that oral-pharyngeal dysphagia in Parkinson's disease appeared to correlate poorly with clinical severity, several patients demonstrating oral and pharyngeal dysfunction before the clinical onset of dysphagia [1]. Furthermore, Thomas and Haigh have reported dysphagia as the presenting feature of PD [49].

While Lewy bodies have been described in the esophagus in Parkinson's disease [43], the true prevalence and clinical significance of esophageal dysmotility and lower esophageal sphincter dysfunction in Parkinson's disease remains unclear. Thus, while earlier studies have described "esophageal dysmotility" in up to 7% of subjects with PD [25], one recent study, employing a detailed manometric protocol uncovered abnormalities in esophaegal motor function in 15 of 22 symptomatic PD patients [17]. We, and others, in contrast, failed to define an increased incidence of esophageal motor dysfunction in PD patients when compared to appropriate controls [28].

Lower esophageal sphincter function has not been directly studied in PD − of interest, however, is the description of prominent belching during "off" periods in some PD subjects [34]. It is now thought that belching is mediated in part by transient relaxation of the lower esophageal sphincter, the major mechanism of both physiologic and pathologic reflux [55]. This observation would suggest that this aspect of lower esophageal sphincter function may be impaired in Parkinson's disease, but this has not been directly evaluated.

Gastric and small intestinal dysfunction in Parkinson's disease

Nausea is a common complaint among patients with Parkinson's disease, and while, in symptom surveys, vomiting did not appear to be more common in PD than in age- and sex-matched controls, this symptom has been described in PD in some reports [24, 27].

The pathophysiology of these symptoms remains poorly understood. Most typically, patients related the onset of nausea to dopaminergic medications, and it is certainly clear that many have central nausea-inducing effects. It is also possible that these agents could exert effects on gut smooth muscle or the enteric nervous system. What is also not clear is to what extent gastric or small intestinal dysmotility occurs in Parkinson's disease, or relates to gastrointestinal symptomatology. Some indirect evidence does suggest that gastroparesis may be prevalent in PD. Thus, one study, which described a high prevalence of gastroparesis in an elderly population, noted that 55% of these patients had underlying PD [29].

Clinical experience suggests that gastroparesis does, indeed, occur in PD. Delayed gastric emptying has been incriminated as fundamental to impaired delivery of orally-ingested dopaminergic medications to the small intestine, their site of absorption [39, 45]. For this reason, various prokinetic agents have been employed to accelerate gastric emptying and to improve drug delivery. This becomes particularly important, of course, among those Parkinson's patients with prominent "on"−"off" fluctuations [21]. While some of these agents, such as domperidone, also have central anti-nausea effects, it does appear that a prokinetic effect may contribute to predictable drug delivery, and, thus, symptom control. Motor function of the stomach has not been directly studied by either manometric, electrogastrographic or imaging techniques − this is clearly a major gap in our understanding of the pathophysiology of nausea, vomiting and upper abdominal pain in patients with Parkinson's disease.

In view of its relative inaccessibility, it is not surprising that small intestinal motor activity has received even less attention. One study, published in abstract form only, documented both quantitative and qualitative differences in motor patterns of the small intestine among patients with PD [12]. The relationship of these findings to symptomatology was not, however, examined. The prevalence, clinical significance and relevance to symptomatology of small intestinal dysmotility in Parkinson's disease remains, therefore, to be defined. Abdominal pain is a not uncommon symptom among patients with Parkinson's disease; in some instances extensive investigation may prove unproductive and the pain unresponsive to conventional therapy. For some of these patients it appears that the pain may originate from the abdominal musculature, rather than the abdominal viscera; this pain appears to represent a component of the PD process itself. It is tempting to speculate that small intestinal dysmotility could contribute to pain in some others, in a manner analogous to the pain associated with the pseudo-obstruction syndromes.

Constipation and defecatory dysfunction in PD

As described by Parkinson himself, constipation is prevalent in PD. In its most advanced state, colonic dysfunction may progress to frank megacolon and several instances of fatal perforated megacolon have been described [6, 7, 16, 36, 44]. Along with dysphagia, therefore, constipation and anorectal dysfunction represent the two major clinical gastrointestinal problems for patients with Parkinson's disease. On the basis of both symptomatology and clinical investigation, it would appear that patients with Parkinson's disease exhibit both slow colon transit and defecatory dysfunction [28, 32]. The former is traditionally represented, in terms of symptoms, by infrequent defecation, the latter by difficult defecation, a sensation of complete evacuation, and prolonged straining. Edwards and colleagues, in a study that described both delayed colon transit and defecatory dysfunction among patients with Parkinson's disease, found, however, that these symptoms were poor predictors of the underlying physiologic defects, whether it be slow transit or anorectal/pelvic floor dysfunction. Furthermore, there was considerable overlap between these two groups, with several patients exhibiting both slow transit and defecatory dysfunction [28]. On anorectal manometry, PD patients with defecatory dysfunction may demonstrate a distinctive abnormality, namely, a "paradoxical" or "hypercontractile" response on testing of the rectosphincteric reflex. On balloon inflation, one sees, in these patients, not the expected relaxation of the internal anal sphincter, but, rather, a markedly hypercontractile response [2, 28]. More detailed manometric studies, which included simultaneous electromyographic recordings from the external anal sphincter and pelvic floor musculature, revealed that internal anal sphincter relaxation was, indeed, intact in these patients, but was masked by a delayed, prolonged and markedly hypercontractile response originating in either the external anal sphincter or puborectalis muscle, or both [4].

Depression, common among PD patients, may present with visceral symptomatology and with "constipation" in particular. The clinician needs to be alert to the patient apparently obsessed by inadequate defecation but whose primary problem is depression and not colonic or anorectal dysfunction. Appropriate anti-depressant therapy will lead to a dramatic improvement in these instances of "obsessive" constipation.

Pathophysiology

The precise pathophysiology of the various gastrointestinal symptoms and functional abnormalities described in Parkinson's disease remain uncertain. Several factors may be relevant. Traditionally, these symptoms were largely ascribed to the side effects of anti-Parkinsonian medications. Certainly, anti-cholinergic agents, popular in the past, can delay gastrointestinal transit and may, indeed, have been relevant in some patients, to the precipitation of constipation or delayed gastric emptying. As mentioned above, dopaminergic compounds may certainly induce nausea through central effects and could, in theory, at least, affect gastrointestinal transit through effects on dopamine receptors in the enteric nervous system or in enteric muscle. It is becoming clear, however, that, for the most part, gastrointestinal symptoms appear to be directly related to the Parkinson's disease process itself. Other factors, such as diet and mobility have also been examined, and do not appear to play a major role in the induction of gastrointestinal symptomatology [24].

The relationship to the Parkinson's disease process may itself be complex. For some symptoms, the relationship appears reasonably straightforward. Thus, for symptoms such as oropharyngeal dysphagia or defecatory dysfunction, which originate from skeletal muscles innervated by the somatic nervous system, one can readily correlate abnormal function in these muscles to that which occurs in other skeletal muscles. These symptoms have, in general, been shown to parallel the severity and duration of Parkinson's disease, and have been shown to deteriorate during "off" periods in those patients with prominent "on"/"off" fluctuations [4]. There is also some evidence that these visceral symptoms may respond acutely to the parenteral administration of the dopaminergic agent apomorphine [26]. Indeed, apomorphine has been used on an as needed basis to facilitate micturition and defecation in patients with severely disordered bladder and anorectal function [19, 47]. What has been less clear cut, however, has been the clinical response of either dysphagia or constipation to prolonged oral dopaminergic medication. Indeed, it has proven difficult, at best, to demonstrate a significant improvement in either swallowing or defecatory dysfunction in relation to the institution or modification of dopaminergic medication.

Evidence is now accumulating to suggest that the Parkinson's disease process may involve the enteric nervous system in a manner analogous to the central nervous system. Several reports have documented Lewy bodies, similar in morphology to those seen in the central nervous system, in the enteric nervous system of the esophagus and colon in PD [35, 43, 46, 51−54]. A relationship to dysfunction in these areas has not been established, though one report suggested that these Lewy bodies predominated in vasoactive intestinal peptide-containing neurons [46]. Furthermore, Singaram and colleagues have recently documented severe depletion of dopaminergic neurons in the colon in some patients with Parkinson's disease, constipation and megacolon [46]. Of importance, the density of dopamine-containing neurons appeared normal in patients with idiopathic non-Parkinson's disease-related megacolon. This is obviously an intriguing finding, and provides, for the first time, some direct evidence for the parallel involvement of the enteric and central nervous systems in Parkinson's disease. How these findings relate to abnormal transit or gastrointestinal symptoms is far from clear. One could speculate, indeed, based on the suggestion that dopamine is an inhibitory neurotransmitter in the gastrointestinal tract, that these patients should demonstrate augmented rather than suppressed motor activity [50].

Exciting possibilities exist in relation to research in this area. Firstly, the enteric nervous system may provide a more accessible target for studies of neural function, morphology and biochemistry in Parkinson's disease. Secondly, if these findings can be replicated in endoscopic or laparoscopic biopsy, these enteric neural abnormalities could permit, for the first time, the diagnosis of Parkinson's disease, in vivo; which is, at present, possible only at autopsy. Finally, studies of the relationships between dopamine depletion, repletion, symptoms, gastrointestinal function and enteric neural morphology could facilitate the delineation of the clinical correlates of enteric neural dysfunction.

Autonomic dysfunction may also be relevant to the pathophysiology of gastrointestinal symptomatology and dysfunction in Parkinson's disease [18]. Autonomic dysfunction in relation to Parkinson's disease has, of course, been best documented in the Shy-Drager syndrome and related autonomic neuropathies. Autonomic dysfunction, however, is also prevalent among patients with PD, per se. How this relates to the prevalence of gastrointestinal symptoms has not been defined. Furthermore, Wakabayashi and colleagues have described the presence of Lewy bodies in autonomic ganglia in patients with Parkinson's disease, thereby providing a possible pathological basis for autonomic dysfunction [54].

Management of gastrointestinal symptoms in Parkinson's disease

Little data exists to guide therapy in patients with Parkinson's disease and gastrointestinal dysfunction. In clinical practice the tendency has been to extrapolate to Parkinson's disease data derived from non-Parkinsonian patients with gastrointestinal symptoms. Thus, PD patients with constipation tend to be treated with stool softening agents, laxatives, enemas and prokinetic agents. Recently, some evidence from controlled clinical trials has, indeed, provided support for the use of these agents in PD. Thus, both psyllium [3] and the prokinetic agent cisapride [33] have been shown to accelerate colon transit and alleviate constipation in patients with Parkinson's disease. Interestingly, fiber supplementation has also been shown to improve the delivery of dopaminergic agents in Parkinson's disease and, thereby, promote more predictable symptom control [5]. These approaches, though apparently effective in patients with mild to moderate constipation, are unlikely to prove effective in more severely constipated subjects. It is extremely important, in these constipated patients, to maintain stool output and thus avoid impaction and potentially fatal megacolon. Enemas are often warranted and indeed indicated to alleviate defecatory dysfunction. As mentioned, there is some evidence to suggest that the dopaminergic agent apomorphine may acutely alleviate distressing defecatory dysfunction; this approach has not, however, been subjected to a controlled clinical trial.

In the management of dysphagia, guidelines for management follow those developed for oropharyngeal dysphagia, in general. Thus, particular attention should be paid to the detection and avoidance of aspiration. Attention to detail may prove most rewarding, and here, expert support from colleagues in speech pathology may prove invaluable – dietary modifications may considerably facilitate swallowing. These patients may also benefit from instruction in a number of maneuvers to facilitate bolus transfer and minimize the risk of aspiration. Some patients with dysphagia may progress to a stage where they are unable to safely maintain an adequate oral intake of nutrients, and may, in particular, experience difficulty in ensuring reliable delivery of medications. In these instances, the technique of percutaneous endoscopic gastrostomy has proved invaluable and has become an important component of the management of patients with advanced Parkinson's disease. Gastroparesis, if present, may, of course, compromise effective use of the gastrostomy for nutrition or drug delivery, and a surgically placed jejunostomy may become necessary.

While, as mentioned above, prokinetic agents have been shown to improve delivery of dopaminergic agents in Parkinson's disease, and, perhaps, also to alleviate nausea, this approach has not been subjected to large scale clinical trials. As measures of gastric emptying rate or some other parameter of gastric motor function have not been directly evaluated, it is difficult to divine from these studies whether the beneficial effect of these agents has been exerted centrally on the chemo-receptor trigger zone, or peripherally as a prokinetic effect.

Summary

Gastrointestinal dysfunction is common and clinically important in patients with Parkinson's disease. Evidence continues to accumulate to indicate that these symptoms reflect, for the most part, the direct involvement of the gastrointestinal tract by the Parkinson's disease process. Gastrointestinal symptomatology may arise not only as a consequence of the effects of PD on skeletal muscles in the oropharynx, anorectum and pelvic floor but also through the direct involvement of the autonomic and enteric nervous systems in the PD process. While many aspects of gastrointestinal dysfunction in Parkinson's disease continue to be delineated, therapeutic approaches to gut symptoms in this common disorder [9] remain in their infancy.

References

1. Ali, G. N., K. L.Wallace, R. Schwartz et al.: Mechanisms of oral-pharyngeal dysphagia in patients with Parkinson's disease. Gastroenterology 110 (1996) 383–392.
2. Ashraf, W., R. F. Pfeiffer, E. M. M. Quigley: Anorectal manometry in the assessment of anorectal function in Parkinson's disease: a comparison with chronic idiopathic constipation. Mov. Dis. 9 (1994) 655–663.
3. Ashraf, W., R. F. Pfeiffer, F. Park et al.: An objective assessment of constipation in Parkinson's disease: response to psyllium. Gastroenterology 108 (1995) A564.
4. Ashraf, W., Z. K. Wszolek, R. F. Pfeiffer et al.: Anorectal function in fluctuating (on–off) Parkinson's disease: evaluation by combined anorectal manometry and electromyography. Mov. Dis. 10 (1995) 650–657.
5. Astarloa, R., M. A. Mena, V. Sanchez et al.: Clinical and pharmacologic effects of a diet rich in insoluble fiber on Parkinson's disease. Clin. Neuropharmacol. 15 (1992) 375–380.
6. Avots-Avotins, K. V., D. E. Waugh: Colon volvulus and the geriatric patient. Surg. Clin. North Am. 62 (1982) 249–259.
7. Bak, M. P., S. J. Boley: Sigmoid volvulus in elderly patients. Am. J. Surg. 151 (1986) 71–75.
8. Bateson, M. C., F. B. Gibberd, R. S. E. Wilson: Salivary symptom in Parkinson's disease. Arch. Neurol 29 (1973) 274–275.
9. Bennett, D. A., L. A. Beckett, A. M. Murray et al.: Prevalence of Parkinsonian signs and associated mortality in a community population of older people. New Engl. J. Med. 334 (1996) 71–76.
10. Bird, M. R., M. C. Woodward, E. M. Gibson et al.: Asymptomatic swallowing disorders in elderly patients with Parkinson's disease: a description of findings on clinical examination and videofluoroscopy in sixteen patients. Age Ageing 23 (1994) 251–254.
11. Born, L. J., R. Harned, L. F. Rikkers et al.: Cricopharyngeal dysfunction in Parkinson's disease; role in dysphagia and response to myotomy. Mov. Dis. 11 (1996) 53–58.
12. Bozeman, T., S. Anuras, T. Hutton et al.: Small intestinal manometry in Parkinson's disease. Gastroenterology 99 (1990) 1202.
13. Bushmann, M., S. Dobmeyer, L. Leeker et al.: Swallowing abnormalities and their response to treatment in Parkinson's disease. Neurology 39 (1989) 1309–1314.
14. Byrne, K. G., R. Pfeiffer, E. M. M. Quigley: Gastrointestinal dysfunction in Parkinson's disease. J. Clin. Gastro. 19 (1994) 11–16.
15. Calne, D. B., D. G. Shaw, A. S. Spiers et al.: Swallowing in Parkinsonism. Br. J. Radiol. 43 (1970) 456–457.
16. Caplan, I. H., H. G. Jacobson, B. M. Rubinstein et al.: Megacolon and volvulus in Parkinson's disease. Radiology 85 (1965) 73–79.
17. Castell, J. A., Q. Li, M. R. Gideon et al.: Esophageal dysfunction in Parkinson's disease. Gastroenterology 106 (1995) A60.
18. Chokroverty, S., K. D. Barron, F. M. Katz et al.: The syndrome of primary orthostatic hypotension. Brain 92 (1969) 743–768.
19. Christmas, T. J., P. A. Kempster, C. R. Chapple et al.: Role of subcutaneous apomorphine in parkinsonian voiding dysfunction. Lancet 2 (1988) 1451–1453.

20. Dantas, R. O., I. J. Cook, W. J. Dodds et al.: Biomechanics of cricopharyngeal bar. Gastroenterology 99 (1990) 1269−1274.
21. Djaldetti, R., M. Koren, I. Ziv: Effect of cisapride on response fluctuations in Parkinson's disease. Mov. Dis. 10 (1995) 81−84.
22. Eadie, M. J., J. H. Tyrer: Alimentary disorders in parkinsonism. Aust. Ann. Med. 14 (1965) 13−22.
23. Eadie, M. J., J. H. Tyrer: Radiological abnormalities of the upper part of the alimentary tract in parkinsonism. Aust. Ann. Med. 14 (1965) 23−27.
24. Edwards, L., R. F. Pfeiffer, E. M. M. Quigley et al.: Incidence of gastrointestinal symptoms in Parkinson's disease. Mov. Dis. 6 (1991) 151−156.
25. Edwards, L. E., R. F. Pfeiffer, E. M. M. Quigley et al.: Gastrointestinal dysfunction in Parkinson's disease. Frequency and pathophysiology. Neurology 42 (1992) 726−732.
26. Edwards, L. L., E. M. M. Quigley, R. K. Harned et al.: Defecatory function in Parkinson's disease: response to apomorphine. Ann. Neuro. 33 (1993) 490−493.
27. Edwards, L., E. M. M. Quigley, R. K. Harned et al.: Gastrointestinal symptoms in Parkinson's disease: 18-month follow-up study. Mov. Dis. 8 (1993) 83−86.
28. Edwards, L. L., E. M. M. Quigley, R. K. Harned et al.: Characterization of swallowing and defecation in Parkinson's disease. Am. J. Gastroenterology 89 (1994) 15−25.
29. Evans, M. A., E. J. Triggs, M. Cheung et al.: Gastric emptying rate in the elderly: implications for drug therapy. J. Am. Geriatr. Soc. 29 (1981) 201−205.
30. Jacob, P., P. J. Kahrilas, J. A. Logemann et al.: Upper esophageal sphincter opening and modulation during swallowing. Gastroenterology 97 (1989) 1469−1478.
31. Johnston, B. T., Q. Li, J. A. Castell et al.: Swallowing and esophageal function in Parkinson's disease. Am. J. Gastroenterol. 90 (1995) 1741−1746.
32. Jost, W. H., K. Schimrigk: Constipation in Parkinson's disease. Klin. Wochenschr. 69 (1991) 906−909.
33. Jost, W. H.: The effects of cisapride on colonic transit time in PD patients. Wien. Klin Wochensch. 106 (1994) 673−676.
34. Kempster, P. A., A. J. Lees, P. Crichton et al.: Off-period belching due to a reversible disturbance of esophageal motility in Parkinson's disease and its treatment with apomorphine. Mov. Dis. 4 (1989) 47−52.
35. Kupsky, W. J., M. M. Grimes, J. Sweeting et al.: Parkinson's disease and megacolon: concentric hyaline inclusions (Lewy bodies) in enteric ganglion cells. Neurology 37 (1987) 1253−1255.
36. Lewitan, A., L. Nathanson, W. R. Slade: Megacolon and dilatation of the small bowel in Parkinsonism. Gastroenterology 17 (1952) 367−374.
37. Li, Q., M. R. Gideon, J. A. Castell et al.: Manometric evaluation of sinemet effect on esophageal function in Parkinson's disease. Gastroenterology 101 (1995) A530.
38. Lieberman, A. N., L. Horowitz, P. Redmond et al.: Dysphagia in Parkinson's disease. Am. J. Gastroenterol. 74 (1980) 157−160.
39. Marsden, C. D.: Problems with long-term levodopa therapy for Parkinson's disease. Clin. Neuropharmacol. 17 (Suppl 2) (1994) 532−544.
40. Palmer, E.: Dysphagia in Parkinsonism. JAMA 229 (1974) 1349.
41. Parkinson, J.: An essay on the shaking palsey. Whittingham and Rowland, London 1817.
42. Penner, A., L. Druckerman: Segmental spasms of the esophagus and their relation to Parkinsonism. Am. J. Dig. Dis. 9 (1942) 282−287.
43. Qualman, S. J., H. M. Haupt, P. Yang et al.: Esophageal Lewy bodies associated with ganglion cell loss in achalasia: similarity to Parkinson's disease. Gastroenterology 87 (1984) 848−856.
44. Rosenthal, M. J., C. E. Marshall: Sigmoid volvulus in association with parkinsonism: report of four cases. J. Am. Geriatr. Soc. 35 (1987) 683−684.
45. Sage, J. I., M. H. Mark: Pharmacokinetics of continuous-release carbidopalevodopa. Clin. Neuropharmacol. 17 (Suppl 2) (1994) 51−56.

46. Singaram, C., W. Ashraf, E. A. Gaumnitz et al.: Depletion of dopaminergic neurons in the colon in Parkinson's disease. Lancet 346 (1995) 861−864.
47. Sotolongo, J. R.: Voiding dysfunction in Parkinson's disease. Semin. Neurol. 8 (1988) 166−169.
48. Stroudley, J., M. Walsh: Radiological assessment of dysphagia in Parkinson's disease. Br. J. Radiol. 64 (1991) 890−893.
49 Thomas, M., R. A. Haigh: Dysphagia, a reversible cause not to be forgotten. Postgrad. Med. J. 71 (1995) 94−95.
50. Valenzuela, J. E.: Dopamine as a possible neurotransmitter in gastric relaxation. Gastroenterology 71 (1976) 1019−1022.
51. Wakabayashi, K., H. Takahashi, S. Takeda et al.: Parkinson's disease: the presence of Lewy bodies in Auerbach's and Meissner's plexuses. Acta Neuropathol. (Berl.) 76 (1988) 217−221.
52. Wakabayashi, K., H. Takahashi, E. Ohama et al.: Tyrosine hydroxylase − immunoreactive intrinsic neurons in the Auerbach's and Meissner's plexuses of humans. Neurosci. Lett. 96 (1989) 259−263.
53. Wakabayashi, K., H. Takahashi, K. Obata et al.: Immunocytochemical localization of synaptic vesicle-specific protein in Lewy body-containing neurons in Parkinson's disease. Neurosc. Lett. 138(2) (1992) 237−240.
54. Wakabayashi, K., H. Takahashi, E. Ohama et al.: Lewy bodies in the visceral autonomic nervous system in Parkinson's disease. Adv. Neurol. 60 (1993) 609−612.
55. Wyman, J. B., J. Dent, R. Heddle et al.: Control of belching by the lower esophageal sphincter. Gut 31 (1990) 639−646.

Alteration of alimentary function in primary autonomic failure

C. J. Mathias

Introduction

The gastro-intestinal tract, along with a number of associated organs such as the salivary glands, is richly innervated by the autonomic nervous system. The salivary glands have a classical supply, with the cholinergic (parasympathetic) system of particular importance. The gut has additional components, comprising the enteric nervous system, with intrinsic plexuses (Meissners and Auerbachs) along with a complex array of various substances and neurotransmitters, including numerous peptides and amines. The neuranatomy and neurochemistry of the alimentary tract is closely linked to its functions [4, 23]. Thus, in the generalised forms of primary autonomic failure there is often derangement of alimentary function. Disturbances in salivation, swallowing and bowel motility, along with post-prandial hypotension will be described, following a brief outline of the primary autonomic failure syndromes.

Classification of primary autonomic failure

The generalised autonomic disorders can be classified under primary where the aetiology is not known, and secondary with the lesion defined (as in spinal cord transection), where the biochemical basis has been elucidated (as in dopamine beta hydroxylase deficiency) or when there is a clear association with a disease process (such as diabetes mellitus) (Table 1) [10]. Drugs and neurally mediated syncope are categorised separately. The primary autonomic failure syndromes fall into two main groups, based on their onset. The acute/sub-acute variety consists of pure pandysautonomias (with both sympathetic and parasympathetic involvement of varying degree), the acute cholinergic dysautonomias (with only cholinergic involvement), and dysautonomias occurring in combination with other neurological features, often suggesting peripheral nerve involvement. The chronic autonomic failure syndromes are more common and fall into two main categories; those without additional neurological features (pure autonomic failure; PAF), and those with neurological features (the Shy-Drager syndrome; SDS/multiple system atrophy; MSA) [11]. The SDS is often used synonymously and interchangeably with MSA; some feel that the latter implies, but does not necessitate, autonomic failure. In this review the term SDS will be used as the description refers to patients with autonomic impairment. Within

Table 1: *Classification of disorders affecting autonomic function (adapted from 10, 16).*

Primary autonomic failure (Aetiology unknown)

   Acute/subacute Dysautonomias

- Pure pandysautonomia
- Pure cholinergic dysautonomia
- Dysautonomia with other neurological features

   Chronic Autonomic Failure Syndromes

- Pure autonomic failure
- Multiple system atrophy/Shy-Drager syndrome
    - parkinsonian form   (MSA-P or SDS-P)
    - cerebellar form   (MSA-C or SDS-C)
    - mixed form   (MSA-M or SDS-M)

Secondary autonomic failure

- With defined lesions
    - spinal cord transection
- With specific biochemical defect
    - dopamine beta-hydroxylase deficiency
- With recognised disorder
    - diabetes mellitus

Drugs/chemicals/toxins

- With direct autonomic effects
    - tricyclic antidepressants
    - botulinum toxin
- Indirectly by causing an autonomic neuropathy
    - alcohol

Neurally mediated syncope

- Vasovagal syncope
- Carotid sinus hypersensitivity

---

the SDS there are three major sub-groups, based on their neurological features, with parkinsonian features (SDS-P), with cerebellar features (SDS-C) and with a combination of these features (SDS-M). The majority of SDS-P and SDS-C, in due course progress into the mixed features form. Autonomic failure also may occur with classical idiopathic Parkinson's disease (IPD), but this differs in many respects from the parkinsonian syndromes of SDS/MSA and will not be considered further.

Salivary gland dysfunction

In the acute dysautonomias, hypostomia and xerostomia is common; the latter is a particular feature of pure cholinergic dysautonomia. It is less likely to occur in the chronic syndromes, especially in SDS. In xerostomia, artificial saliva is often helpful. In some SDS dribbling of saliva may occur; this is more likely to be due to the motor deficit and associated swallowing disturbances than to excessive salivary secretion. The problem can be reduced with anticholinergic drugs, although in severe cases other approaches, including irradiation of salivary glands may be needed.

Disorders of swallowing

In the acute dysautonomias, dysphagia may be an early feature, because of disordered motility of the lower third of the oesophagus which has smooth muscle and an autonomic innervation. Radiological and endoscopic techniques, along with oesophageal manometry are useful investigations. Cholinomimetics, such as carbachol and bethanechol, may be helpful. In chronic autonomic failure, there are marked differences between PAF and SDS. Oro-pharyngeal dysphagia does not occur in PAF, while it is common in SDS, especially as the disease progresses [11]. There do not appear to be obvious differences between the parkinsonian and the cerebellar forms, although this needs further study. Whether the abnormalities differ from those observed in IPD is not known. Videocinefluoroscopy is a valuable investigation as it allows the early phases of swallowing to be assessed with foods of different consistency and volume. This information often enables the provision of suitable advice to aid the patient and help in decisions on intervention. It is of particular importance in determining the risk of tracheal aspiration, which SDS are prone to because of associated vocal cord paresis. If dysphagia is severe, or if there is an enhanced risk of tracheal aspiration, a percutaneous feeding gastrostomy may need to be considered.

Gastric and small intestinal motility

This may be affected in the acute dysautonomias. In the chronic forms usually there are no clinical problems. In both PAF and SDS gastric fullness may be troublesome after a meal; however, gastric emptying studies using radionucleide techniques suggest an initial rapid emptying phase, following by a later, slower phase [15]. There is no clear evidence that they have a form of the 'dumping syndrome', which can complicate surgical procedures to improve gastric drainage especially when combined with a truncal vagotomy.

Large bowel and anal sphincter malfunction

Constipation is a prominent feature in both the acute and chronic syndromes. In pure cholinergic dysautonomias and acute pandysautonomias it may be severe. Along with impaired small bowel motility, intestinal obstruction may be suspected; in some this has resulted in an unnecessary exploratory laparotomy. In the chronic forms, constipation is a common autonomic feature. As these patients are often over 50, other causes of altered large bowel activity, including malignancies may need to be considered. A combination of approaches, which includes an increase in fibre intake and the use of laxatives, may be needed to prevent or reduce constipation. Diarrhoea is infrequent, but may complicate severe constipation, as a result of overflow. This may result in faecal incontinence, which occasionally may be caused by anal sphincter dysfunction. Electromyographic studies in the SDS characteristically indicate anal sphincter denervation with subsequent reinnervation [3], although there may be no direct functional deficits. This pattern of abnormality favours involvement of Onufs' nucleus within the sacral spinal cord.

Post-prandial hypotension

This has been well-characterised in the chronic autonomic failure syndromes, and both PAF and SDS are affected [15]. Following food ingestion, substantial hypotension can occur within 15 minutes and may persist for 3 hours, even with the subject supine and horizontal [17]. Sitting or standing after food ingestion often results in an exacerbation of postural hypotension [13]. The degree of fall appears to be dependent upon the composition of food, as it is greatest with carbohydrate, less with lipid, and minimal with a protein meal [15]. The complex interactions between the autonomic, gastro-intestinal and cardiovascular systems which follow food ingestion are impaired in autonomic failure, with postprandial hypotension as a key clinical problem in some. Carbohydrate stimulates the release of insulin, which is one among a variety of peptides with vasodilatatory effects that may cause or contribute to post-prandial hypotension [14]. Differences in gastro-intestinal/pancreatic hormonal responses to meals of different composition may be an explanation for the variability in responses in daily life.

In normal subjects, food results in a marked increase in splanchnic blood flow; superior mesenteric artery blood flow, for instance, can double from 0.5 to 1.0 litre per minute [8]. Normally, this is counteracted by increased sympathetic activity to the heart and other vascular regions, including skeletal muscle; compensatory measures such as an increase in cardiac output and regional vasoconstriction help maintain blood pressure. In chronic autonomic failure, similar changes in splanchnic blood flow occur post-prandially. However, there are no compensatory changes in cardiac function and in other vascular beds presumably because of sympathetic denervation; the lack of such changes probably accounts for the marked blood pressure fall post-prandially [9]. In PAF, who often have a more severe peripheral sympathetic denervation, there is often a greater

Table 2: *Management approaches in post-prandial hypotension.*

Non-Pharmacological
- Small, frequent meals
- Avoid   — refined carbohydrates
          — alcohol
- Rest after meals

Pharmacological
- Caffeine
- Indomethacin
- Octreotide

post-prandial fall in blood pressure, which may be linked additionally to differences in gut peptide secretion, as described for insulin [1].

The degree of post-prandial hypotension, and its ability to aggravate postural hypotension can be investigated readily in the laboratory by determining the supine blood pressure response to a standard meal and incorporating the responses to postural change before and after the meal; there are advantages in using liquid meals of mixed composition [12, 13]. In some, post-prandial hypotension may be severe enough that the subject actually avoids eating, and can lose a substantial amount of weight. Reducing post-prandial hypotension is thus an important aspect of management, and has been closely linked to advances in understanding the pathophysiological basis of the problem. Practical advice is important. Smaller meals eaten more frequently maintain the caloric intake and cause less of a fall in blood pressure than larger, fewer meals of equivalent calories [19]. Changing the composition of food to avoid refined carbohydrate is helpful. Many are aware of the intolerance to even small amounts of alcohol, which can substantially lower blood pressure [5]. Resting in a semi-recumbent position after meals should be encouraged (Table 2).

Pharmacological approaches include the use of caffeine, indomethacin, and octreotide. Caffeine, either in tablet form or in the form of strong coffee, has been reported to help, and may act by blocking vasodilatatory adenosine receptors [18]. It does not seem effective in severely affected patients [2]. Indomethacin probably acts by reducing the formation of vasodilatatory prostaglandins [21], but it has a number of side effects, including gastric ulceration, and is not an ideal choice. The peptide release inhibitor, octreotide, which is a somatostatin analogue, is currently the most effective drug to reduce post-prandial hypotension. It probably acts by inhibiting release of vasodilatatory peptides, but has a rapid pressor effect, albeit transient, suggesting that other mechanisms may be involved [6, 20]. Following food ingestion, octreotide prevents the rise in superior mesenteric artery blood flow and has no discernable cardiac or peripheral vascular effects, indicating that an action mainly on the splanchnic bed probably accounts for its benefits [8]. It is given subcutaneously in relatively small doses of 50–100 microgrammes, once or twice a day, half an hour before the main meals. Side effects include abdominal colic and diarrhoea. In chronic autonomic failure it also reduces postural hypotension and improves exercise tolerance [7, 1, 22]; the reasons for these beneficial effects are not entirely clear.

Summary

Alimentary function is often affected in primary autonomic failure. There may be impairment of salivation, swallowing and gastro-intestinal motility, especially involving the large bowel. Disruption of autonomic-gastrointestinal-cardiovasacular interactions often occur. This review focuses on the key features of alimentary dysfunction occurring in primary autonomic failure and outlines the major investigation and management approaches used.

References

1. Armstrong, E., C. J. Mathias: The effects of the somatostatin analogue, octreotide, on postural hypotension, before and after food ingestion in primary autonomic failure. Clinical Autonomic Research 2 (1991) 135–40.
2. Armstrong, E., L. Watson, T. C. Hardman et al.: Effects of oral caffeine on post-prandial and postural hypotension in chronic autonomic failure. Journal of the Autonomic Nervous System 31 (1990) 174–175.
3. Beck, R. O., C. J. Fowler, C. J. Mathias: Genito-urinary dysfunction in disorders of the autonomic nervous system. In: D. N. Rushton (Ed.): Handbook of Neuro-Urology, Chapter 11, pp. 281–301. Marcel-Dekker, New York 1994.
4. Bishop, A. E., J. M. Polak: The gut and the autonomic nervous system. In: R. Bannister, C. J. Mathias (Eds.): Autonomic Failure. A Textbook of Clinical Disorders of the Autonomic Nervous System, 3rd Edition, pp. 160–177. Oxford University Press, Oxford 1992.
5. Chaudhuri, K. R., S. Maule, T. Thomaides et al.: Alcohol ingestion lowers supine blood pressure, causes splanchnic vasodilatation and worsens postural hypotension in primary autonomic failure. Journal of Neurology 241 (1994) 145–152.
6. Hoeldtke, R. D., T. M. O'Doriso, G. Boden: Treatment of autonomic neuropathy with a somatostatin analogue, SMS 201-995. Lancet ii (1986), 602–605.
7. Hoeldtke, R. D., B. C. Israel: Treatment of orthostatic hypotension with octreotide. Journal of Clinical Endocrinology and Metabolism 68 (1989) 1051–1059.
8. Kooner, J. S., W. S. Peart, C. J. Mathias: The peptide release inhibitor, octreotide (SMS 201-995) prevents the haemodynamic changes following food ingestion in normal human subjects. Quarterly Journal of Experimental Physiology 74 (1989) 569–572.
9. Kooner, J. S., S. J. Raimbach, L. Watson et al.: Relationship between splanchnic vasodilatation and post-prandial hypotension in patients with primary autonomic failure. Journal of Hypertension 7 (suppl. 6) (1989) 40–41.

10. Mathias, C. J.: Disorders of the autonomic nervous system. In: W. G. Bradley, R. B. Daroff, G. M. Fenichel et al. (Eds.): Neurology in Clinical Practice 2nd Edition, Volume II, Chapter 82, pp. 1953–1981. Butterworth – Heinemann, Boston, 1996.

11. Mathias, C. J., A. C. Williams: The Shy-Drager Syndrome and Multiple System Atrophy. In: D. Calne (Ed.): Neurodegenerative Disorders, Chapter 43, pp. 743–767. W. B. Saunders, Philadelphia 1994.

12. Mathias, C. J., R. Bannister: Investigation of autonomic disorders. In: R. Bannister, C. J. Mathias (Eds.): Autonomic Failure. A Textbook of Clinical Disorders of the Autonomic Nervous System, 3rd Edition, pp. 255–290. Oxford University Press, Oxford 1992.

13. Mathias, C. J., E. Holly, E. Armstrong et al.: The influence of food on postural hypotension in three groups with chronic autonomic failure: clinical and therapeutic implications. Journal of Neurology, Neurosurgery and Psychiatry 54 (1991) 726–730.

14. Mathias, C. J., D. F. da Costa, P. Fosbraey et al.: Hypotensive and sedative effects of insulin in autonomic failure. British Medical Journal 295 (1987) 161–163.

15. Mathias, C. J., R. Bannister: Postcibal hypotension in autonomic disorders. In: R. Bannister, J. C. Mathias (Eds.): Autonomic Failure. A Textbook of Clinical Disorders of the Autonomic Nervous System, 3rd Edition, pp. 489–509. Oxford University Press, Oxford 1992.

16. Mathias, C. J.: Autonomic neuropathy – aspects of diagnosis and management. In: A. K. Asbury, P. K. Thomas (Eds.): Peripheral Nerve Disorders II, Chapter 5, pp. 95–117. Butterworth–Heinemann, Oxford 1995.

17. Mathias, C. J., D. F. da Costa, P. Fosbraey et al.: Cardiovascular, biochemical and hormonal changes during food induced hypotension in chronic autonomic failure. Journal of the Neurological Sciences 94 (1989) 255–269.

18. Onrot, J., M. R. Goldberg, I. Biaggioni et al.: Haemodynamic and humoral effects of caffeine in autonomic failure. Therapeutic implications for post-prandial hypotension. New England Journal of Medicine 313 (1985) 549–554.

19. Puvi-Rajasingham, S., C. J. Mathias: Effect of meal size on post-prandial blood pressure and on postural hypotension in primary autonomic failure. Clinical Autonomic Research 6, (1996), 111–114.

20. Raimbach, S. J., P. Cortelli, J. S. Kooner et al.: Prevention of glucose-induced hypotention by the somatostatin analogue, Octreotide (SMS 201-995) in chronic autonomic failure-haemodynamic and hormonal changes. Clinical Science 77 (1989) 623–628.

21. Robertson, D., D. Wade, R. M. Robertson: Post-prandial alterations in cardiovascular haemodynamics in autonomic dysfunction states. American Journal of Cardiology 48 (1981) 1048–1052.

22. Smith, G. D. P., L. P. Watson, D. V. Pavitt et al.: Effect of the somatostatin analogue, octreotide, an exercise-induced hypotension in human subjects with chronic sympathetic failure. Clinical Science 89 (1995) 367–373.

23. Wingate, D. L.: Autonomic dysfunction and the gut. In: R. Bannister, C. J. Mathias (Eds.): Autonomic Failure. A Textbook of Clinical Disorders of the Autonomic Nervous System, 3rd Edition, pp. 510–528. Oxford University Press, Oxford 1992.

Effect of altered control of the autonomic nervous system on gastrointestinal function

M. Camilleri

Introduction

The extrinsic neural control of the gut is one of the three important modulators of its motor function [4]. The cranial and sacral parasympathetic outflow is generally excitatory to the gastrointestinal smooth muscle. On the other hand, the thoracolumbar sympathetic outflow is usually inhibitory to smooth muscle and excitatory to sphincters. The neurotransmitter in the parasympathetic supply and at the prevertebral sympathetic ganglia is acetylcholine; on the other hand, the postganglionic sympathetic fiber supplying the gastrointestinal tract releases norepinephrine at its terminal synapse.

The extrinsic neural control is not merely efferent to the gut, but is extremely important in conveying afferent information from the gastrointestinal tract [11]. Thus, visceral afferents mediate sensations such as hunger, pain, intestinal distention, and the desire to defecate, to mention a few. These afferent pathways course along the vagal and splanchnic afferents to the brain and spinal cord. It has been estimated that the majority of vagal fibers at the level of the diaphragm are afferent. Visceral afferent fibers arising from the gastrointestinal tract also provide the first-order neuron in the three-neuron chain leading to conscious perception. The first-order neuron has its cell body in the dorsal root ganglion from which axons course to both the prevertebral ganglia and the dorsal horn of the spinal cord. The former fibers are thought to be involved in local reflex responses that persist even after dorsal rhizotomy, suggesting that the prevertebral ganglia constitute an important relay station for some of the homeostatic functions of the intestine, such as viscerovisceral reflexes [13]. The second axon from the dorsal root ganglion cell synapses with a second-order neuron in the dorsal horn of the spinal cord. This second neuron crosses the spinal cord and ascends in the spinothalamic and spinoreticular tract towards the brain stem. The third-order neuron arises in the nuclei of the thalamus or reticular formation and projects towards the somatosensory cortex and the anterior cingulate gyrus. Some of the reflex responses mediated at the levels of the prevertebral ganglia or spinal cord are susceptible to the descending influence of fibers that arise in the cortex and brain stem, which modulate peripheral reflexes and perhaps also inhibit some of the sensations arising in the gastrointestinal tract [10].

Neurologic disorders affecting gastrointestinal motor function

There are several common neurologic disorders that may result in abnormalities in motor function of the gastrointestinal tract [4]. These disorders may affect either the sympathetic or parasympathetic nervous system or both. Common examples seen in clinical practice include parkinsonism, multiple sclerosis, brain stem stroke, and autonomic neuropathies, typically, those associated with diabetes mellitus. Less commonly, primary autonomic system degenerations may also occur and result in motor, secretory, or sensory dysfunction in the gut. The common clinical presentations of these extrinsic neurologic disorders are transfer dysphagia, gastric stasis, constipation, and fecal incontinence. Symptoms of sympathetic or parasympathetic dysfunction are useful indicators to the possibility of autonomic nervous dysfunction (Table 1).

However, it is becoming increasingly clear that disturbances of the extrinsic neural control may occur in the absence of an identified neurologic syndrome and result in clinical presentations with gastrointestinal motor dysfunction. Thus, for example, we had shown in a series of patients with severe, apparently functional gastrointestinal disease that a thermoregulatory sweat test demonstrated large areas of anhydrosis suggesting a sympathetic dysfunction in association with their clinical syndrome [7]. Subsequently, Altomare and colleagues identified a sympathetic cholinergic defect as a common problem in patients with severe constipation [2]. More recently, Aggarwal and colleagues [1] have suggested that constipation-predominant irritable bowel syndrome is associated with vagal dysfunction, whereas diarrhea-predominant irritable bowel syndrome is associated with sympathetic dysfunction. These preliminary intriguing observations need to be followed with more formal analysis of the sensitivity and specificity of the tests used and optimizing the conditions under which the autonomic nervous system is assessed (see Table 2 for summary of tests, interpretation and pitfalls). For example, tests of sympathetic adrenergic function are critically dependent upon the state of hydration of the patient, and the

Table 1: *Symptoms and signs suggestive of autonomic dysfunction.*

Sympathetic	Parasympathetic
Failure of pupils to dilate in the dark	Fixed dilated pupils
Fainting, orthostatic dizziness	Lack of pupillary accommodation
Constant heart rate with orthostatic hypotension	Decreased gut motility
Absent piloerection	Dry eyes and mouth
Absent sweating	Dry vagina
Impaired ejaculation	Impaired erection
Paralysis of dartos muscle	Difficulty with emptying urinary bladder Recurrent urinary tract infections

potential interference of medical therapy taken for other conditions should not be underestimated [8]. The most common pitfall in clinical practice is the use of interfering medications which include the concomitant use of benzodiazepines (as night sedatives or anxiolytics), tricyclic antidepressants (for depression or peripheral neuropathy), and alpha-2 adrenergic agonists (for hypertension) or alpha-1 adrenergic antagonists (for bladder outlet obstruction).

On the other hand, it is clear that certain neurologic syndromes presenting as gastroparesis or chronic intestinal dysmotility will be associated with significant evidence of extrinsic neural defects [3, 9]. We have recently reported [5] on 50 patients with these clinical syndromes in association with diverse conditions, including postgastric surgery, diabetes mellitus, and a number of miscellaneous neurologic syndromes; in these patients we identified disturbances in sympathetic and parasympathetic innervation to the viscera.

Autonomic function testing

In a recent review [8], we tabulated the tests available for assessing autonomic function and discussed the pros and cons of these methods. Table 2 is reproduced from that review. The tests of autonomic function can be subdivided into: 1. sympathetic adrenergic tests; 2. sympathetic cholinergic tests; 3. vagal tests. Regrettably, there are very few tests that specifically assess the autonomic innervation in the gastrointestinal viscera. These tests have been described elsewhere [4] and are being reviewed in another chapter (Altomare) and, therefore, only brief commentary will be provided here.

Sympathetic adrenergic tests

Among the sympathetic adrenergic tests, the ones most widely used in our center are the blood pressure response to a head-up tilt at 80° to the horizontal. The blood pressure response to tilt is entirely dependent upon sympathetic adrenergic function, and there should normally be a drop of less than 25 mmHg systolic and 15 mmHg diastolic. The Valsalva maneuver has several components which include a sympathetic adrenergic component that maintains the blood pressure response. However, the change in pulse rate during phase 4 of the Valsalva maneuver is clearly a vagally-mediated parasympathetic response. Thus, the Valsalva maneuver cannot be regarded as a pure sympathetic test. Doppler flow studies of the superior mesenteric artery provide an approach to evaluate abdominal sympathetic adrenergic function.

A test of the sympathetic postganglionic adrenergic fiber that is seldom used is the plasma norepinephrine response to intravenous edrophonium. In this test, the short-acting anticholinesterase, edrophonium, is administered intravenously

Table 2: *Commonly performed autonomic nervous function tests.*

Test	Physiologic functions tested	Rationale	Comments or pitfalls
Sympathetic function			
Thermoregulatory sweat test (% surface area of anhydrosis)	Pre- and postganglionic cholinergic	Stimulation of hypothalamic temperature control centers	Cumbersome, whole body test
Quantitative sudomotor axon reflex test (sweat output, latency)	Postganglionic cholinergic	Antidromic stimulation of peripheral fiber by axonal reflex	Needs specialized facilities
Heart rate and blood pressure responses			
Orthostatic tilt test	Adrenergic	Baroreceptor reflex	Impaired responses if intravascular volume is reduced
Postural adjustment ratio	Adrenergic	Baroreceptor reflex	Impaired responses if intravascular volume is reduced
Cold pressor test	Adrenergic	Baroreceptor reflex	Impaired responses if intravascular volume is reduced
Sustained hand grip	Adrenergic	Baroreceptor reflex	Impaired responses if intravascular volume is reduced
Plasma norepinephrine response to: Postural changes	Postganglionic adrenergic	Baroreceptor stimulation	Moderate sensitivity, impaired response if intravascular volume is reduced

I. V. edrophonium	Postganglionic adrenergic	Anticholinesterase 'stimulates' postganglionic fiber at prevertebral ganglia	False negatives due to contributions to plasma norepinephrine from many organs
Parasympathetic function			
Heart rate (R-R) variation with deep breathing	Parasympathetic	Vagal afferents stimulated by lung stretch	Best cardiovagal test available, but not a test of abdominal vagus
Supine/erect heart rate	Parasympathetic	Vagal stimulation by change in central blood volume	Cardiovagal test
Valsalva ratio (heart rate, max/min)	Parasympathetic	Vagal stimulation by change in central blood volume	Cardiovagal test
Gastric acid secretion or plasma pancreatic polypeptide response to modified sham feeding or hypoglycemia	Parasympathetic	Stimulation of vagal nuclei by sham feeding or hypoglycemia	Abdominal vagal test, critically dependent on avoidance of swallowing food during test
Nocturnal penile tumescence	Pelvic parasympathetic	Integrity of S_{2-4}	Plethysmographic technique requiring special facilities
Cystometrographic response to bethanechol	Pelvic parasympathetic	Increase in intravesical pressure suggests postganglionic denervation supersensitivity	Tests parasympathetic supply to bladder, not bowel

to stimulate the postganglionic sympathetic adrenergic neuron to release norepinephrine into the plasma, and this can be detected by sampling blood every 1 or 2 minutes over a period of 10 minutes. The vascular beds that release norepinephrine include the pulmonary circulation, kidneys, and the gastrointestinal viscera. Therefore, this test cannot be regarded as a pure gastrointestinal sympathetic test.

Sympathetic cholinergic tests

Among the sympathetic cholinergic tests, the thermoregulatory sweat test and quantitative sudomotor axon reflex test are available in our center. The thermoregulatory sweat test identifies the area of the body with anhydrosis (normally, < 5% body surface area should be anhydrotic) and indicates an abnormality in the sweat pathway anywhere from the hypothalamus to the postganglionic sympathetic fiber. The quantitative sudomotor axon reflex test involves iontophoresing acetylcholine into one area of the skin and measuring the sweat output into an adjacent but physically separated area. This test stimulates an axon reflex if the postganglionic cholinergic sympathetic neuron is intact and thereby induces sweat output from the neighboring sweat glands.

Vagal tests

Among vagal tests, the most commonly performed is the R-R interval response to deep breathing, and this is sometimes formalized as the 30 to 15 ratio indicating the R-R intervals to be selected for comparison between the test period and control. Although widely used, this test is susceptible to variation among gender and age, and breathing deeply 6 times per minute may be difficult to standardize. In the author's experience this test is somewhat oversensitive in the identification of the abdominal vagal dysfunction, although, theoretically, a cardiovagal deficit should be an accurate method to assess abdominal vagal function in most neuropathic processes which are usually length-dependent and, therefore, affect abdominal branches of the vagus before the cardiac branches are involved. For this reason, a specific abdominal vagal function test is useful in clinical practice, and we have applied the plasma pancreatic polypeptide response to modified sham feeding for this purpose [5, 15]. An alternative approach to stimulate the vagal nuclei in the brain stem is by insulin-induced hypoglycemia. The simplicity of the sham feeding test and the relative safety with avoidance of hypoglycemia render the sham feeding test more acceptable in our clinical laboratory.

In order to illustrate the use of these tests, two short case histories [12, 15] will be presented.

Case 1: A 20 year-old female college student presented approximately one week after the onset of infectious mononucleosis with nausea, vomiting, constipation, bloating, distension, as well as a dry mouth, dry eyes, failure to sweat, difficulty with emptying the urinary bladder, recurrent urinary infections, recurrent vaginal infections, and dyspareunia. Over the next three years, she was admitted to the hospital at least ten times for acute episodes of pseudo-obstruction requiring nasogastric decompression, and she also needed home total parenteral nutrition. Investigations demonstrated normal blood pressure response to tilt and to the Valsalva maneuver, but abnormal R-R interval response to deep breathing, pancreatic polypeptide response to sham feeding, sweat test, and quantitative sudomotor axon reflex test. Pharmacologic tests proved cholinergic denervation hypersensitivity of the pupil and urinary bladder. The constellation of clinical symptoms and autonomic dysfunctions were highly suggestive of a selective cholinergic dysautonomia, probably related to infection with the Epstein-Barr virus.

Case 2: A 53 year-old man had sudden onset of inability to feed because of recurrent nausea, vomiting and early satiety. Exploratory laparotomy excluded mechanical obstruction. He required home parenteral nutrition for 6 months before being seen at our center. Autonomic testing demonstrated an abnormal thermoregulatory sweat test (42% anhydrosis), but normal postganglionic sympathetic function including the quantitative sudomotor axon reflex test, plasma norepinephrine response to intravenous edrophonium, and plasma norepinephrine in the lying and standing position. In view of these findings, a central sympathetic lesion was suspected, and a brain magnetic resonance scan demonstrated a brain stem tumor.

Algorithm for the investigation of patients with suspected GI motility disorders

The clinical history is obviously key to identifying the region of the gut that is affected in each individual patient. This will also lead to the most logical investigation according to the region affected.

Transfer dysphagia

In patients with transfer dysphagia, there is a disturbance in the pharyngoesophageal junction that results in recurrent aspiration or difficulties in transferring the bolus of food or fluid from the pharynx to the esophagus. The investigation of choice in our practice is a video barium swallow seeking evidence of incoordination between the pharynx and esophagus, penetration of barium into the upper airway, and excluding alternative diagnoses such as structural abnormalities of the upper gut. Although it is increasingly applied as a clinical tool, measurement of pharyngoesophageal contractions by manometry or solid-state transducer rarely adds much to the information obtained from a careful video barium swallow performed by an expert radiologist. It may be necessary to use foods of different consistencies during stress tests in order to elicit the functional aberration in patients with transfer dysphagia.

Upper gastrointestinal dysmotility

In patients presenting with syndromes suggesting upper gastrointestinal dysmotility such as nausea, vomiting, early satiety, abdominal bloating, or pain, the clinical history should also be useful to identify patients with suspected autonomic dysfunction. Such symptoms include postural dizziness, lack of sweating, failure of erection or ejaculation, difficulties with emptying the urinary bladder or recurrent urinary infections, and dryness of the eyes, mouth and vagina. The symptoms referable to the sympathetic and parasympathetic nervous system are listed in Table 1.

The first investigation in patients with suspected upper gut dysmotility is the scintigraphic gastric and small bowel transit test (Fig. 1). Novel methods have been devised to make these tests more cost effective. Thus, scans taken immediately after ingestion of the meal, as well as 2, 4, and 6 hours later have been shown [14] to provide high diagnostic accuracy when compared to more detailed but costlier transit profiles and computer-generated data. If the gastric and small bowel transit test is abnormal and the patient has a known underlying disease process, it is usually unnecessary to pursue any further investigation,

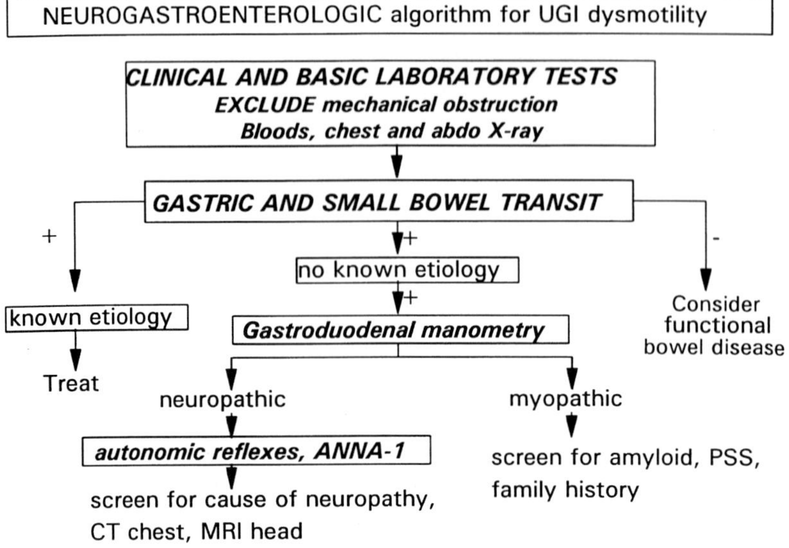

Fig. 1: *Algorithm for management of patients with suspected upper gut dysmotility.*

and the appropriate nutritional and pharmacological treatments can be pursued. On the other hand, if there is no known underlying disorder, gastrointestinal manometry and tests of extrinsic neural control of the viscera may be extremely helpful to identify the etiology of the dysmotility. The presence of symptoms on systems review that suggests autonomic dysfunction helps to select patients for autonomic testing if these are not widely available. If the autonomic tests confirm the presence of an extrinsic neural defect, it is then crucial to screen the patient for the cause of that autonomic dysfunction, such as diabetes, amyloidosis, porphyria, heavy metal poisoning, or a paraneoplastic process. The latter is associated with an autoimmune ganglionitis in association with small cell lung cancer [10], a syndrome for which a screening serologic test is available seeking for an antibody directed against myenteric plexus neurons called the antineuronal enteric antibody or anti-Hu antibody. The selection of patients for these tests may also be facilitated in some centers by the availability of gastrointestinal manometric studies. Manometry differentiates between the low amplitude contractile activity typical of a myopathic process and the normal amplitude, but irregular or incoordinated phasic pressure activity that typifies a neuropathic process [4].

Severe constipation

In patients presenting with severe constipation, the algorithm (Fig. 2) for management is similar and requires a colonic transit test, usually with a radiopaque

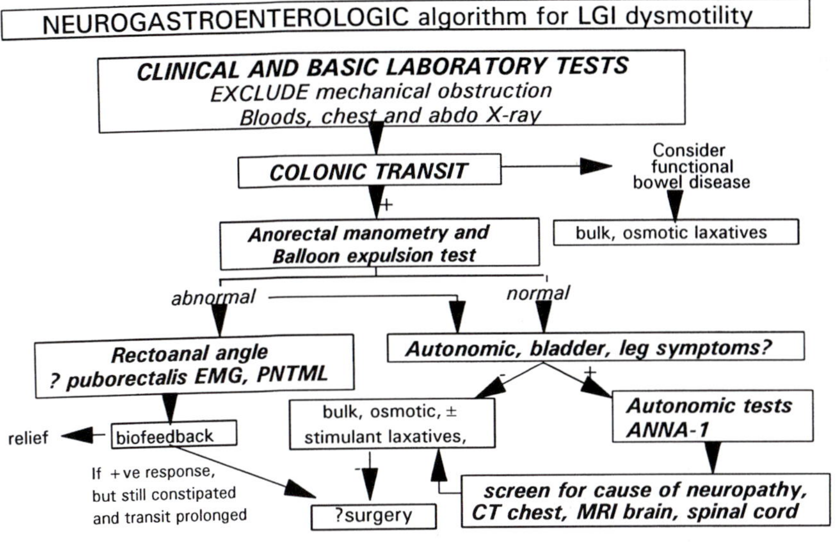

Fig. 2: *Algorithm for management of patients with suspected lower gut dysmotility.*

marker method or, more recently, with a scintigraphic approach [16]. The presence of colonic transit delay may be due to either a colonic motor dysfunction or an obstruction to defecation. Hence, it is crucial to perform screening tests for anismus and pelvic floor dyssynergia such as by anorectal manometry and balloon expulsion from the rectum. Pelvic floor dysfunction may result from a pudendal neuropathy or sacral S2 to S4 radiculopathy resulting in failure of relaxation of the puborectalis muscle and persistence of the relatively acute rectoanal angle during attempts to defecate.

Fecal incontinence

In patients presenting with fecal incontinence, the rectal examination clearly will show whether weakness involves the anal sphincter tone at rest (a function of the internal anal sphincter) or at squeeze (the external anal sphincter with its extrinsic parasympathetic denervation). Anal vector manometry and endosonography of the anal canal are helpful in identifying weakness and asymmetry within the anal sphincters that may be the cause of incontinence. In clinical practice, it is rarely necessary to perform EMG studies of the sphincters or puborectalis, or to measure the pudendal nerve terminal motor latency to prove the denervation.

Autonomic dysfunctions as modifiers of response to prokinetic therapy

In a medium-term, placebo-controlled trial [6] and in a subsequent one-year open trial of cisapride at a dose of 20 mg, three times per day, in patients with gastroparesis or chronic intestinal dysmotility, we demonstrated that the presence of abdominal vagal dysfunction results in a reduced symptomatic benefit of cisapride treatment when compared to other patients with idiopathic or sympathetic denervation. Conversely, there was a beneficial role of sympathetic denervation in the symptomatic response to cisapride. These studies require confirmation by other centers.

Conclusion

The autonomic nervous system is intricately involved in the control of gastrointestinal motor and sensory function. The use of autonomic testing has been intercalated in the diagnostic approach to the patient with suspected upper or lower gastrointestinal motor disturbances. Identification of the level of the extrinsic neural lesion may be useful to facilitate the diagnostic process and indicate which patients require costly imaging of the central nervous system or spinal cord. Autonomic tests also indicate the pathogenesis of some patients with altered gastrointestinal motility and identify the underlying cause, such as clinically unsuspected amyloidosis, porphyria, or heavy metal poisoning, in patients presenting with gastrointestinal symptoms. This discipline has brought together the neurologists and gastroenterologists at our center to better identify the mechanism leading to gastrointestinal symptoms in patients with dysmotilities.

Summary

This chapter reviews the anatomy and pharmacology of the autonomic nervous system involved in the extrinsic innervation of the gastrointestinal tract. Common extrinsic neurologic disorders such as brain stem stroke, diabetes with autonomic neuropathy, multiple sclerosis, parkinsonism, and spinal cord injury may alter gastrointestinal motility. The main gastroenterologic manifestations are transfer dysphagia, gastric stasis, constipation and fecal incontinence. However, patients without overt neurologic disorders may present with suspected gastrointestinal dysmotility as a result of an extrinsic neural deficit. In this chapter, we discuss an algorithm for the investigation of such patients: transit tests are used as screening procedures for the identification of dysmotility and are followed by autonomic function tests which appraise the parasympathetic supply to viscera and differentiate pre- and postganglionic sympathetic lesions. This strategy facilitates selection of patients for further imaging of the nervous system. The commonly performed autonomic function tests are discussed in some detail and a couple of examples from a tertiary referral practice are selected to illustrate the use of autonomic testing to pinpoint the level and nature of the extrinsic neural defect resulting in gastrointestinal motor dysfunction. A role for extrinsic autonomic disturbances has been postulated in irritable bowel syndrome, but remains far from proven. Finally, there is some evidence that the presence of vagal dysfunction reduces the symptomatic response of patients with gastroparesis or chronic intestinal dysmotility to the orally administered prokinetic agent, cisapride. By way of contrast, it appears that sympathetic denervation may be associated with increased symptomatic benefit as compared to patients with upper gut dysmotility resulting from idiopathic disorders or vagal denervation.

References

1. Aggarwal, A., T. Cutts, T. Abell et al.: Predominant symptoms in irritable bowel syndrome correlate with specific autonomic nervous system abnormalities. Gastroenterology 106 (1994) 945–950.

2. Altomare, C., M. Pilot, M. Scott et al.: Detection of subclinical autonomic neuropathy in constipated patients using a sweat test. Gut 33 (1992) 1539–1543.
3. Bharucha, A., M. Camilleri, P. Low et al.: Autonomic dysfunction in gastrointestinal motility disorders. Gut 34 (1993) 397–401.
4. Camilleri, M.: Disorders of gastrointestinal motility in neurologic diseases. Mayo Clin. Proc. 65 (1990) 825–846.
5. Camilleri, M., R. Balm, P. Low: Autonomic dysfunction in patients with chronic intestinal pseudo-obstruction. Clin. Auton. Res. 3 (1993) 95–100.
6. Camilleri, M., R. Balm, A. Zinsmeister: Determinants of response to a prokinetic agent in neuropathic chronic intestinal motility disorder. Gastroenterology 106 (1994) 916–923.
7. Camilleri, M., R. Fealey: Idiopathic autonomic denervation in eight patients presenting with functional gastrointestinal disease: A causal association? Dig. Dis. Sci. 35 (1990) 609–616.
8. Camilleri, M., M. Ford: Functional gastrointestinal disease and the autonomic nervous system: a way ahead? (Editorial) Gastroenterology 106 (1994) 1114–1118.
9. Camilleri, M., J. Malagelada, V. Stanghellini et al.: Gastrointestinal motility disturbances in patients with orthostatic hypotension. Gastroenterology 88 (1985) 1852–1859.
10. Lennon, V., D. Sas, M. Busk et al.: Enteric neuronal autoantibodies in pseudoobstruction with small-cell lung carcinoma. Gastroenterology 100 (1991) 137–142.
11. Mayer, E., G. Gebhart: Basic and clinical aspects of visceral hyperalgesia. Gastroenterology 107 (1994) 271–293.
12. Sodhi, N., M. Camilleri, J. Camoriano et al.: Autonomic function and motility in intestinal pseudoobstruction caused by paraneoplastic syndrome. Dig. Dis. Sci. 34 (1989) 1937–1942.
13. Szurszewski, J., S. Miller: Physiology of prevertebral ganglia. In: L. Johnson (Ed.): Physiology of the Gastrointestinal Tract, 3rd ed., pp. 795–877. Raven Press, New York 1993.
14. Thomforde, G., M. Camilleri, S. Phillips, L. Forstrom: Evaluation of an inexpensive screening scintigraphic test of gastric emptying. J. Nucl. Med. 36 (1995) 93–96.
15. Vassallo, M., M. Camilleri, B. Caron et al.: Gastrointestinal motor dysfunction in acquired selective cholinergic dysautonomia associated with infectious mononucleosis. Gastroenterology 100 (1991) 252–258.
16. von der Ohe, M., M. Camilleri: Measurement of small bowel and colonic transit: indications and methods. Mayo Clin. Proc. 67 (1992) 1169–1179.

Neurodiagnostic tests of degenerative diseases

R. F. Pfeiffer

With the increasing life expectancy brought about by advances in modern medicine, the group of neurodegenerative diseases have assumed increasing importance as factors impacting quality of life. Their economic importance − both in direct medical costs and in hidden costs of lost productivity and independence of living − is astounding and often underappreciated.

One of the great difficulties in dealing with these processes, with their insidious onset and gradual progression, has been in accurately identifying them, particularly early in their course. The hope that the increasing array of neurodiagnostic tests available to the neurologist would lead to definitive diagnostic capabilities with regard to the various neurodegenerative diseases has remained in essence unfilled and their diagnosis remains largely a clinical exercise. Diagnostic studies may provide very suggestive clues to the diagnosis of a neurodegenerative disease or they may exclude others, but they do not provide the diagnosis by themselves. This is especially true with regard to the gastrointestinal aspects of these diseases in that the neurodiagnostic studies typically utilized by neurologists shed little or no light on whether or why an individual with a neurodegenerative disease will develop gastrointestinal dysfunction as a part of the clinical picture.

The armamentarium of diagnostic tests that may be mobilized by the neurologist includes tests of both structure and function. Computed tomography (CT) and magnetic resonance imaging (MRI) provide evidence about structural detail. Of the two, MRI provides more intricate detail of brain parenchymal structural changes and is the more valuable in evaluating neurodegenerative diseases. A wider array of tests of neurological function has been developed and ranges from the well-established (some would say staid) electroencephalography (EEG) and the various evoked potentials (EP's) to still-experimental, more exciting tracer-based studies such as positron emission tomography (PET) and single photon emission computed tomography (SPECT). Functional tests of the neuromuscular system, such as electromyography (EMG) and nerve conduction velocity (NCV) studies, are useful in the evaluation of some neurodegenerative diseases − especially motor neuron disease − but are generally more valuable in the evaluation of peripheral nervous system diseases.

In evaluating an individual with a suspected neurodegenerative disease it is important that these various neurodiagnostic studies be performed prudently and judiciously. Blanket use of the procedures is both expensive and wasteful. Although PET is still considered by many to be an experimental procedure and is not readily available in most locations, PET findings in the various neurodegenerative diseases will be included in this survey since the potential for PET to improve diagnostic capabilities in this group of diseases is considerable.

In this essay some of the most common neurodegenerative diseases will be addressed and the utility of various neurodiagnostic tests in the evaluation of the individual diseases will be discussed.

Parkinson's disease

One of the most common neurodegenerative disorders, Parkinson's disease (PD) is characterized clinically by the tetrad of rigidity, bradykinesia, rest tremor, and postural instability, along with a wide variety of secondary clinical signs. In its fully developed form, PD can be diagnosed with relative ease and accuracy on clinical grounds alone, especially if there is also a positive response to levodopa. However, in its early stages or if the clinical appearance is not entirely typical, accurate diagnosis can become distressingly difficult. In fact, even in the best of hands the diagnosis of PD is incorrectly made approximately 20% of the time [18]. In light of this, the presence of a sensitive and specific diagnostic test would be invaluable. Unfortunately, none currently exists. Available neurodiagnostic studies, including PET, may demonstrate changes that are suggestive, but not ones that are unequivocally diagnostic of PD.

On MRI, findings such as cortical atrophy and deep white matter changes may be present, as well as signal hypointensity in the globus pallidus on T2-weighted images [8]. However, these are non-specific findings that do not separate PD from other parkinsonian syndromes or even from normal aging [16]. Narrowing of the substantia nigra pars compacta (SNC) has been reported to be characteristic of MRI in PD. The SNC can be visualized as the area of higher signal intensity sandwiched between the low intensity signals of the red nucleus and the substantia nigra pars reticulata (SNR) on midbrain MRI cuts [9]. However, this finding is not always discernible in individual patients and, in any case, does not differentiate PD from other parkinsonian syndromes [35].

PET has provided a rich source for investigative effort in PD. Glucose metabolism, as measured by fluorodeoxyglucose (FDG), may show global reduction in PD while regional increases, particularly in the globus pallidus contralateral to the most affected limbs, have also been described [22]. However, these changes are of insufficient magnitude or specificity to be of any practical diagnostic value in the individual patient. Dopaminergic function can be more specifically studied with compounds such as fluorodopa (FD), raclopride (RAC), and nomifensine (NMF). Fluorodopa accumulates in dopaminergic neurons. Striatal FD uptake serves as a measure of nigrostriatal dopaminergic neuron integrity and is a presynaptic phenomenon. Raclopride, in contrast, is a dopamine D2 receptor antagonist and, thus, striatal RAC binding is a measure of post-synaptic neuronal integrity. Other dopamine receptor ligands have also been studied. Nomifensine binds to the dopamine transporter, which is responsible for dopamine reuptake into the presynaptic dopaminergic neuron, and is, therefore, another measure of presynaptic nigrostriatal dopaminergic neuronal function.

In PD there is a striking reduction in striatal FD accumulation which correlates with motor performance [33]. The reduction in striatal FD is most pronounced in the putamen [2]. It may even be possible to detect changes in FD uptake prior to the development of clinical symptoms [33]. However, reductions in striatal FD uptake are not specific for PD and are also seen in other parkinsonian syndromes. In untreated PD striatal RAC binding is slightly increased [30], but in individual patients this may not be discernible and in advanced, treated PD RAC binding may actually be reduced [3]. A reduction in NMF-derived activity in the striatum has also been described in PD, but is not consistently present [24].

SPECT represents a more economical and more readily available approach to functional neuroimaging. Recent studies with SPECT have shown that the dopamine transporter marker, β-CIT, may be able to accurately separate patients with PD from normal controls and that the reduction in β-CIT activity correlates with disease severity [32]. Whether these findings will be specific for PD, allowing its separation from other parkinsonian syndromes, remains to be determined.

Multiple system atrophy

Multiple system atrophy (MSA) has been defined as a syndrome characterized clinically by varying combinations of parkinsonian, autonomic, cerebellar, and pyramidal features. The pathology of MSA involves not only the basal ganglia but also a variety of brainstem, cerebellar, and even spinal cord structures. Levodopa responsiveness is generally minimal or absent in MSA. Terms that have been utilized in the past to describe what are now felt to be different clinical facets or presentations of MSA include Shy-Drager syndrome (SDS), olivopontocerebellar atrophy (OPCA), and striatonigral degeneration (SND) [27].

Decreased signal intensity in the putamen on T2-weighted images with high field strength (1.5 Tesla) MRI is characteristic of the atypical parkinsonian syndromes, including MSA, but is not usually seen in PD [16]. There is strong suggestive evidence that this hypointensity of the putamenal signal is due to iron accumulation [16]. Reduced signal intensity in the globus pallidus and narrowing of the SNC are also seen in MSA, as in PD.

PET demonstrates reduction in striatal FD uptake in MSA that may be subtly different from that seen in PD in that both putamen and caudate are equally involved in MSA, while the caudate is relatively spared in PD [4]. Striatal RAC binding, however, may differentiate between MSA and PD in that it may be reduced in MSA, in contrast to the increased binding described in untreated early PD [30, 3]. Glucose metabolism, as measured by FDG, may also be abnormal in MSA with frontal hypometabolism noted in some studies [10]. In the OPCA form of MSA marked reductions in FDG in cerebellar and brainstem structures has been described [13].

Progressive supranuclear palsy

The clinical presentation of progressive supranuclear palsy (PSP) is one of rigid-akinetic, levodopa-unresponsive parkinsonism upon which a progressive supra-nuclear gaze palsy is superimposed, although sometimes not until the advanced stages of the illness. Other extrapyramidal and pyramidal signs may also appear. Neuropathologically it is characterized by involvement of the basal ganglia and various brainstem nuclei.

The neuroradiologic picture of PSP is, in many aspects, similar to that of MSA. Some differences exist, however. In both CT and MRI studies midbrain atrophy has been described [31, 20]. Putamenal hypointensity on T2-weighted MRI is less prevalent in PSP than in MSA [6]. FGD PET demonstrates a characteristic frontal hypometabolism that is probably due to dysfunction in subcortical structures [7]. Abnormalities with other PET ligands are similar to those seen with MSA. PSP is one of the few neurodegenerative diseases where electrophysi-ological studies may be of some value. Routine EEG often shows diffuse slowing, a very nonspecific abnormality, but sleep studies have demonstrated a variety of abnormalities such as hyposomnia with frequent awakenings and reduced REM periods [1].

Alzheimer's disease

Alzheimer's disease (AD) is the most common cause of dementia and looms as a massive medical and socioeconomic problem in the 21st century. Its primary clinical feature is progressive dementia, but extrapyramidal and other motor features may also develop.

MRI has been extensively investigated as a potential tool in the diagnosis of AD, but the investigations have met with little success. Conventional MRI cannot reliably separate AD from other forms of dementia, although it may be useful in identifying some entities that can produce or masquerade as neurodegenerative dementia, such as normal pressure hydrocephalus and subdural hematoma. Sophisticated volumetric studies may do a better job of identifying AD but are currently not practical for routine clinical use [16].

PET studies with FDG demonstrate reduced glucose metabolism most prominently in parietal and temporal cortex [33, 29], but with more advanced AD, the frontal lobes also are affected [33].

Huntington's disease

Huntington's disease (HD) is an autosomal dominant disorder characterized by a combination of progressive dementia, often accompanied by behavioral changes, and extrapyramidal dysfunction, usually consisting of chorea. The defective gene is on the short arm of chromosome 4 and consists of an expanded trinucleotide repeat [19].

Neuroimaging procedures in HD typically demonstrate abnormalities that, while highly typical for HD, are not absolutely specific for it. Both CT and MRI demonstrate atrophy of the head of the caudate with progressive flattening of the lateral walls of the frontal horns along with ventricular enlargement [16, 37, 36]. MRI demonstrates the caudate atrophy more clearly and earlier than CT [16]. Reduction of putamenal volume on MRI has been noted to be an even more specific marker for HD [15]. Pallidal and putamenal signal hypointensity on MRI T2-weighted images are seen with high field strength (1.5 Tesla) studies [25].

FDG PET studies consistently demonstrate caudate hypometabolism [21, 40]. As with the CT and MRI changes, this hypometabolism is not specific for HD and may be seen with some other choreiform disorders [33]. These FDG PET findings are a more sensitive indicator of HD than the structural studies and can be seen prior to the development of caudate atrophy. FDG PET may even demonstrate changes in asymptomatic individuals [14].

Wilson's disease

Wilson's disease is characterized by a dizzying array of symptoms and signs that may include hepatic, neurologic, ocular, psychiatric, hematologic, and musculoskeletal manifestations [26]. It is an autosomal recessive disorder in which the defective gene has recently been proposed to encode for a copper transporting P-type ATPase which is expressed in liver and kidney [5, 39]. It is located on chromosome 13 [12].

In the presence of neurologic dysfunction, the diagnosis of WD can be firmly established in most instances by a combination of tests, including serum ceruloplasmin, 24-hour urinary copper, and slit-lamp ophthalmoscopic exam to determine if Kayser-Fleisher rings are present [26]. In individuals presenting with only hepatic manifestations a liver biopsy to document elevated hepatic copper content is usually necessary [26].

Neuroimaging studies can also be valuable adjunctive tests in the diagnosis of WD. MRI abnormalities are said to be present in 100% of individuals with WD who have neurologic dysfunction [38, 28]. Increased signal intensity on T2-weighted images, sometimes surrounding a zone of decreased intensity, can be found in the basal ganglia, thalamus, and brainstem [23]. Sometimes the hyperintense lesions are better seen on spin-density weighted sequences [11].

PET has not been extensively utilized in the evaluation of WD, although changes in both FDG [17] and FD [34] imaging have been described.

Other diseases

Specific diagnostic tests exist for several other neurodegenerative diseases that will not be discussed here in detail. Motor neuron disease (amyotrophic lateral sclerosis) is characterized by specific EMG/NCV abnormalities, while neuroacanthocytosis is identified by the presence of excessive acanthocytes on properly prepared blood smears. Hallervorden–Spatz disease displays strikingly reduced signal intensity in the globus pallidus and SNR on MRI, presumably due to the iron deposition in these structures that is a hallmark of this disease.

Summary

The ability to accurately and expeditiously diagnose the various neurodegenerative disease processes, especially in their earliest stages, remains an elusive goal for the neurologist. Neurodiagnostic tests have not been able thus far to provide definitive diagnostic information in most instances. They have become valuable diagnostic aids, but clinical history and examination still retain their position as the indispensable means to the diagnosis of neurodegenerative diseases.

Neurodiagnostic tests that evaluate central nervous system (CNS) structure and function, as described in this essay, provide virtually no useful information regarding the function or dysfunction of the CNS centers controlling or modifying gastrointestinal and urologic function in the various neurodegenerative diseases. This remains an area ripe for further study and discovery.

References

1. Aldrich, M., N. Foster, R. White et al.: Sleep abnormalities in progressive supranuclear palsy. Ann. Neurol. 25 (1989) 577–581.
2. Brooks, D., V. Ibanez, G. Sawle et al.: Differing patterns of striatal [18F]-dopa uptake in Parkinson's disease, multiple system atrophy, and progressive supranuclear palsy. Ann. Neurol. 28 (1990) 547–555.
3. Brooks, D., V. Ibanez, G. Sawle et al.: Striatal D2 receptor status in patients with Parkinson's disease, striatonigral degeneration, and progressive supranuclear palsy, measured with [11C]-raclopride and positron emission tomography. Ann. Neurol. 31 (1992) 184–192.
4. Brooks, D., E. Salmon, C. Mathias et al.: The relationship between locomotor disability, autonomic dysfunction, and the integrity of the striatal dopaminergic system in patients with multiple system atrophy, pure autonomic failure, and Parkinson's disease, studied with PET. Brain 113 (1990) 1539–1552.
5. Bull, P., G. Thomas, J. Rommens et al.: The Wilson disease gene is a putative copper transporting P-type ATPase similar to the Menkes gene. Nature Genet. 5 (1993) 327–337.
6. Cardoso, F., J. Jankovic: Progressive Supranuclear Palsy. In: D. Calne (Ed.): Neurodegenerative Diseases, pp. 769–786. W. B. Saunders, Philadelphia 1994.
7. D'Antona, R., J. Baron, Y. Samson et al.: Subcortical dementia: Frontal cortex hypometabolism detected by positron tomography in patients with progressive supranuclear palsy. Brain 108 (1985) 785–789.
8. Drayer, B.: Imaging of the aging brain. Part II. Pathologic conditions. Radiology 166 (1988) 797–806.
9. Duguid, J., R. De La Paz, J. Degroot: Magnetic resonance imaging of the midbrain in Parkinson's disease. Ann. Neurol. 20 (1986) 744–747.
10. Eidelberg, D.: Positron Emission Tomography Studies in Parkinsonism. In: J. Cedarbaum, S. Gancher (Eds.): Parkinson's Disease. Neurologic Clinics 10 (1992) 421–433.
11. Engelbrecht, V., G. Schlaug, H. Hefter et al.: MRI of the Brain in Wilson's Disease: T2 Signal Loss Under Therapy. J. Computer Assisted Tomography 19 (1985) 635–638.
12. Frydman, M., B. Bonné-Tamir, L. Farrer et al.: Assignment of the gene for Wilson's disease to chromosome 13. Proc. Natl. Acad. Sci. USA 82 (1985) 1819–1821.
13. Gilman, S., D. Markel, R. Koeppe et al.: Cerebellar and brainstem hypometabolism in olivopontocerebellar atrophy studied with positron emission tomography. Ann. Neurol. 23 (1988) 223–230.
14. Grafton, S., J. Mazziotta, J. Paul et al.: A comparison of neurological, metabolic, structural, and genetic evaluations in persons at risk for Huntington's disease. Ann. Neurol. 28 (1990) 614–621.
15. Harris, G., G. Pearlson, C. Peyser et al.: Putamen volume reduction on magnetic resonance imaging exceeds caudate changes in mild Huntington's disease. Ann. Neurol. 31 (1992) 69–75.
16. Hauser, R., C. Olanow: Magnetic resonance imaging of neurodegenerative diseases. J. Neuroimag. 4 (1994) 146–158.
17. Hawkins, R., J. Mazziotta, M. Phelps: Wilson's disease studied with FDG and positron emission tomography. Neurology 37 (1987) 1707–1711.
18. Hughes, A., S. Daniel, L. Kilford et al.: The accuracy of clinical diagnosis of idiopathic Parkinson's disease: a clinicopathologic study. J. Neurol. Neurosurg. Psychiatry 55 (1992) 181–184.
19. Huntington's Disease Collaborative Research Group: A novel gene containing a trinucleotide repeat that is expanded and unstable on Huntington's disease chromosomes. Cell 72 (1993) 971–983.
20. Jankovic, J., D. Friedman, F. Pirozollo et al.: Progressive supranuclear palsy: Motor, neurobehavioral, and neuro-ophthalmic findings. In: M. Streifler, A. Korczyn, E. Melamed et al. (Eds.):

Parkinson's Disease: Anatomy, Pathology, and Therapy. Advances in Neurology, Vol. 53, pp. 293−303. Raven Press, New York 1990.

21. Kuhl, D., M. Phelps, C. Markham et al.: Cerebral metabolism and atrophy in Huntington's disease determined by 18-FDG and computed tomographic scan. Ann. Neurol. 12 (1982) 425−434.

22. Leenders, K.: Cerebral Energy Metabolism and Blood Flow in Parkinson's Disease. In: W. Martin (Ed.): Functional Imaging in Movement Disorders, pp. 115−130. CRC Press, Boca Raton 1990.

23. Mahalhaes, A., P. Caramelli, J. Menezes et al.: Wilson's disease: MRI with clinical correlation. Neuroradiology 36 (1994) 97−100.

24. Martin, W.: Parkinson's Disease and Aging: Presynaptic Nigrostriatal Function. In: W. Martin (Ed.): Functional Imaging in Movement Disorders, pp. 103−113. CRC Press, Boca Raton 1990.

25. Mazziotta, J.: PET and Huntington's Disease. In: W. Martin (Ed.): Functional Imaging in Movement Disorders, pp. 177−192. CRC Press, Boca Raton 1990.

26. Pfeiffer, R., M. Ebadi: Wilson's Disease. In: M. Stern, W. Koller (Eds.): Parkinsonian Syndromes, pp. 321−340. Marcel Dekker, New York 1993.

27. Quinn, N.: Multiple system atrophy. In: C. Marsden, S. Fahn (Eds.): Movement Disorders 3, pp. 262−281. Butterworth−Heinemann, Oxford 1994.

28. Roh, J., T. Lee, B. Wie et al.: Initial and follow-up brain MRI findings and correlation with the clinical course in Wilson's disease. Neurology 44 (1994) 1064−1068.

29. Salmon, E., G. Franck: Positron emission tomographic study in Alzheimer's disease and Pick's disease. Arch. Gerontol. Geriatr. 1 (1989) 241−247.

30. Sawle, G., D. Brooks, V. Ibanez et al.: Striatal D2 receptor density is inversely proportional to dopa uptake in untreated hemi-Parkinson's disease. J. Neurol. Neurosurg. Psychiatry 53 (1990) 177.

31. Schonfield, S., L. Golbe, J. Sage et al.: Computed tomographic findings in progressive supranuclear palsy: Correlation with clinical grade. Movement Disord. 2 (1987) 263−278.

32. Seiby, L., K. Marek, D. Quinlan et al.: Decreased Single-Photon Emission Computed Tomographic [^{123}I] β-CIT Striatal Uptake Correlates with Symptom Severity in Parkinson's Disease. Ann. Neurol. 38 (1995) 589−598.

33. Snow, B.: Positron Emission Tomography. In: D. Calne (Ed.): Neurodegenerative Diseases, pp. 427−444. W. B. Saunders, Philadelphia 1994.

34. Snow, B., M. Bhatt, W. Martin et al.: The nigrostriatal dopaminergic pathway in Wilson's disease studied with positron emission tomography. J. Neurol. Neurosurg. Psychiatry 54 (1991) 12−17.

35. Stern, M., B. Graffman, B. Skolnick et al.: Magnetic resonance imaging in Parkinson's disease and parkinsonian syndromes. Neurology 39 (1989) 1524−1526.

36. Stober, T., W. Wussow, K. Schimrigk: Bicaudate diameter − the most specific and simple CT parameter in the diagnosis of Huntington's disease. Neuroradiology 26 (1984) 25−28.

37. Terrence, C., J. Delaney, M. Alberts. CT for Huntington's disease. Neuroradiology 13 (1977) 173−175.

38. Thuomas, K., S. Aquilonius, K. Bergstrom et al.: Magnetic resonance imaging of the brain in Wilson's disease. Neuroradiology 35 (1993) 134−141.

39. Yamaguchi, Y., M. Heiny, J. Gitlin: Isolation and Characterization of a Human Liver cDNA as a Candidate Gene for Wilson Disease. Biochem. Biophys. Res. Commun. 197 (1993) 271−277.

40. Young, A., J. Penney, D. Markel et al.: PET scan investigations of Huntington's disease: Cerebral metabolic correlates of neurologic features and functional decline. Ann. Neurol. 20 (1986) 296−303.

Diagnostic tests of the autonomic nervous system

D. F. Altomare

Introduction

Disorders of Autonomic Nervous System (ANS) function are usually characterized by widespread abnormalities of both the sympathetic and the parasympathetic system, most frequently involving sweating ability, the eyes, the cardiovascular, urinary, sexual and digestive systems.

Many of the patients referred to gastroenterologists and gastrointestinal surgeons complain of symptoms secondary to alteration in function of a part of the gastrointestinal (GI) tract, classified as functional diseases because no organic cause can be recognized. These include such affections as irritable bowel syndrome, idiopathic constipation, chronic idiopathic pseudobstruction, gastroesophageal reflux, chronic diarrhoea, etc. which can often be referred to a primary (idiopathic) or secondary autonomic failure.

An understanding of the mechanisms at the basis of these diseases is essential in order to choose the appropriate medical or surgical treatment, and, although a large number of biochemical, functional and pharmacological tests have been proposed for investigating autonomic integrity, only a few combine sensitivity and reliability without requiring sophisticated or expensive equipment and therefore are available to all neurologists, gastroenterologists and surgeons.

In this chapter we review some of the tests available and describe a new sensitive and inexpensive test of autonomic integrity (the Sweat Spot Test) and its clinical applications in gastroenterology.

Autonomic system failure and the gut

An intact sympathetic and parasympathetic nerve supply to the GI tract is essential for normal function (motility, secretion and absorption), hence any damage to one or both branches of the ANS is likely to be followed by various gut motility and secretory disturbances. The regulation of bowel nervous system, in fact, is the result of a very complex integration of factors including smooth muscle electrical and contractile properties, autonomic nervous supply, integrity of the little gut brain represented by the enteric nerve system with its numerous neurotransmitters and the indirect influence on them that the Central Nervous System (CNS) can exert.

The idea that some functional gut diseases like chronic idiopathic constipation, irritable bowel syndrome, gastroparesis etc. may owe their pathogenesis to an impaired extrinsic autonomic control of gut motility comes from the common observation that most of the patients suffering from diseases involving the ANS, like degenerative diseases (Parkinson's disease, Shy-Drager syndrome, Riley-Day syndrome), infectious diseases (Epstein Barr virus mononucleosis, Herpes-Zoster-varicella virus) neoplastic diseases (brain stem neoplasia), traumatic (spinal injury, surgical vagotomy or sympathectomy) and metabolic diseases (diabetes), complain of various motility disturbances, the most common being constipation. Furthermore, many patients suffering from severe idiopathic constipation also complain of other motility disturbances involving the bladder [14], oesophagus, stomach, ileum [20] and probably gallbladder, suggesting multiple organ involvement in a systemic disease [25].

Impairment of the ANS was proposed as a cause of bowel motility dysfunction as early as 1928 [4]. Abnormal cardiovascular reflexes were demonstrated in patients with gastro-oesophageal reflux [8] and gastroparesis is a well known clinical manifestation of diabetic neuropathy. Recently, slow transit constipation was presumed to be a pan-enteric motor disorder on the basis of association with other gut motility disturbances [22, 15], and an attempt to detect ANS abnormalities in constipated patients was carried out by Waldron et al. [26]. Using only cardiovascular tests described by Ewing and Clarke [10], they found 1 abnormal test in 4 of the 8 patients studied. Camilleri and colleagues were able to correlate neurogenic orthostatic hypotension with fasting manometry abnormalities in the antrum and proximal small bowel, suggesting an associated impaired autonomic nerve supply to the upper GI tract and cardiovascular system [5]. The same authors detected some degree of idiopathic autonomic denervation (both sympathetic and parasympathetic) in a group of 8 patients suffering from upper GI tract motility abnormalities [6].

Using a sweat test which will be described below [1], our group demonstrated that a subclinical form of autonomic failure was detectable in 11 of 23 non diabetic patients with severe slow transit constipation and in none of the control group.

The prevalence of autonomic dysfunction in constipated patients was recently investigated by Surrenti et al. [24] using autonomic tests assessing the cardiovagal, sympathetic adrenergic and cholinergic (quantitative sudomotor test) functions. Using a standardized scoring system to diagnose dysautonomia, they were able to identify only one case of autonomic dysfunction in 19 patients with slow transit constipation, and 3 out of 51 patients complaining of constipation from other causes. However, autonomic tests were used only in 28 patients with symptomatic dysautonomia out of 70 constipated patients. The limited sensitivity of the tests used and the strict cut-off score required in that study may have left some cases undetected. This is also suggested by the fact that only 4 of the 28 patients with symptoms of autonomic failure had positive tests. This may explain why these data are in disagreement with the results of our study which aimed to detect early and even asymptomatic autonomic impairment.

Bharucha et al. [3] reviewed the records of 113 patients with a gastrointestinal motility disorder and found a correlation between the autonomic score, obtained by evaluating tests of sympathetic and parasympathetic function, and motility scores, obtained by analyzing gastrointestinal manometry under fasting and fed conditions. Using these tests, autonomic dysfunction was detected in a varying percentage (from 27% to 69%) of patients with gastrointestinal motility disorders.

Clinical evaluation of autonomic function

The tests for evaluating autonomic function overlap the boundaries of different disciplines and their evaluation often requires a physician with experience of disorders of the ANS. Many tests can be used to investigate the integrity of the autonomic nervous system, but they are not always reliable or easy to perform.

Three main groups of tests can be distinguished [7]:

Sympathetic adrenergic function tests

Functional tests
The orthostatic tilt test, postural adjustment ratio and sustained handgrip test investigate the changes in blood pressure and heart rate as an adrenergic response to stimulated barocepters. Blood pressure changes during the Valsalva manoeuvre also indicate sympathetic adrenergic response to stimulated baroceptors. In the cold-pressor test peripheral vasoconstriction increases blood pressure and induces bradycardia.

Biochemical tests
Plasma norepinephrine response to postural changes is related to the spillover of this cathecholamine from post ganglionic sympathetic fibres. Its level is reduced in post-ganglionic adrenergic failure whereas it is normal in pre-ganglionic failure, although in this case it does not increase after 15 min standing upright.

Changes in vasopressin serum levels after induced hypotension are used to assess the afferent branch of the sympathetic adrenergic system.

Pharmacological tests

Increase in plasma norepinephrine in response to iv edrophonium, a short-acting anticholinesterase that stimulates post-ganglionic release of norepinephrine. Changes in blood pressure and heart rate to iv phenylephrine (α_1-adrenoceptor agonist), isoproterenol (β-adrenoceptor agonist), clonidine (α_2-adrenoceptor agonist), yohimbine (α_2-adrenoceptor antagonist).

The sensitivity, reliability and reproducibility of these tests are limited by many factors like the patient's degree of hydration and the presence of cardiovascular disease. Some also require expensive facilities which are not always available or are uncomfortable. Pharmacological tests are not without risk for the patient.

Parasympathetic tests

Vagal function tests can be subdivided into cardiovagal tests, like heart rate variation during deep breathing, supine/erect heart rate and Valsalva R-R ratio, and gastrointestinal vagal tests like postprandial gastrointestinal response to hypoglycemia and sham feeding using the chew-and-spit technique. In the first group of tests, the interval between successive R waves on an ECG is recorded in response to vagal stimulation due to changes in central blood volume or lung stretch. In the abdominal vagal tests, plasma levels of pancreatic polypeptide are measured in response to hypoglycemia or sham feeding. The main limit of these tests is their sensitivity. They are often negative if autonomic neuropathy is not clinically evident [11] and, for this reason, are of limited help in detecting subclinical autonomic neuropathies. Their response may be influenced by age, gender and cardiovascular symptoms like arrhythmia.

Investigation of sacral parasympathetic function requires more specialized equipment to perform combined cystometrography and electromyography, penile tumescence and internal anal sphincter function studies or sacral root stimulation.

Sympathetic cholinergic function tests (sweating tests)

Sweating is controlled by two different neural pathways [9] (Fig. 1):

The main pathway is an essential part of the thermoregulatory system and controls most of the sweat glands, whereas the sweat glands of the palms of the hands and the soles of the feet and part of the glands on the skin of the brow are controlled by the second pathway. In response to increased temperature, the thermoregulatory centre in the anterior hypothalamus is activated. The neural activity, via the preganglionic neurons in the lateral horn of the gray matter of the spinal cord and the postganglionic neurons of the sympathetic chain T1−L2, activates the sweat glands. Acetylcholine is the neurotransmitter for the entire pathway. This is the only part of the sympathetic system where acetylcho-

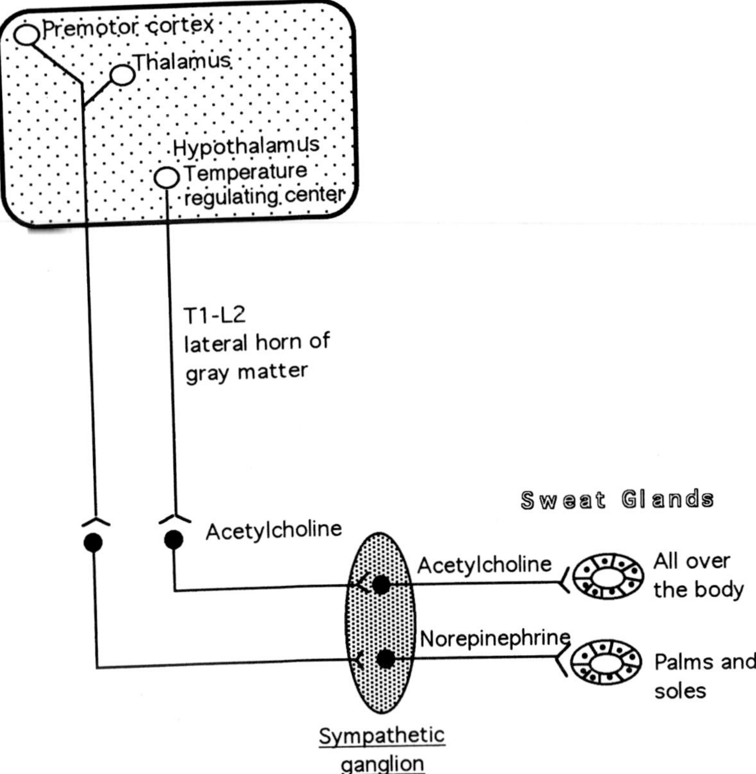

Fig. 1: *Neural control of sweating in humans.*

line (rather than noradrenaline) is the neurotransmitter of post-ganglionic fibres. The other pathway is part of an integrated response to emotional or stress situations. This may be associated with other signs of adrenergic stimulation like piloerection, vasoconstriction, increased pulse and respiratory rate. The "cold sweat" experienced with strong emotions is due to peripheral vasoconstriction with sweat. The neural stimulus originates in the premotor cortex and/ or thalamus and, via the sympathetic ganglia reaches the sweat glands in the soles of the feet and palms of the hands.

Investigations of sweating abnormalities have been carried out using different tests, the most common being:

The quantitative sudomotor axon reflex test (QSAT, measure of postganglionic cholinergic fibres) which measures the sweat output ($\mu l/cm^2$), latency and duration in the leg and forearm after iontophoresis of acetylcholine.

The thermoregulatory sweat test (TST) (% of surface area of anhydrosis) using alizarine or quinizarine painted all over the body (preganglionic sympathetic fibres).

The measurement of *Galvanic current resistance* of the skin before and after sweating (preganglionic sympathetic fibres).

All these tests require sophisticated and expensive equipment with specialized operators. Moreover, QSAT gives widely varying results depending on the skin area and patient's gender. TST is difficult to quantify and requires cumbersome equipment while the Galvanic measure is poorly reproducible and better applied to a skin area damaged by spinal lesions.

The *Sweat Spot Test* (SST) can be considered a new, inexpensive, time saving and reproducible sweat test, which is reliable for quantitative analysis of the severity of nerve damage. The test is really a new version of old tests developed for the study of sweating abnormalities [12] and was designed by Ryder and co-workers for the diagnosis of diabetic neuropathy using intradermal acetylcholine [23]. The test has been further modified by our group to investigate the integrity of preganglionic fibres using thermal stimulus and has been clinically applied in patients with idiopathic slow transit constipation [1] and in the selection of those with ischaemic limb to be submitted to lumbar sympathectomy [2].

An attempt to overcome the poor sensitivity of most of the tests described was done by Low at the Mayo Clinic using a scoring system obtained in an autonomic reflex screen including the thermoregulatory sweat test or quantitative sudomotor test and sympathetic and vagal cardiovascular tests [18].

Performing the sweat spot test
Material required: 2% alcohol iodine solution, a fine sterile emulsion of 100 gr of maize starch in 100 gr of arachis oil, a 1% solution of acetylcholine (Miochol−Cooper vision ltd or Acetilcolina cloruro mg 20 − Farmigea S.p.A. PISA Italy), 2 fine paint-brushes (to be used for application of the solutions on the skin), an insulin-syringe with a 25 G needle, an empty slide mount and a water soluble ink fine pen.

Photographic equipment: A macro lens or a teleconverter can be applied to a common camera for focusing the image at 15−20 cm distance, mounted on a tripod with a 100 W beam directed at an angle of 45° toward the image, and a 400 ASA color film (black and white is more expensive to develop).

Procedure: A standard site on the dorsum of the foot is defined by a line between the protuberance of the first tarsometatarsal joint and the cleft between the second and third toes. This area of the skin is painted with iodine solution and allowed to dry. An empty slide mount is then placed longitudinally on this site, its medial inner border on the line and its proximal medial corner at the first tarsometatarsal joint.

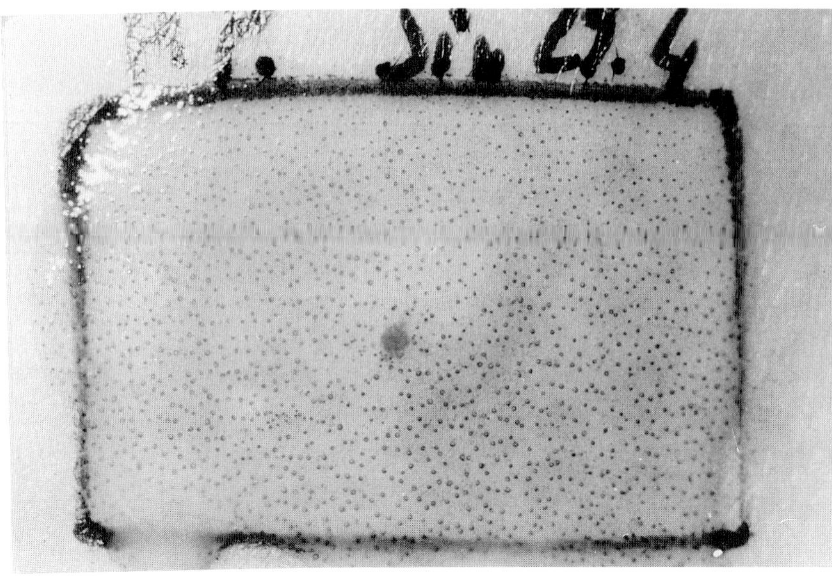

Fig. 2: *Normal appearance of the Ach Sweat-Spot test. Note the even distribution of little dots corresponding to the gland pores after intradermal injection of acetylcholine.*

The inner perimeter of the slide mount is then marked with a pen and the patient's initials and the date are noted on the top border. The skin is then painted with a thin layer of thoroughly mixed emulsion using the second brush.

Pre-ganglionic fibre assessment: a thermal stimulus (produced by a 100 W light taken at a distance of about 10 cm from the skin) is applied for 5 min. If the sympathetic pathway is normal, the sweat from the stimulated sweat glands activates a colorimetric reaction between the iodine and the starch so that each pore can be seen as a little black dot.

Post-ganglionic fibre assessment: An intradermal injection of 0.1 ml of the acetylcholine solution is made at the centre of the marked area. In 2−3 min an even distribution of fine black dots, corresponding to the gland pores, will appear (Fig. 2).

A normal response is characterized by the appearance of an even distribution of the fine black dots whereas in the case of autonomic denervation, the distribution will be patchy and the number of working sweat glands reduced (Fig. 3).

Denervated glands to not respond to the thermal stimulus or even to the acetylcholine injection, probably because of loss of specific receptors and atrophy of the glands. Furthermore, acetylcholine is known to be cotransmitted with the Vasoactive Intestinal Polipeptide (VIP) at the junction with sweat glands, VIP probably being responsible for the local vasodilation necessary for a normal

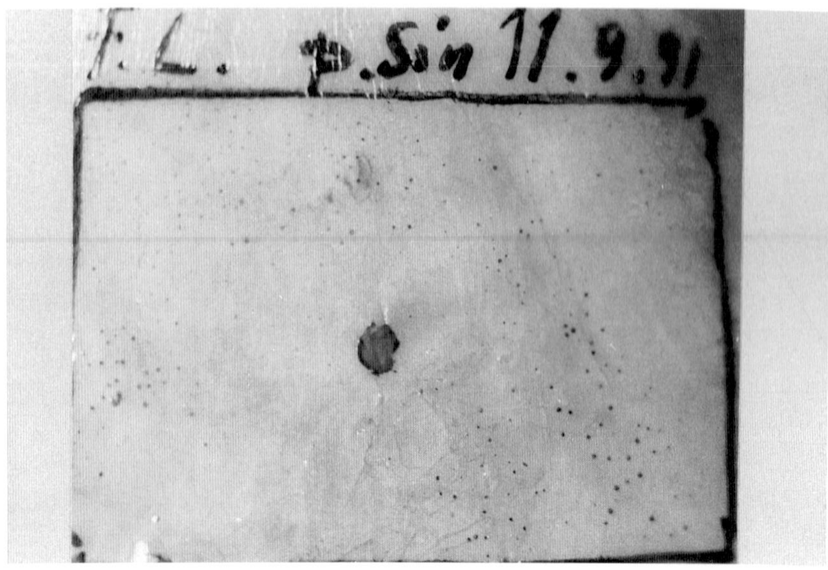

Fig. 3: *Patchy distribution and reduced total number of working sweat glands (autonomic neuropathy) in a patient with severe slow transit constipation.*

response. It is possible that a full response requires the combined action of both neurotransmitters and that in the event of nerve degeneration, acetylcholine alone does not provide an adequate stimulus.

Evaluation of the test

The skin area is photographed. The negative is mounted on a slide and projected on a screen. The image is magnified ten times (short side 24 cm) and focused. A 20 × 20 grid (with each square measuring 2.5 cm) designed on a transparent sheet (for overhead projection) is put on the image. The centre of the grid coincides with the site of injection. The number of dots in each square is counted including those touching the upper and left border of the square. Those touching the right and lower side are ignored.

Normal values of the SST: In Ryder's experience, a finding of 5 or more squares (> 8.3% of the squares counted) with less than 6 dots was considered clearly abnormal, while patients with 2−4 abnormal squares were considered borderline. Using the ROC curve analyses, we found that the highest efficiency for separating normal from abnormal subjects was a percentage of 0.033 abnormal squares (which correspond to 2/60) and/or a mean SST (which is calculated by dividing the sum of dots counted with the number of squares) below 12. The two methods of evaluation strictly correlated. Using these quantification methods, different degrees of severity of sweating impairment can be detected (Fig. 4).

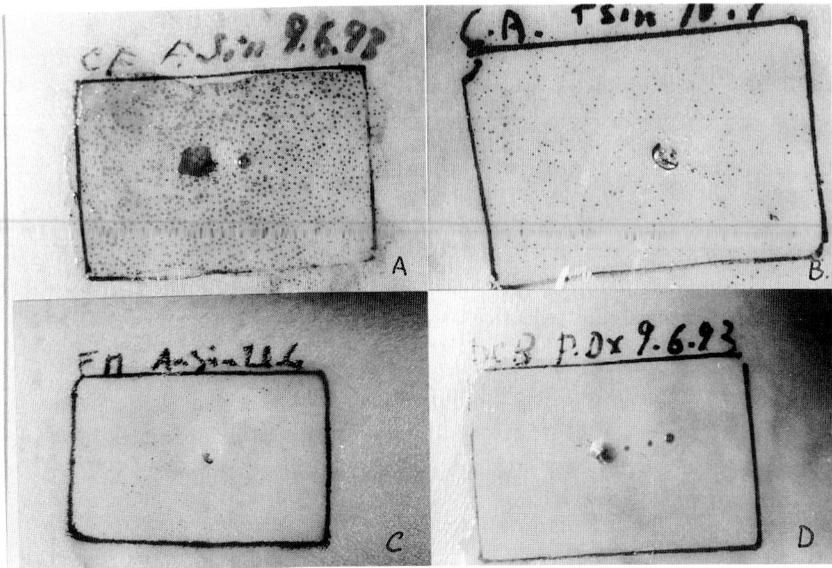

Fig. 4: *Different degrees of autonomic denervation of the sweat glands: A = normal response, B = moderate autonomic denervation, C = severe autonomic denervation, D = complete denervation.*

Validation of the SST

Interobserver variation: We tested the interobserver variation of the SST by performing a K statistic analysis on the agreement among 3 different observers who examined the same series of tests independently. K value was 0.81 with a $p < 0.0001$.

Influences of age or gender: No effect of age was demonstrated on the SST score in Ryder's experience using two way analysis of variance and multiple regression, while we found greater abnormalities in the oldest patients with chronic constipation. This finding was not detected in the age and sex matched control group, since it could have been the expression of the duration of the neuropathy itself rather than the effect of age. No effect of gender was demonstrated by Ryder, while in our series of constipated patients, more than 90% were women and so its effect on the SST values could not be evaluated.

Sensitivity: the longest autonomic nerve fibres are believed to be more early damaged in diseases involving the ANS and therefore the choice of the skin of the feet as the standard site for the SST should enhance its sensitivity. This is particularly true in diabetic neuropathy, where sweating abnormalities in the lower extremities precede manifestation in other sites. The higher sensitivity of the SST (which explores peripheral autonomic function) was demonstrated by Ryder to be more sensitive than classic cardiovascular tests (which assess central autonomic function) and pupillary tests, in diabetic patients with impotence, in our experience the Valsalva ratio was normal in 7 of 8 chronic constipated patients in whom the SST showed sympathetic denervation, while no patients with normal SST had a positive Valsalva ratio.

Clinical applications of the Sweat Spot Test
So far this test has been clinically used in the diagnostic evaluation of the following diseases:

Diabetic neuropathy: Ryder et al. [23] specifically designed this test for detecting diabetic neuropathy in 24 diabetics complaining of impotence and found it much more sensitive than the traditional battery of cardiovascular and pupillary tests.

Slow transit constipation: We tested the hypothesis that some cases of idiopathic slow transit constipation could be related to a degree of autonomic failure and found that 11 of the 23 patients studied (47%) had abnormal Ach SST and 5 had a borderline response [1].

These data have been confirmed in a further group of patients with colonic inertia examined in our Institute: in 21 patients with slow transit constipation, 9 (43%) showed abnormal Ach SST (post ganglionic fibres) and 8 (38%) abnormal thermal SST (preganglionic fibres). These findings were associated with delayed small bowel transit (H_2-breath test) in 5 cases and orthostatic hypotension in 4 (unpublished data).

These findings may have clinical relevance in the selection of constipated patients with colonic inertia to submit to total colectomy. In fact there is an increasing evidence in the literature that patients with colonic inertia are a heterogeneous population. Among patients with chronic slow transit constipation with severe abdominal symptoms, some need a partial or total removal of the colon despite normal histology, but constipation or the abdominal symptoms may nevertheless persist in a group of these patients [13−17]. Although some patients who fail to improve after subtotal colectomy have associated unrecognized defecation problems, others might have whole GI tract involvement in a systemic idiopathic autonomic neuropathy (even subclinical), causing associated unrecognized motility disturbances in other parts of the GI tract (stomach, small bowel, rectum). Recently, an interesting study on the long term results of total colectomy for intractable constipation was carried out by Redmore et al. [22]. They were able to distinguish two groups of patients with different prognosis: those with colonic inertia alone, who had 90% success rate after total colectomy and those who had colonic inertia associated with other clinical or subclinical gastrointestinal motility disturbances, such as delayed small bowel transit, oesophageal diskinesia or bradygastria, who had only 12.5% success rate after a median follow-up of 7.5 years. Although no tests of autonomic function were performed in these patients, it seems highly probably that the latter group could be affected by a subclinical autonomic neuropathy. Furthermore, a selective neural sweating deficit of post-ganglionic sympathetic cholinergic fibres has recently been demonstrated using nicotine injection (axon reflex sweating) in a group of severely constipated patients with normally functioning sweat glands (after methacholine stimulation) [21]. The criteria for selecting these patients for colectomy should therefore include tests of autonomic function like the SST and cardiovascular tests, besides the physiological colo proctological investigations proposed by Wexner [27].

Lumbar sympathectomy: The SST was used to select patients who would have benefit from lumbar sympathectomy [2]: many patients with an ischaemic limb already have autosympathectomy due to diabetes, the ischemia itself or other causes, and lumbar sympathectomy cannot be expected to improve blood flow to the extremities in these cases. Furthermore, the procedure can produce incomplete denervation to the limb, mainly after chemical sympathectomy. These factors may be responsible for the poor predictability of success of lumbar sympathectomy.

We found that only patients with normal innervation or minor sympathetic denervation (SST ≥ 8) improved after lumbar sympathectomy.

Furthermore, postoperative SST verification showed that two patients who had been expected to benefit from the procedure and did not improve, did not actually have sympathetic denervation in the skin area tested.

Other functional gastrointestinal diseases: Autonomic disfunctions have been implicated in the pathogenesis of many other functional diseases of the GI tract, like irritable bowel syndrome, chronic diarrhea, gastroparesis, chronic intestinal pseudobstruction, oesophageal reflux and achalasia. In these cases the role of the SST, in association with other autonomic tests or alone, in detecting autonomic failure remains to be clarified.

Limits of the SST
The main criticism that could be raised at the use of the SST for assessing autonomic integrity in patients with gastrointestinal functional diseases is that this test only explores the cholinergic sympathetic system, fibres which are not present in the GI tract [7]. However, the most common diseases affecting the ANS usually involve the whole nervous system. The main pattern of autonomic dysfunction includes generalized autonomic failure (which is the most common form, caused by diabetes, multiple systemic atrophy, Guillan-Barré syndrome, paraneoplastic syndromes, etc.), distal sympathetic neuropathy which involves adrenergic and cholinergic fibres with vasomotor and sudomotor alterations, pure cholinergic (cardiovagal symptoms and anhydrosis without orthostatic hypotension) and pure adrenergic (orthostatic hypotension) neuropathies [19]. No specific diseases of the sympathetic cholinergic fibres alone are known, so that

damage to this section of the ANS may well reflect systemic nervous damage to the ANS.

Sympathetic denervation of the GI tract can be expected to increase motility as an effect of unbraked vagal tone in the absence of the sympathetic tone, causing diarrhea instead of constipation, but increased motility does not necessarily result in increased propulsive activity. In fact, increased mixing and segmental activity has been reported in constipation [15] and irritable bowel syndrome [16].

Sweating tests have been extensively used in association with cardiovascular tests for assessing ANS function in patients with functional gastrointestinal disease [6, 24, 26].

Advantages of the SST
The advantages of the SST can be summarized as follows:

a. The test may be positive even in the absence of clinical symptoms of autonomic failure like orthostatic hypotension, impotence, urinary incontinence. It can therefore be used for early detection of otherwise asymptomatic autonomic failure.

b. Except for research purposes, the response can easily be gauged by the experienced naked eye at the bedside, without needing to analyze the photo.

c. Progression or therapeutic regression of the neuropathy can be assessed by later testing of the same area.

d. Pre- and post-ganglionic sympathetic pathways can be explored with the same equipment and technique in less than 15 min.

e. The test is inexpensive, time saving, reproducible, easy for a non-specialized operator to perform and is not influenced by age or gender.

Conclusions

A reliable test of autonomic integrity has implications in the diagnosis and therapy of many diseases and should therefore not only be highly sensitive and quantifiable, but also easy to perform and time saving and should not require sophisticated or expensive equipment or specialized operators. In this respect, the SST may be considered a step forward in comparison with the classic sweat tests and deserves a role in the assessment of ANS beside some of the most reproducible classic cardiovascular tests.

Acknowledgments: the Author wishes to thank Elisabetta Martinelli, MD, for assistance in preparing the paper, Marie-Anne Pilot, PhD, for her helpful comments, and Mary Pragnell, BA, for correcting the manuscript.

References

1. Altomare, D. F., M.-A. Pilot, M. Scott et al.: Detection of subclinical autonomic neuropathy in constipated patients using a sweat test. Gut 33 (1992) 1539—1543.
2. Altomare, D. F., R. Lovreglio, M. Regina et al.: Acetylcholine sweat-spot test: an easy way to select patients for lumbar sympathectomy. Lancet 344 (1994) 976—978.
3. Bharucha, A. E., M. Camilleri, P. A. Low et al.: Autonomic dysfunction in gastrointestinal motility disorders. Gut 34 (1993) 397—401.
4. Bockus, H. L., J. Bank, S. A. Wilkinson: Neurogenic mucous colitis. Am. J. Med. Sci. 176 (1928) 813—828.
5. Camilleri, M., J. R. Malagelada, V. Stanghellini et al.: Gastrointestinal motility disturbances in patients with orthostatic hypotension. Gastroenterology 88 (1985) 1852—1859.
6. Camilleri, M., R. D. Fealey: Idiopathic autonomic denervation in 8 patients presenting with functional gastrointestinal disease. A causal association? Dig. Dis. Sci. 35 (1990) 609—616.
7. Camilleri, M.: Functional gastrointestinal disease and the autonomic nervous system: a way ahead? Gastroenterology 106 (1994) 1114—1118.
8. Chakraborty, T. K., A. L. Ogilvie, R. C. Heading et al.: Abnormal cardiovascular reflexes in patients with gastro-oesophageal reflux. Gut 30 (1989) 46—49.
9. Chalmers, T. M., C. A. Keele: The nervous and chemical control of sweating. Br. J. Dermatol. 64 (1952) 43—54.
10. Ewing, D. J., B. F. Clarke: Diagnosis and management of diabetic autonomic neuropathy. Br. Med. J. 285 (1982) 916—918.
11. Fisher, B. M., B. M. Frier: Usefulness of cardiovascular tests of autonomic function in asymptomatic diabetic patients. Diabetes Res. Clin. Pract. 6 (1989) 157—160.
12. Kahn, D., S. Rothman: Sweat response to acetylcholine. J. Dermat. Invest. 5 (1942) 413—444.
13. Kamm. M. A., P. R. Hawley, J. E. Lennard-Jones: Outcome of colectomy for severe idiopathic constipation. Gut 29 (1988) 969—973.
14. Kerrigan, D. D., M. G. Lucas, W. M. Sun et al.: Idiopathic constipation associated with impaired urethrovesical and sacral reflex function. Br. J. Surg. 76 (1989) 748—751.
15. Kumar, D., D. Waldron, N. S. Williams et al.: Slow transit constipation: a pan-enteric motor disorder? Gastroenterology 96 (1989) A277.
16. Kumar, D., L. D. Wingate: The irritable bowel syndrome: paroxysmal motor abnormalities. Lancet (1985) ii 973—977.
17. Leon, S. H., S. Krishnamurthy, M. D. Shuffer: Subtotal colectomy for severe idiopathic constipation: a follow-up study of 13 patients. Dig. Dis. Sci. 32 (1987) 1249—1254.
18. Low, P. A.: Composite autonomic scoring scale for laboratory quantification of generalized autonomic failure. Mayo Clinic Proc. 68 (1993) 748—752.
19. Low, P. A.: Laboratory evaluation of autonomic failure. In: P. A. Low (Ed.): Clinical autonomic disorders; evaluation and management, pp. 157—165. Little Brown, Boston 1993.
20. Panagamuwa, B., D. Kumar, J. Ortiz et al.: Motor abnormalities in the terminal ileum of patients with chronic idiopathic constipation. Br. J. Surg. 81 (1994) 1685—1688.
21. Raethien, I., M. A. Pilot, P. Anand et al.: Selective autonomic deficits in slow transit constipation. Gut 35 (1994) S28.
22. Redmond, J. M., G. W. Smith, I. Barofsky et al.: Physiological test to predict long-term outcome of total abdominal colectomy for intractable constipation. Am. J. Gastroent. 90 (1995) 748—753.
23. Ryder, R. E. J., R. Marshall, K. J. Johnson et al.: Acetylcholine sweat-spot test for autonomic denervation. Lancet (1988) i 1303—1305.
24. Surrenti, E., D. M. Rath, J. H. Pemberton et al.: Audit of constipation in a tertiary referral gastroenterology practice. Am. J. Gastroenterology 90 (1995) 1471—1475.

25. Waiter, A., G. Devroede, A. Duranceau et al.: Constipation with colonic inertia. A manifestation of systemic disease? Dig. Dis. Sci. 28 (1983) 1025−1033.
26. Waldron, D. J., N. S. Williams, D. Kumar et al.: Is intractable constipation associated with a systemic autonomic neuropathy? (Abstract). Br. J. Surg. 76 (1989) 645.
27. Wexner, S. D. O., N. Daniel, D. G. Jagelman: Colectomy for constipation: physiologic investigation is the key to success. Dis. Colon Rectum 34 (1991) 851−856.

Urinary manifestation of neuro-degenerative diseases

C. J. Fowler

Introduction

A consideration of bladder symptoms in patients with neuro-degenerative disease is important for two reasons:

1. The contribution such symptoms can make to the correct neurological diagnosis.
2. Medical management of incontinence is often very successful in these patients, to their considerable relief.

Neurological control of the bladder

Figure 1 shows the sites within the nervous system which are thought to be the main regions important in neurological control of the bladder. There is a substantial body of evidence to suggest that there exists in the dorsal tegmentum of the pons in humans as well as experimental animals, nuclei which control the bladder, known as the pontine micturition centres [3, 6]. In health the bladder exists in one of two mutually exclusive conditions, in the storage or in the voiding mode. The neural programs which control the bladder in each of these conditions reside in the pontine micturition centres and the effect of supra pontine centres is to switch control by the pontine micturition centres from one state into another. Although the role of medial areas of the frontal lobes is well established in terms of bladder control [2] the influence of the basal ganglia and cerebellum is much less certain. The efferent and afferent innervation of the lower urinary tract mostly travel through the most caudal spinal roots, the sacral roots 2−4.

Spinal cord disease

It is immediately apparent from Figure 1 that the integrity of the spinal cord and the connections between the pons and the sacral cord are critical for physiological bladder control. Following a cord lesion both the processes of storage and voiding are likely to be affected. For storage the bladder requires constant inhibition of the parasympathetic outflow to the detrusor muscle and following

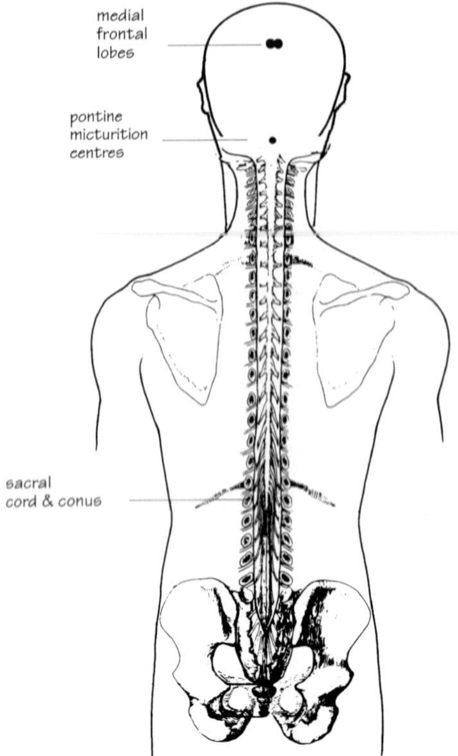

Fig. 1: *Sites within the central nervous system which are important for bladder control.*

the loss of this the bladder typically develops "detrusor hyperreflexia", a term which describes involuntary contractions of the bladder that occur on filling due to a neurological lesion. Following a chronic spinal cord lesion the innervation of the bladder becomes reorganised and instead of the reflexes operating transpinally (vertically), a new reflex emerges at a sacral level (horizontally). The afferent impulses of the reflex arc which then determine bladder emptying are unmyelinated C-fibres [7]. It appears that the C-fibres in humans which become functionally significant following a spinal cord lesion are sensitive to capsaicin [12], an observation which has implications for the management of patients with detrusor hyperreflexia of spinal origin.

In addition to disturbances of storage, spinal cord disease disrupts co-ordinated voiding. The relaxation of the striated muscles of the sphincter and pelvic floor which usually precedes the onset of a detrusor contraction is lost, and there is a tendency for the sphincters to contract whilst the bladder itself is also contracting − a condition known as detrusor sphincter dyssynergia.

In practical terms the cause of bladder symptoms in spinal cord disease is usually apparent as the vast majority of patients have evidence of an upper motor neuron lesion when their lower limbs are examined. The reason for this is evident from Figure 1, the origin of the innervation of the lower limbs arising from L2–S1.

Parkinsonism, akinetic rigid syndrome and cerebellar ataxia

The role of bladder symptoms in the diagnosis of conditions presenting with parkinsonism, akinetic rigid syndrome or cerebellar ataxia is of great interest. The differential diagnosis of these disorders includes idiopathic Parkinson's disease (IPD), Cortical Lewy-Body Disease (CLBD), Progressive Supranuclear Palsy (PSP) and Multiple System Atrophy (MSA). Although unfortunately there is currently no effective treatment for any of these conditions, it is important that the patient be given a confident neurological diagnosis and sphincter EMG has proved to be very valuable in this context. Disturbance of bladder control is a common feature of many advancing neurological diseases but characteristically in MSA urinary incontinence is particularly troublesome at an early stage. In a series of 62 patients with MSA, bladder dysfunction was the initial complaint in 25% and in 37% of men erectile failure was the sole initial symptom [4]. Prompt recognition of the correct diagnosis should lead to appropriate medical treatment of incontinence and urological surgery be avoided.

Sphincter EMG in the differential diagnosis of parkinsonism

The selective sparing of a group of anterior horn cells in the sacral spinal cord in patients dying with amyotrophic lateral sclerosis was described by Mannen [14]. The special nature of these anterior horn cells had been identified by Onufrowicz [15] and it was proposed that this group of anterior horn cells innervated the striated muscles of the urethral and anal sphincters, thus explaining the preservation of vesicorectal function until relatively late in the progression of amyotrophic lateral sclerosis. This group of cells became known as Onuf's nucleus and Sung et al. [19] demonstrated that patients dying with Shy-Drager syndrome appeared to have selective loss of these anterior horn cells in contrast to patients with amyotrophic lateral sclerosis. Sakuta et al. [19] showed electromyographic changes of chronic reinnervation in the motor units of the striated muscle of the sphincter in patients with MSA. Kirby et al. (1986) [13] reported on the urodynamic and neurophysiological findings in a number of patients with MSA, showing changes of extreme chronic reinnervation in the motor units of the urethral sphincter. Since in idiopathic Parkinson's disease the anterior horn cells in Onuf's nucleus are not affected sphincter EMG was proposed as a means of distinguishing between IPD and MSA in patients with bladder symptoms [8].

Method for sphincter EMG

The motor units of the striated muscle of both the urethral and anal sphincter fire tonically at a steady rate, making them ideally suited to capture using a trigger and delay line and motor unit analysis. The duration of motor units was found to be the most robust measure of chronic reinnervation in these patients as there seems to be little compacting to give high amplitude potentials, the motor units instead becoming exceedingly prolonged. To perform the test 10 different motor units are captured and the mean of their duration calculated. If a mean upper limit of 8.5 msec is taken there is inevitably some overlap between control "normal" and patients with only modest changes of chronic reinnervation [10]. A cut off point of 10 msec is probably reasonable as a good discriminating level between "normal" and "reinnervation". Palace and her colleagues from The National Hospital for Neurology and Neurosurgery [16] describe the value of sphincter EMG in a series of 127 patients suspected of MSA. Taking an upper limit of 10 msec, 89 patients (70%) were demonstrated to have an abnormal sphincter EMG. The weakness of this study is that because this was a report of clinical experience and the test was usually only carried out in patients in whom a diagnosis of MSA was considered likely, the number of patients with a normal result is relatively small. When the final diagnosis was considered 2 years later, it was found that 70% of those with an abnormal sphincter EMG were subsequently diagnosed as having Multiple System Atrophy. Furthermore 81% of those diagnosed as having MSA had had an abnormal sphincter EMG.

MSA and the bladder

Assisted by sphincter EMG in recognising MSA it has become clear how easy it is to confuse patients with early MSA and bladder symptoms, with those who have idiopathic Parkinson's disease and coincidental urological problems. Patients were categorised as having definite, probable or possible MSA according to established criteria [21] and yet a further group of patients was identified on the basis of their urogenital symptoms. These patients could not, according to the neurological criteria, be considered to have MSA, mostly because they had shown a good L-Dopa response. However, their early bladder symptoms were typical of the condition as was their subsequent clinical course and their sphincter EMG was abnormal. From this group it has been possible to establish urological criteria which favour the diagnosis of MSA as opposed to IPD. A study is now in progress to establish the discriminating power of these criteria since these would be of obvious value to both urologists and neurologists who do not have access to sphincter EMG.

The literature

From reading the literature it is clear that a number of studies, some of which are regarded as being definitive on the subject of the bladder and Parkinson's disease [18], have included patients with MSA. It appears that disturbed bladder function can occur in patients with idiopathic Parkinson's disease either through coincidental urological problems such as prostatic outflow obstruction or possibly as a result of the disease itself causing hyperreflexia. This could either be due to loss of inhibitory input from the basal ganglia or possibly as an effect of the anti-parkinsonian medication. However, although urinary frequency and urgency may be troublesome and common in patients with IPD [9], incontinence is not such a problem, unlike with MSA [4]. The urological literature has inevitably described patients with severe bladder disturbance with parkinsonism [1, 17, 5] and it seems highly likely that much of it has been invalidated by the inclusion of patients with MSA.

PSP and MSA

Although the evidence that sphincter EMG is valuable in distinguishing between patients with IPD and MSA, uncertainty surrounds the value of the investigation in distinguishing between patients with PSP and MSA. In our own series 9 patients with PSP, 2 had highly abnormal sphincter EMG with a prolonged mean duration of the motor units. One was a man of 62 with an axially pronounced akinetic rigid syndrome and supra nuclear palsy but also severe urinary incontinence which came on at much the same time as his bladder symptoms. The other was a lady of 79 who presented with a disturbance of gait. Her postural reflexes were severely impaired and her speech was hypophonic. She had marked axial rigidity and a supra nuclear gaze palsy. At about the time of the onset of her neurological picture she also developed urinary incontinence and was demonstrated to have hyperreflexia and incomplete bladder emptying and sphincter EMG was highly abnormal. A recent paper by Valldeoriola [20] compared the results of sphincter EMG in 12 patients with PSP, 6 with IPD and 6 with MSA. The difference between the patients with IPD and MSA as observed by others was confirmed, but 2 of their 12 patients with PDP had markedly abnormal sphincter EMG, and there were two with a lesser abnormality. One of these patients although they fulfilled accepted criteria for the diagnosis of PSP, had marked incontinence. It has been argued from this that sphincter EMG is not of value in distinguishing between PSP and MSA.

Medical management of incontinence

Once the neurological basis for a patient's bladder symptoms has been identified and the diagnosis of a progressive neuro-degenerative disease is made, medical rather than surgical management of incontinence is advisable. This can be highly effective as long as the degree of incomplete bladder emptying is recognised. Figure 2 shows the management protocol used at the National Hospital for Neurology and Neurosurgery for patients with neurogenic bladder disorders [11]. The central investigation for this is measurement of the post micturition residual volume. If the patient has established neurological disease and is complaining of urgency or frequency, detrusor hyperreflexia can reasonably be assumed and can be effectively treated with anticholinergics, either taken orally or instilled intravesically. However these measures are unlikely to

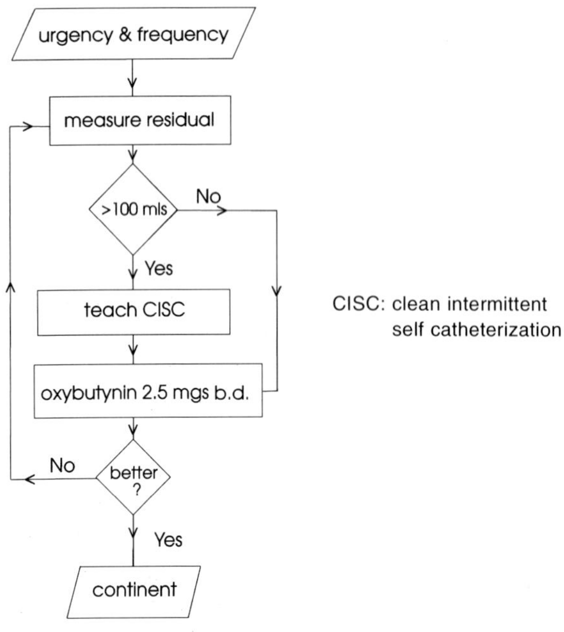

Fig. 2: *Management protocol for neurogenic bladder disorders.*

be effective in the presence of incomplete bladder emptying. Using intermittent self-catheterisation and oxybutynin a high proportion of patients with MSA can be restored to continence for several years during the early stages of their condition before becoming severely disabled [4]. With time and neurological deterioration, these medical means may no longer be effective and a point is often reached at which an in-dwelling catheter becomes necessary.

Intravesical capsaicin has been demonstrated to be of value in patients with detrusor hyperreflexia due to spinal cord disease [12] because of its mechanism of disrupting the unmyelinated C-fibre reflex, but it has not yet been tried in any patients with MSA or IPD and on theoretical grounds, if the hyperreflexia in those conditions is occurring from loss of inhibition on the pontine micturition centre, it seems probable it would not be effective.

Often although incontinence can be lessened using a combination of intermittent self-catheterisation and anticholinergics, there may be a persisting problem with night time frequency. This is particularly likely in patients with autonomic failure in whom urine production is increased when they are recumbent. The synthetic antidiuretic hormone, Desmopressin spray ("Desmospray") taken at night can both reduce night time urinary frequency as well as lessen postural hypotension.

Conclusion

Attention to the urinary symptoms of patients with neuro-degenerative diseases is worthwhile both because of the clues they may give about the true nature of the disease and in particular early recognition of MSA. Furthermore patients early in the course of developing a neurodegenerative disorder can have continence restored by medical means and potentially harmful surgical procedures avoided.

References

1. Andersen, J. T., S. Hebjorn, C. Frimodt-Moller et al.: Disturbances of micturition in Parkinson's Disease. Acta Neurologica Scandinavica 53 (1976) 161–170.
2. Andrew, J., P. W. Nathan: Lesions of the anterior frontal lobes and disturbances of micturition and defaecation. Brain 87 (1964) 233–262.
3. Barrington, F. J. F.: The relation of the hind-brain to micturition. Brain 44 (1921) 23–53.
4. Beck, R. O., C. D. Betts, C. J. Fowler: Genito-urinary dysfunction in Multiple System Atrophy: clinical features and treatment in 62 cases. Journal of Urology 151 (1994) 1336–1341.
5. Berger, Y., J. G. Blaivas, E. R. DeLaRocha et al.: Urodynamic findings in Parkinson's Disease. Journal of Urology 138 (1987) 836–838.

6. de Groat, W. C.: Central neural control of the lower urinary tract. In: G. Bock, J. Whelan (Eds.): Neurobiology of Incontinence. John Wiley & Sons, Chichester 1990.

7. de Groat, W., T. Kawatani, T. Hisamitsu: Mechanisms underlying the recovery of urinary bladder function following spinal cord injury. Journal of Autonomic Nervous System 30 (1990) S71−S78.

8. Eardley, I., N. P. Quinn, C. J. Fowler et al.: The value of urethral sphincter electromyography in the differential diagnosis of parkinsonism. British Journal of Urology 64 (1989) 360−362.

9. Fitzmaurice, H., C. J. Fowler, D. Rickards et al.: Micturition disturbance in Parkinson's Disease. British Journal of Urology 57 (1985) 652−656.

10. Fowler, C. J.: Pelvic floor neurophysiology. In: J. Osselton (Ed.): Clinical Neurophysiology. Butterworth Heinemann, Oxford 1995.

11. Fowler, C. J.: Investigation of the neurogenic bladder. Journal of Neurology, Neurosurgery and Psychiatry 60 (1996) 6−13.

12. Fowler, C. J., R. O. Beck, S. Gerrard et al.: Intravesical capsaicin for treatment of detrusor hyperreflexia. Journal of Neurology, Neurosurgery, and Psychiatry 57 (1994) 169−173.

13. Kirby, R. S., C. J. Fowler, J. Gosling et al.: Urethro-vesical dysfunction in progressive autonomic failure with multiple system atrophy. Journal of Neurology, Neurosurgery and Psychiatry 49 (1986) 554−562.

14. Mannan, T., M. Iwata, Y. Toyokura et al.: Preservation of a certain motor neurone group in amyotrophic lateral sclerosis: its clinical significance. Journal of Neurology, Neurosurgery and Psychiatry 4 (1977) 464−469.

15. Onufrowicz, B.: On the arrangement and function of the cell groups of the sacral region of the spinal cord in man. Arch. Neuro. Psychopath. 3 (1900) 387−412.

16. Palace, J., V. Chandiramani, C. J. Fowler: Value of sphincter EMG in the diagnosis of Multiple System Atrophy. Neurogastroenterology & Motility (1996) in press.

17. Pavlakis, A. J., M. B. Siroky, I. Goldstein et al.: Neurologic findings in Parkinson's Disease. Journal of Urology 129 (1983) 80−83.

18. Staskin, D. S., Y. Vardi, M. A. Siroky: Post-prostatectomy incontinence in the parkinsonian patient: the significance of poor voluntary sphincter control. Journal of Urology 140 (1988) 117−118.

19. Sung, J. H., A. R. Mastri, E. Segal: Pathology of the Shy-Drager syndrome. J. Neuropathol. Exp. Neurol. 38 (1978) 253−268.

20. Valldeoriola, F., J. Valls-Sole, E. Tolosa et al.: Striated anal sphincter denervation in patients with progressive supranuclear palsy. Movement Disorders 10 (1995) 550−555.

21. Wenning, G., Y. Shlomo, M. Magalhaes et al.: Clinical features and natural history of multiple system atrophy. Brain 117 (1994) 835−845.

Cardiac dysautonomia in patients with symptomatic small volume prostatic benign hyperplasia

W. Artibani, F. Bellavere, A. Calpista, F. Carraro, A. Ruffato,
R. Piazza, E. Pescatori

Introduction

Roos et al. published in 1989 [9] an interesting paper on the mortality and reoperation rate after open and transurethral resection of the prostate (TURP) for benign prostatic hyperplasia (BPH). This was a retrospective study of 54,000 prostatectomies, based on insurance claims data in Manitoba, Oxford and Denmark. An increased risk of death from cardiovascular disease was reported 90 days, 1, 5 and 8 years after TURP compared with open operation.

This observation raised a lot of debate among the urologic community. The easier criticism was the possible existence of a main selection bias related to comorbidity, assuming that patients undergoing TURP had more comorbidity than those undergoing open prostatectomy.

In a second study published in 1990 [5] Malenka reexamined the data base for Manitoba using an extensive set of chart-based indicators to measure health status. Even including the issue of comorbidity in the analysis, the final results were unchanged being the risk of dying 5 years postoperatively 1.5 times greater for patients undergoing TURP than open prostatectomy.

Longterm mortality after TURP has therefore become a hot topic. A large cooperative prospective randomized clinical trial on the treatment of BPH is in progress under the patronage of the American Urological Association, being the issue of longterm mortality after TURP central to the study [7].

The following comments from Neal [8] seem to be plenty of common sense and they are not easy to disagree with: "The idea that a TURP lasting 40 minutes could cause a fatal heart attack 8 years later is not easy to accept. ... Is it really possible that factors such hypovolemia, hypothermia, hypotension, glycine absorption, hyperammonemia, hyponatremia or sepsis could cause subtle metabolic disturbances leading to permanent cardiac damage?" Nevertheless some possible explanations have been proposed. Evans et al. [4] very elegantly demonstrated hemodynamic evidence for cardiac stress during TURP related to rapid central cooling, and prevention of cardiac stress keeping the patients warm.

A different way to look at the problem is to focus on patients who are candidate to TURP, rather than to accuse TURP itself. Patients undergoing TURP usually have small prostates and it seems reasonable to wonder whether a 10 grams BPH is the same disease as a 100 grams BPH [10]. In fact, small BPH may be more precociously and intensively symptomatic and the outflow obstruction has been shown to be more frequent and more pronounced, even though most studies have not shown any statistical correlation between prostate size and symptoms severity or degree of obstruction. A small BPH can be very disabling while a very large BPH can develop without generating symptoms.

Hinman Jr. [5] suggested the hypothesis that, using his own words, "might patients with symptomatic small prostates have greater sympathetic activity than those with relaxed large prostates, activity that also stimulates the heart?" A way of looking at this hypothesis is to consider the role of the so-called cardiac autonomic dysfunction or cardiac dysautonomia [3]. Cardiac dysauto-nomia is an important expression of autonomic neuropathy and can be the cause of unexpected death mainly due to painless myocardial infarction. Experts on diabetic autonomic neuropathy have identified cardiac dysautonomia as a very poor prognostic indicator in diabetes. This cardiac dysfunction can be accurately diagnosed and may be present independently from diabetes [1−3].

Aim and design of the study

The aim of this study was to test the hypothesis that patients with symptomatic small volume BPH may have cardiac autonomic dysfunction. This was a prospective study comparing the results of cardiovascular autonomic tests in patients with small volume BPH candidate to TURP, to the results obtained in age-matched asymptomatic subjects.

Material and methods

The inclusion criteria were the following: a patient candidate to TURP on the basis of routine clinical evaluation, aged 45 to 65 years, with a sonographic volume of the prostate less than 40 grams.

The exclusion criteria included: hypertension under medical treatment, diabetes, history of cardiac disease and previous myocardial infarction.

The following cardiovasular autonomic tests were used: LS, SL2, DB, VR and power spectral analysis. They consist in the analysis of beat to beat variations after different manoeuvers. LS (lying to standing) measures the R-R interval at beats 15 and 30 after standing and is expressed at the 30/15 ratio. SL2 (standing

Table 1: *Patients characteristics.*

	mean	SD
age (years)	56.3	11.7
sonographic volume of the prostate (g)	29.2	5.9
I-PSS	14.5	5.6
L	3.3	1.3

legenda:
I-PSS: international prostatic symptoms score.
L: quality of life index.

to lying) is a test proposed by Bellavere et al. [2] measuring the immediate heart rate response to lying down. DP (deep breathing) measures the differences between maximum and minimum heart rates over one minute when breathing deeply at 6−8 breaths per minute. VR (Valsalva ratio) measures the reaction following a standardized forced expiration against resistance, expressing it as the ratio of the longest R-R interval after the manoeuvre to the shortest R-R interval during the manoeuvre.

Power spectral analysis of heart-rate variations [1] provides the possibility of examining the functioning of autonomic pathways through breakdown into two frequency bands and of their effects on heart-rate cyclic variability.

50 BPH patients and 15 age-matched asymptomatic subjects were enrolled in the study. The patients' characteristics are presented in Table 1.

Statistical evaluation: the comparison of group means was conducted with the Student t test for paired and unpaired data, with 0.05 as the significant level (2 sided).

Results

The results are reported in Tables 2 and 3. They showed a statistically significant difference between control group and BPH patients regarding LS, SL2, DB and the low frequency band of power spectral analysis.

Adopting the normal values proposed by Ewing, 34% of BPH patients had a clearly abnormal (below 2 SD) DB test and 12% a clearly abnormal LS test.

Comment

Patients with symptomatic small volume BPH candidate to TURP showed altered cardiovascular tests in comparison with a normal control group. These results were unexpected and very exciting.

Table 2: *Differences in LS, SL2, DB and VR between study group and control group.*

	control group M (SD)		symptomatic BPH M (SD)		P	
number	15		50			
age	56.3	(11.7)	59.2	(5.4)	0.18	ns
LS	1.229	(0.156)	1.101	(0.063)	0.000015	***
SL2	1.356	(0.133)	1.285	(0.104)	0.034	*
DB	23.5	(9.3)	18.6	(6.7)	0.029	*
VR	1.75	(0.31)	1.60	(0.27)	0.089	ns

legenda:
LS = Lying to standing.
SL2 = Standing to lying.
DB = Deep breathing.
VR = Valsalva ratio.

Table 3: *Power spectral analysis on lying.*

		control group M (SD)		symptomatic BPH M (SD)		P	
low frequency	LF	551	(660)	257	(259)	0.012	*
	Lfu	57.9	(21.7)	59.3	(24.8)	0.84	ns
high frequency	HF	243	(278)	211	(445)	0.79	ns
	Hfu	33.1	(16.9)	28.8	(18.9)	0.43	ns
ratio	LF/HF	2.96	(3.02)	6.54	(14.39)	0.34	ns

The clinical relevance of our observations is at present impossible to say, and we are strictly following this cohort of patients.

However, we have now a working hypothesis to explain a fatal heart attack 8 years after TURP for small symptomatic BPH.

References

1. Bellavere, F., I. Balzani, G. De Masi et al.: Power spectral analysis of heart-rate variations improves assessment of diabetic autonomic neuropathy. Diabetes 41 (1992) 633.
2. Bellavere, F., D. J. Ewing: Autonomic control of the immediate heart rate response to lying down. Cli. Sci. 62 (1982) 57.
3. Bellavere, F., M. Ferri, L. Guarini et al.: Prolonged QT period in diabetic autonomic neuropathy: a possible role in sudden cardiac death? Br. Heart J. 59 (1988) 379.
4. Evans, J. W., M. Singer, S. S. Coppinger et al.: Prevent cardiac stress during TURP — Keep the patients warm. J. Urol. (1993) AUA abstr 436, 322A.
5. Hinman, F. Jr.: Neural control of the prostate and surgical outcome. AUA Today (1991).

6. Malenka, D. J., N. Ross, E. S. Fisher et al.: Further study of the increased mortality following transurethral prostatectomy: a chart-based analysis. J. Urol. 144 (1990) 224.
7. Mebust, W. K.: Transurethral prostatectomy: AUA Update Series, Lesson 18 (1994) 142.
8. Neal, D. E.: Prostatectomy — An Open or Closed Case. Br. J. Urol. 66 (1990) 449.
9. Roos, N. P., J. E. Wennberg, D. J. Malenka et al.: Mortality and reoperation rate after open and transurethral resection of the prostate for benign prostatic hyperplasia. New Engl. J. Med. 320 (1989) 1120.
10. Steg, A.: Transurethral versus open prostatectomy. Do these procedures apply to the Same patients and the same disease? Eur. Urol. 20 (1991) 173.

Management of gastrointestinal alterations in Parkinson's disease

F. Stocchi

Sir James Parkinson in his classic 1817 monograph already described gastrointestinal dysfunction in the patients with shaking palsy: "… food is with difficulty retained in the mouth until masticated; and then as difficultly swallowed … the saliva fails of being directed to the back part of the fauces, and hence is continually draining from the mouth … the bowels which all along had been torpid, now in most cases, demand stimulating medicines of very considerable power: the expulsion of the faeces from the rectum sometimes requiring mechanical aid" [27]. Nowadays many authors had clearly described systemic symptoms in patients with Parkinson's disease (PD) and other parkinsonisms [9, 10, 11]. These symptoms and dysfunction not only are very distressing for the patients but interfere with the treatment of their disease. In this chapter gastrointestinal dysfunction in parkinsonism, the interference with treatment and tricks to overcome the problems are reviewed.

The majority of the parkinsonian patients depend for their motility and daily living from the blood level of dopaminergic drugs. These drugs have a short half life, consequently each single tablet ensures the patient few hours of freedom which are obtained after the tablet has been absorbed and has produced a sufficient blood level to be effective. Thus, before being effective, the tablet must be swallowed by the patient, it must pass through the oesophagus and the stomach. Then, with gastric contents absorbed from the small gut, it then enters the blood stream and from the blood into the brain through the blood brain barrier (Fig. 1). Therefore any dysfunction of the gastrointestinal system may contribute to erratic absorption of dopaminergic drugs with delayed or unpredictable clinical response to oral medications.

Swallowing abnormalities and oesophageal alterations

Dysphagia and a variety of swallowing abnormalities are well-recognised complications of PD (Table 1) Logemann et al. reported abnormal lingual control of swallowing [20]. Blonsky et al. described lingual festination in which the elevated tongue prevented passage of the bolus into the pharynx [3]. Longemann et al. and Robbins et al. discussed a delayed swallowing reflex and noted aspiration [19]. Bushmann et al. reported a repetitive and involuntary reflux

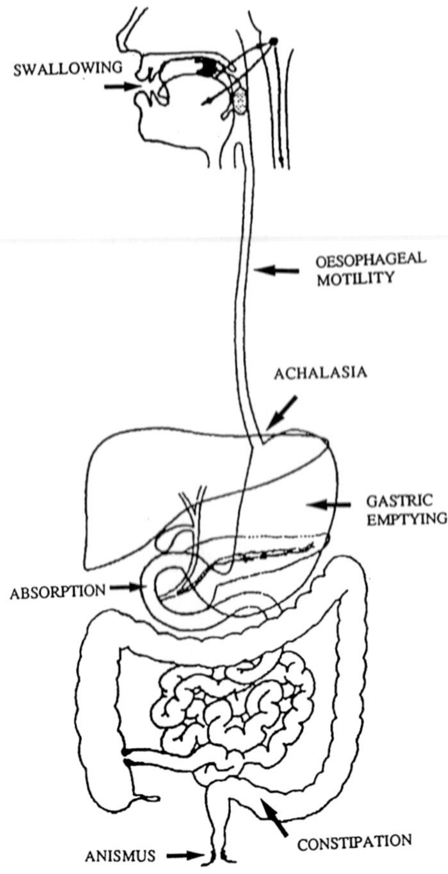

Fig. 1: *Gastrointestinal dysfunction which may interfere with treatment of parkinsonism.*

Table 1: *Swallowing abnormalities.*

- Disturbed lingual peristalsis
- Piecemeal swallowing
- Vallecular and piriform sinus residue
- Coating of pharyngeal walls
- Decreased relaxation of pharynx after swallow
- Increased oral transit time
- Bolus falling over base of tongue
- Vestibular aspiration
- Decreased laryngeal elevation
- Decreased oral mobility
- Drooling saliva

from the vallecula and piriform sinuses into the oral cavity. They also observed that some patients have great difficulty swallowing pills with retention in the vallecula for long periods of time [5]. Dopaminergic drugs may improve swallowing, although not consistently for all patients [6]. On the contrary anticholinergics may impair swallowing.

The main oesophageal alterations in parkinsonian patients consist in non peristaltic contractions, belching, segmental spasms, oesophageal dilatation, gastrooesophageal reflux [12]. Belching can be relatd to "ON−OFF" fluctuations [14], therefore it disappears when the patients turn "ON" (motile state). Bramble et al. suggested that cholinergic rather than dopaminergic mechanisms are more important in the control of oesophageal motility in parkinsonian patients. They showed that intravenous atropine produced marked disruption of co-ordination in response to swallows in patients with PD when compared with control subjects [4]. Therefore anticholinergic drugs may worsen co-ordination in response to swallows.

Patients with swallowing or/and oesophageal alterations may benefit from the use of liquid formulation of levodopa (levodopa methyl-esther, dispersible madopar) [29] or from the subcutaneous injections of the dopamine receptor agonist apomorphine [26]. Anticholinergic drugs should be withdrawn but, in some patients with severe drooling of saliva, peripheral anticholinergic belladonna folium may be useful. However drooling saliva is not related to salivary hypersecretion but rather to pooling of saliva within the mouth as a consequence of impaired deglutition [8].

Some patients present motor dysfunctions resembling oesophageal achalasia, which may be treated with the usual modalities or, as recently reported, with botulinum toxin injection into the cardia.

Stomach

Levodopa (L-dihydroxyphenilalanine) is a large neutral amino acid (LNAA) and furthermore is not absorbed from the stomach, which nonetheless plays an important role controlling the access of levodopa to its absorptive sites in the small bowel. It has been demonstrated that in parkinsonian patients a levodopa tablet may remain in the stomach for a very long time without clinical effect. Factors that delay gastric emptying also delay and blunt peak plasma levodopa levels and may cause a delay or a complete failure of the clinical response to the dose [2]. When levodopa is taken after meals it may be poorly absorbed probably for the delayed gastric emptying related to meal characteristics such as bulk caloric contents, and composition [7, 13]. Lipids but also some drugs like dopamine agonists or anticholinergics delay gastric emptying. Excessive gastric acidity also delays gastric emptying but neutralisation of stomach contents may lead to incomplete dissolution of the levodopa tablets and thus incomplete absorption [17]. Gastric emptying may be also delayed by PD itself or by constipation because of the cologastric reflex.

Many authors have shown that the direct infusion of liquid levodopa into the duodenum ensures a more reliable and predictable response to the drug [28]. Moreover the levodopa plasma levels after intraduodenal infusion are much more stable than after intragastric infusion [16]. These studies indicate the relevant role of the stomach in the pathophysiology of motor fluctuations in parkinsonian patients. Levodopa is absorbed only from the small bowel (mainly in the duodenum, but there is some absorption in the jejunum and ileum) which contains large neutral amino acid (LNAA) transporters and because of their high capacity, the competition between levodopa and other dietary LNAAs (e. g., valine, leucine and isolucine) is limited although it may occur [31].

Other common gastric symptoms in parkinsonian patients are epigastric fullness, bloating and vomiting.

Liquid levodopa may improve patients with motor fluctuations ensuring a better absorption. Levodopa methyl-esther and dispersible madopar are absorbed more quickly than standard levodopa preparation especially when the drug is taken after meals [29]. Subcutaneous infusion of dopamine agonists (apomorphine and lisuride) [30] are very effective in controlling motor fluctuations bypassing the gastrointestinal tract. Parkinsonian patients should be taught to eat small meals and avoid protein during the day and to take the drugs when fasting. Domperidone and cisapride may be helpful in some patients.

Bowel

Both symptoms and radiological signs suggestive of small intestine motor dysfunction in PD have been reported but the frequency and the functional significance of some of these findings remain uncertain (Table 2).

As far as large bowel is concerned, symptoms and signs are more evident and their frequency is high in the PD population (Table 3) [15, 18]. Constipation is

Table 2: *Small bowel dysfunctions.*

- Distension
- Colic
- Diarrhoea secondary to bacterial overgrowth
- Malnutrition secondary to bacterial overgrowth

Table 3: *Large bowel dysfunctions.*

- Distension
- Colic
- Constipation
- Spurious diarrhoea
- Anismus
- Megacolon
- Sigmoid volvulus

by far the most frequent symptom referred by PD patients and may be the result of several dysfunctions. For stool expulsion to occur, faecal material must first be propelled through the colon by colonic muscle contraction and then expelled through the coordinated actions of the rectum, anal sphincters, and pelvic floor muscles, as well as the musculature of the abdominal wall and diaphragm [23]. In parkinsonism constipation is due to colon inertia or to outlet-type dysfunction or both [1, 21, 22]. In colonic inertia the ineffective musculature induces a slow transit of feces through the colon [1, 25]. The outlet-type dysfunction is mainly due to the inability of the patients to relax the pelvic floor and therefore to straighten the anorectal angle [23, 24]. Sometimes paradoxical anal sphincter muscle contraction resembling anismus type pelvic outlet obstruction may occur too [24]. Therefore continuing to use laxatives in patients who cannot achieve effective defecation due to pelvic floor dystonia will only produce adverse effects from the laxatives and further increase the patients' frustration. The difficulty to relax the pelvic floor is a common symptom in severe parkinsonian patients and it generally responds to dopaminergic drugs [23]. Paradoxical EMG activity in anal sphincter muscles tends to persist even in "ON" phase. However, a definite improvement in pelvic outlet obstruction has been demonstrated with proctography after apomorphine administration [23]. Therefore the patients should make attempts to defecate when "ON" or use rapidly acting drugs (levodopa methyl-esther or apomorphine) before starting defecation. Unfortunately some patients still experience difficulty defecating when motor disability had otherwise been reversed by dopaminergic drugs. In these patients the injection of botulinum toxin in the puburectalis muscle and/ or in the external and sphincter may be useful. Botulinum toxin injection may be used also in those patients with painful anismus type dystonia.

Laxatives are useful in patients with normal pelvic floor relaxation.

References

1. Arhan, P., G. Devroede, G. Jehannin et al.: Segmental colon transit time. Dis. Colon Rectum 24 (1981) 625–629.

2. Baruzzi, A., M. Contin, R. Riva et al.: Influence of meal ingestion time on pharmacokinetics of orally administered levodopa in parkinsonian patients. Clin. Neuropharmacol. 10 (1987) 527–537.

3. Blonsky, E. R., J. A. Logemann, B. Boshes et al.: Comparison of speech and swallowing function in patients with tremor disorders and in normal geriatric patients: a cinefluorographic study. J. Gerontol. 30 (1975) 299–303.

4. Bramble, M. G., J. Cunliffe, W. Dellipiani: Evidence for a change in neurotransmitter affecting oesophageal motility in Parkinson's disease. J. Neurol Neurosurg. Psychiatry 41 (1978) 709–712.

5. Bushmann, M., S. M. Dobmeyer, L. Leeker et al.: Swallowing abnormalities and their response to treatment in Parkinson's disease. Neurology 39 (1989) 1309–1314.

6. Calne, D. B., D. G. Shaw, A. S. D. Spiers et al.: Swallowing in parkinsonism. Br. J. Radiol. 43 (1970) 456–457.

7. Dubois, A.: Diet and gastric digestion. Am. J. Clin. Nutr. 42 (1985) 1002–1005.

8. Eadie, M. J., J. H. Tyrer: Alimentary disorders in parkinsonism. Aust. Ann. Med. 14 (1965) 13–22.

9. Edwards, L. L., E. M. M. Quigley, R. F. Pfeiffer: Gastrointestinal dysfunction in Parkinson's disease: Frequency and pathophysiology. Neurology 42 (1992) 726–732.

10. Edwards, L. L., R. F. Pfeiffer, E. M. M. Quidley et al.: Gastrointestinal symptoms in Parkinson's disease. Mov. Disord. 6 (1991) 151–156.

11. Edwards, L. L., E. M. M.Quigley, R. Hofman et al.: Gastrointestinal symptoms in Parkinson's disease: 18-month follow-up study. Mov. Disord. 8 (1993) 83–86.

12. Gibberd, F. B., J. A. Gleeson, A. A. R. Gossage et al.: Oesophageal dilatation in Parkinson's disease. J. Neurol. Neurosurg. Psychiatry 37 (1974) 938–940.

13. Kelly, K. A.: Motility of the stomach and gastroduodenal junction. In: L. R. Johnson (Ed.): Physiology of the gastrointestinal tract. Raven Press, New York 1981.

14. Kempster, P. A., A. J. Lees, P. Crichton et al.: Off-period belching due to a reversible disturbance of oesophageal motility in Parkinson's disease and its treatment with apomorphine. Mov. Disord. 4 (1989) 47–52.

15. Kupsky, W. J., M. M. Grimes, J. Sweeting et al.: Parkinson's disease and megacolon: concentric hyaline inclusions (Lewy bodies) in enteric ganglionic cells. Neurology 37 (1987) 1253–1255.

16. Kurlan, R., K. P. Rothfield, W. R. Woodward et al.: Erratic gastric emptying of levodopa may cause "random" fluctuations of parkinsonian mobility. Neurology 38 (1988) 419–421.

17. Leon, A. S., H. Speigel: The effect of antacid administration on the absorption and metabolism of levodopa. J. Clin. Pharmacol. 12 (1972) 263–267.

18. Lewitan, A., L. Nathanson, W. R. Slade: Megacolon and dilatation of the small bowel in Parkinsonism. Gastroenterology 17 (1952) 367–374.

19. Logemann, J. A., B. Boshes, E. R. Blonsky et al.: Speech and swallowing evaluation in the diagnosis of neurologic disease. IVth Am. Congress Neurol. 18 (1975) 71–78.

20. Logemann, J. A., E. R. Blonsky, B. Boshes: Lingual control in Parkinson's disease. Trans. Am. Neurol. Assoc. 98 (1973) 276–278.

21. Lubowski, D. Z., M. Swash, M. Henry: Neural mechanisms in disorders of defecation. Baillieres Clin. Gastroenterol. 2 (1988) 210–223.

22. Martelli, H., G. Devroede, P. Arhan et al.: Mechanisms of idiopathic constipation: outlet obstruction. Gastroenterology 75 (1978) 623–631.

23. Mathers, S. E., P. A. Kempster, P. J. Law et al.: Anal sphincter dysfunction in Parkinson's disease. Arch. Neurol. 46 (1989) 1061–1064.

24. Mathers, S. E., P. A. Kempster, M. Swash et al.: Constipation and paradoxical puborectalis contraction in anismus and Parkinson's disease: a dystonic phenomenon? J. Neurol. Neurosurg. Psychiatry 51 (1988) 1503–1507.

25. McLean, R. G., R. C. Smart, D. Gaston-Perry et al.: Colon transit scintigraphy in health and constipation using oral I-131-cellulose. J. Nucl. Med. 31 (1990) 985–989.
26. Muguet, D., E. Broussolle, G. Chazot: Apomorphine in patients with Parkinson's disease. Biomed. Pharmacother. 49 (1995) 197–209.
27. Parkinson, J.: An essay on the shaking palsy. Whittingham and Rowland, London 1817.
28. Ruggieri, S., F. Stocchi, A. Carta et al.: Jejunal delivery of L-dopa methyl ester. The Lancet xii (1989) 45–46.
29. Steiger, M. J., F. Stocchi, L. Bramante et al.: The clinical efficacy of single morning doses of levodopa methyl-esther, dispersible madopar and sinemet plus in Parkinson's disease. Clin. Neuropharmacol. 15 (1992) 501–504.
30. Stocchi, F., S. Ruggieri, F. Viselli et al.: Subcutaneous lisuride infusion. In: J. P. W. F. Lakke, E. M. Delhaas, A. W. F. Rutgers (Eds.): New trends in clinical neurology: parenteral drug therapy in spasticity and Parkinson's disease. The Parthenon Publishing group, USA 1992.
31. Wade, D. N., P. T. Mearrik. D. J. Birkett et al.: Active transport of L-dopa in the intestine. Nature 242 (1973) 463–465.

Management of swallowing disorders

R. Shaker, E. Bardan

Swallowing is a highly coordinated physiologic event that involves sequential
and overlapping contractions of the facial, cervical, oral, pharyngeal, laryngeal,
and esophageal muscular apparatus and results in transit of ingested material
and saliva from the mouth into the stomach.

For descriptive purposes, swallowing could be divided into four consecutive
phases: 1) preparatory, 2) oral, 3) pharyngeal, and 4) esophageal [5, 69]. These
phases merely represent the anatomic regions traversed by the bolus. During
the preparatory phase, for the most part, the bolus remains in the oral cavity,
undergoes physical and some chemical changes. Through the act of mastication
and mixing with saliva it develops suitable physical qualities for transit through
the aerodigestive tract. During this phase the bolus is sized, shaped and positioned on the dorsum of the tongue for initiation of the oral phase of swallowing.

During the oral phase, sequential squeeze of the tongue against the hard and
soft palate generates a peristaltic pressure wave [78] that propels the bolus from
the oral cavity into the pharynx.

During the pharyngeal phase, the pharynx, upper esophageal sphincter (UES)
and larynx [1] become elevated, and three of the four routes connected to the
pharynx, namely nasal cavity, oral cavity and larynx [84, 97, 98], become sealed
off while the fourth route, the upper esophageal sphincter opens and the bolus
is transported into the esophagus by rapid forceful posterior tongue movement
(thrust) continued from the oral phase, as well as the peristaltic contraction of
the pharyngeal constrictors against the soft palate, base of the tongue, and the
larynx. During oropharyngeal swallow the nasopharynx is sealed by contraction of the superior pharyngeal constrictor and elevation of soft palate and
its contact with the posterior pharyngeal wall (vela pharyngeal closure). The
oral cavity is closed by elevation of the tongue base and its contact with the
hard and soft palate [2]. During the oropharyngeal swallow, important biomechanical events involving intrinsic glottic, as well as supra- and infrahyoid
muscles, take place that result in the closure of the airway [16, 79], as well as
in the opening of the upper esophageal sphincter [13, 47] (Fig. 1). These events
include adduction of the true vocal cords and arytenoids (first tier of airway
closure) followed by vertical approximation of the adducted arytenoids to the
base of epiglottis (second tier of closure) (Fig. 2) followed by the descent of the
epiglottis covering the closed glottis thereby closing the laryngeal vestibule

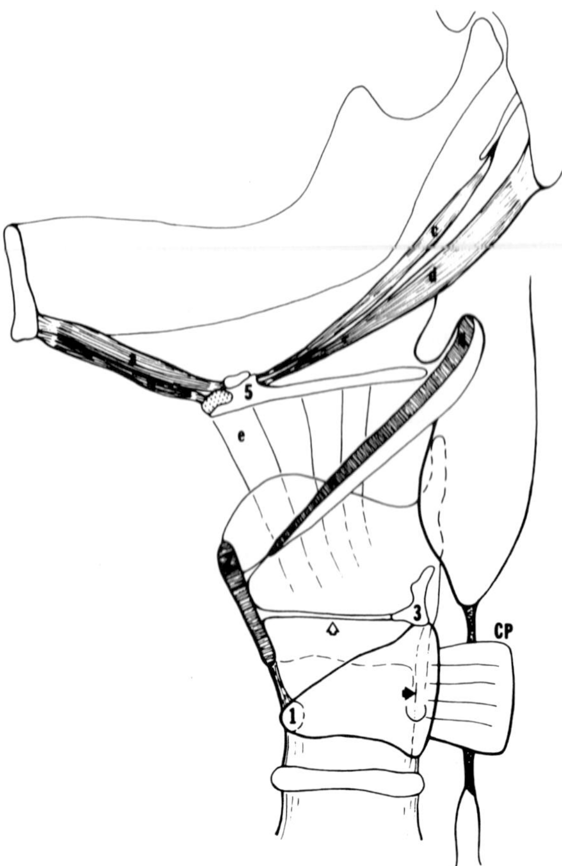

Fig. 1: *Schematic representation of suspension of hyoid and larynx. Hyoid (5) is suspended from mandible and skull by four suprahyoid muscles: anterior pair − geniohyoid (b) and anterior digastric (a); posterior pair − stylohyoid (c) and posterior digastric (d). These muscles generate a superior and anterior movement of hyoid during swallowing. Larynx is attached to hyoid by paired thyroglossus muscles (e) and thyrohyoid membrane (not shown). Larynx consists of following cartilages: epiglottic (4), thyroid (2), cricoid (1), and arytenoid (3). Epiglottis is attached anteriorly to thyroid cartilage, just superior to ventral attachment of vocal cords (open arrow) on thyroid cartilage. Posteriorly, vocal cords attach to vocal process of arytenoids. Arytenoids sit on superior margin of cricoid plate. Posterior border of trachea is indicated by solid arrow. Just below this arrow is a hinge joint between inferior cornu of thyroid cartilage and cricoid cartilage. Shortening of cricothyroid muscle (not shown) approximates anterior thyroid cartilage to anterior rim of cricothyroid muscle. This movement passively tenses vocal cords and tucks introitus of laryngeal vestibule ventrally under free margin of epiglottis. During swallowing, larynx makes a superoanterior excursion because of its attachment to hyoid. Thyrohyoid muscles (e) contract so that larynx approximates and becomes locked to hyoid. Thus, superior movement of the larynx exceeds that of the hyoid. Shortening of the thyrohyoid muscles also rotates epiglottis into a horizontal position. Because of its attachment to cricoid, cricopharyngeus (CP) moves superiorly about 1.5 cm during swallow-induced orad excursion of larynx.*
Reproduced by permission from Dodds et al. [20].

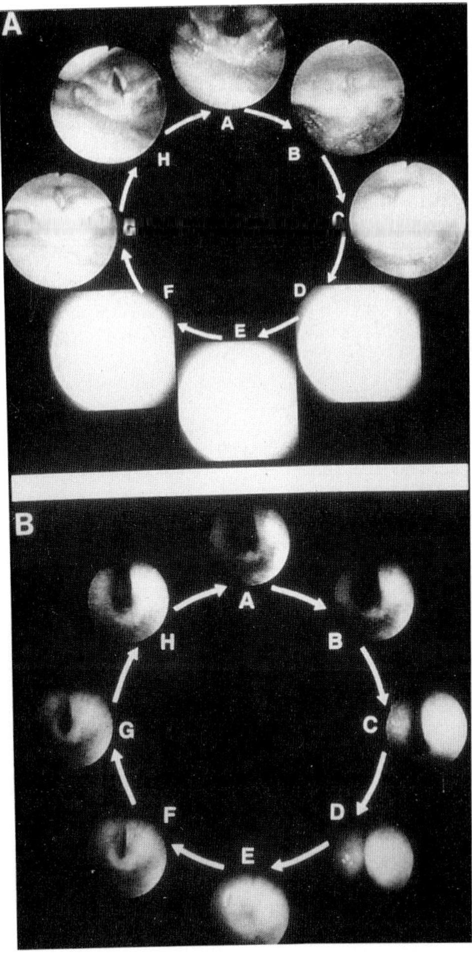

Fig. 2: *Examples of still frames of deglutitive vocal cord closure seen by transnasal videoendoscopy in (A) a normal volunteer and (B) by transtracheal videoendoscopy in a patient with tracheostomy. (A) (A) Glottis immediately before initiation of swallow. Vocal cords are open at their resting position. (B) Complete deglutitive vocal cord and arytenoid adduction. (C) Adducted arytenoids have approximated the base of the epiglottis. (D–F) Obscured view because of pharyngeal contraction and laryngeal elevation. (G) Vocal cords can be seen still adducted following the descent of the larynx and opening of the pharynx after passage of the bolus. (H) Vocal cords are beginning to open at the completion of swallow. (B) (A) Inferior view of glottis at rest. The introitus to the trachea is wide open immediately before the initiation of swallow. (B and C) Vocal cords are in the process of adduction narrowing the introitus. (D) Cords are in contact with each other in the anterior part. However, the posterior gap is still open. (E) Posterior gap is now closed, resulting in complete closure of the introitus to the trachea. (F) Posterior gap is partially reopened while anterior part of the cords are still in contact. (G and H) Cords are further opened returning to resting position. Please note that contrary to the transnasal view, in the transtracheal view, the introitus to the trachea remained visible during the entire period of swallowing.*
Reproduced by permission from Shaker et al. [80].

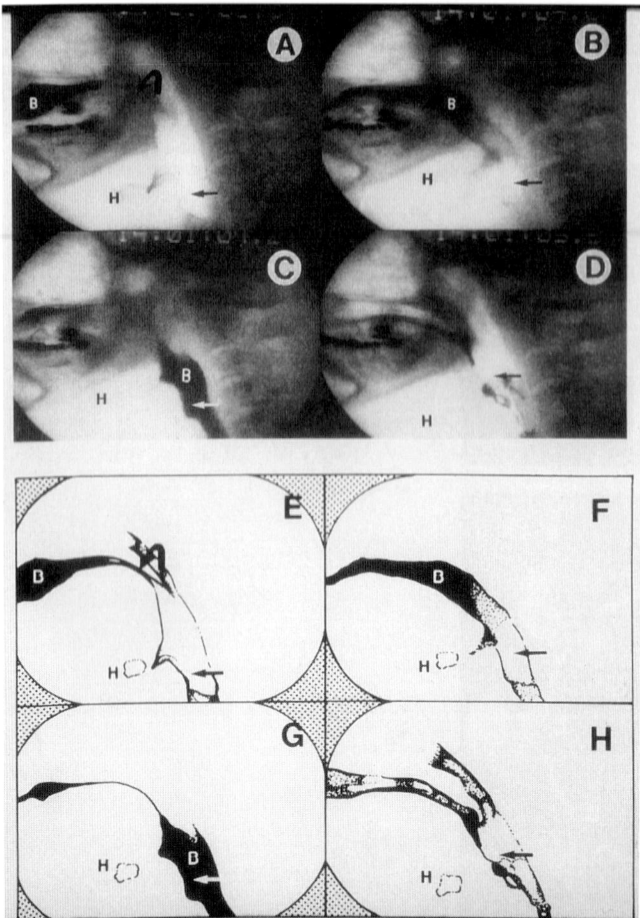

Fig. 3: *Example of the sequence of events during primary swallows. The primary swallow (A–D) resulted in bolus transport from the mouth into the pharynx and esophagus. B, barium bolus; H hyoid bone. Straight arrows indicate pharyngeal lumen. (A and E) Bolus of 5 ml of barium is held in the oral cavity immediately before the onset of swallowing. Tongue base and soft palate are in contact (curved arrow), segregating the oral bolus from the pharyngeal cavity. (B and F) Tongue base is depressed and soft palate has elevated and is in contact with the posterior pharyngeal wall. This resulted in closing off the nasopharynx and allowing the bolus to enter the pharynx. (C and G) Bolus traversing the pharynx while the nasopharynx and oral cavity are sealed off by approximation of the soft palate and posterior pharyngeal wall and apposition of the tongue base and soft palate, respectively. The hyoid bone has moved upward and forward. (D and H) The barium bolus has cleared the pharynx, the oral cavity and nasopharynx are open, and the larynx and hyoid bone have returned to the resting position.*
Reproduced by permission from Shaker et al. Gastroenterology 107 (1994) 396–401.

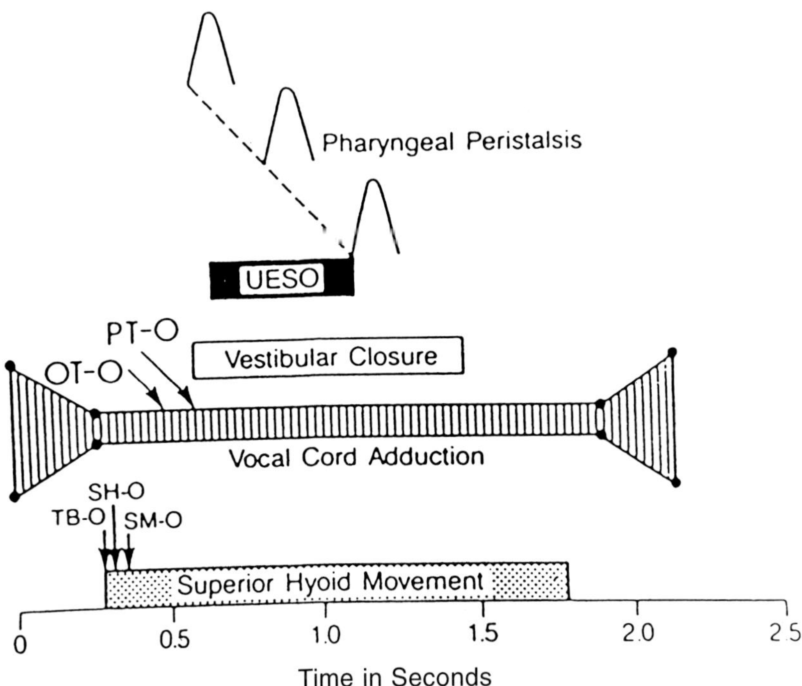

Fig. 4: *Relationship of deglutitive vocal cord kinetics to other events of the oropharyngeal phase of swallowing during 5-ml barium swallows. Bolus transit through the pharynx and across the UES begins and ends while the vocal cords are at maximal adduction. TB-O: onset of tongue base movement; SH-O: onset of superior hyoid movement; SM-O: onset of submental myoelectrical activity; UESO, UES opening; OT-O, onset of bolus movement from the mouth; PT-O: arrival of bolus into pharynx.*
Reproduced by permission from Shaker at al. Semin. Gastrointest. Dis. 3(3) (1992) 115—128.

(third tier of closure) beginning with vocal cords closure or shortly afterwards, the entire larynx is pulled upwards and forward by the contraction of the suprahyoid muscle group. This displacement results in the positioning of the closed larynx under the tongue base away from the path of the bolus, thereby providing additional protection against aspiration it also helps closing the laryngeal vestibule [17, 27, 63] (Fig. 3).

During oropharyngeal swallowing, the UES transiently relaxes and subsequently is pulled upward/forward by the contraction of the same suprahyoid muscles that displace the larynx. This traction results in active opening of the UES which is also modified by the bolus size [13, 47]. The temporal relationship of the events that take place during the oropharyngeal phase of swallowing is shown in Fig. 4. As seen under normal conditions [79], oropharyngeal swallowing begins with the vocal cords closure signifying the activation of airway protection, and ends when the cords return to their resting positions. During this time the respiration is reflexively inhibited [12, 48, 49, 88, 90].

During the esophageal phase of swallowing the bolus is transported further into the esophagus and stomach.

From a functional point of view, events that take place during the oropharyngeal swallowing contribute to the following functions: 1) transit of the bolus, 2) protection of the airway. The transit and protective aspect of the oropharyngeal swallowing are highly coordinated and recent studies have shown that oropharyngeal transit occurs during the full activation of the protective aspect of swallowing [79]. A successful oropharyngeal swallow requires the effective and coordinated actions of the anatomical elements involved in these two functions. Normal oropharyngeal swallowing is therefore defined as complete transit of the ingested material from the mouth into the esophagus without compromising the airway. Oropharyngeal dysphagia may develop when the efficacy and/or coordination of either transport or protective aspect of oropharyngeal swallowing are compromised. The true prevalence of oropharyngeal dysphagia is not known. However, studies have shown a 50−60% prevalence in nursing homes [92] and 10−30% in general medical wards [37, 57]. In addition, a survey study estimated the prevalence of dysphagic symptoms at 6.9% in a midwestern population [91].

Neural control of swallowing

Neural controls of swallowing consist of three major parts: 1) sensory afferent fibers contained in the cranial nerves, 2) central organizing centers, 3) efferent motor fibers contained in the cranial nerves and ansa cervicalis.

Sensory afferent signals

Sensory afferent signals originated from the oral-pharyngeal cavity are carried by the branches of glossopharyngeal (IX) and vagus nerves (X) to the nucleus tractus solitarius (NTS) in the medulla. These afferent sensory fibers also carry sensory information from the pulmonary stretch receptors, as well as chemoreceptors located in carotid and aortic bodies. They are also used for the control of the respiratory system.

Central organizing center

The medulla oblongata houses paired swallowing centers responsible for processing afferent sensory signals and programming the motor swallowing sequences [22−24]. These centers are poorly defined areas and comprised of the nucleus tractus solitarius (NTS), ventromedian reticular formation (VMFR) and nucleus ambiguous (NA). There is increasing evidence that cortical structures have a significant influence on the brain stem swallowing centers [31, 39, 55, 56]. Cortical areas; in preorbital gyrus and lateral precentral gyrus, have been implicated to influence and modulate the deglutition. Cortical projections have been found connecting the cortical and medullary swallowing centers. Although poorly understood, some experimental evidence suggests the presence of a close functional, structural, and physiologic interaction between deglutitive and respiratory centers and their afferent and efferent inputs [65, 66, 90].

Motor efferent signals

Motor output to the muscular apparatus of the oropharynx for swallowing is transmitted by axons whose cell bodies are located in the brain stem swallowing centers. These include motor nucleus of trigeminal (V), facial (VII), and hypoglossal (XII) nerves. It also includes the nucleus ambiguous which not only consists of premotor commanding neurons, but also houses large motor neurons that are distributed to striated muscles innervated by glossopharyngeal (IX) and vagus (X) nerves.

Muscular apparatus of swallowing

A total of 30 paired striated muscles participate in oropharyngeal swallowing. The muscular apparatuses of oral pharyngeal swallowing and their innervation are shown in Table 1. In summary, the tongue is controlled by the cranial nerve XII and ansa cervicalis (C1−C2). Muscles of the palate, pharynx, larynx, and cricopharyngeus are mainly controlled by the vagus nerve. Supra and infrahyoid

Table 1: *Muscular apparatus of oral-pharyngeal swallowing.*

Muscle group	Innervation
Mandibular muscles	Mandibular branch of trigeminal nerve (V3)
Facial muscle	Facial nerve (VII)
Intrinsic tongue muscles	Hypoglossal nerve (XII)
Extrinsic tongue muscles (except palatoglossus, X)	Ansa cervicalis (C1, C2)
Soft palate (except tensor veli palatini, V3)	Vagus (X)
Pharyngeal muscles and cricopharyngeus (except stylopharyngeus, IXn.)	Vagus (X)
Intrinsic laryngeal muscles (except cricothyroid, SLN)	Vagus (X) recurrent laryngeal
Suprahyoid and infrahyoid muscles	V3, ansa cervicalis (C1, C2) and VII

muscles that provide deglutitive orad movement of the hyoid bone, larynx, and upper esophageal sphincter and induce opening of the UES following its relaxation are innervated by ansa cervicalis (C1−C2), V3, and VII.

Symptoms of oropharyngeal dysphagia

Except for silent aspirations that present with frequent pneumonia, most oropharyngeal dysphagia patients seek help because of symptoms. These symptoms reflect the abnormalities in transport or protective functions during oropharyngeal swallowing (Table 2). Dysphagia symptoms are highly specific and should not be labeled as functional or psychogenic. Although subtle, abnormalities may escape detection, every effort needs to be made to arrive at a diagnosis. In a study of 23 referred patients labeled as psychogenic dysphagia Ravich et al. were able to document an explanation for symptoms in 15 (65%) [34]. A frequently reported symptom is a sensation of inadequate clearance of the bolus from the pharynx: "food sticks in the throat". This sensation although may be caused by the presence of large residue in the pyriform sinus or valleculae, it may also be a referred sensation from obstruction of the distal esophagus. The strictures of the proximal esophagus may also present themselves with cervical symptoms. For this reason, in patients with complaint of cervical symptoms evaluation of esophagus must be a part of the dysphagia workup. Since inflammation, abrasion, or tumors of the hypopharyngeal area may produce the same sensation, a careful examination by direct visualization of this area has to be included in the workup. Swallow related coughing and/or choking due to misdi-

Table 2: *Symptoms of oral/pharyngeal dysphagia.*

Inability to keep the bolus in the oral cavity
Difficulty gathering the bolus in the back of the tongue
Hesitation or inability to initiate the swallow
Food sticking in the throat
Nasal regurgitation
Inability to propel the food bolus caudad into the pharynx
Difficulty swallowing solids
Frequent repetitive swallowing
Frequent throat clearing
Gargly voice after meal
Hoarse voice
Nasal speech and dysarthria
Swallow related cough: before, during, or after swallowing
Avoidance from social dining
Weight loss
Recurrent pneumonia

rection of the bolus into the airway is another common complaint. Invasion of the upper airway by the bolus may occur before initiation of, during or after completion of oropharyngeal swallowing [8] and cause coughing or choking sensation. Predeglutitive aspiration occurs when the bolus is lost from the mouth into the hypopharynx prematurely when swallowing has not yet been triggered and the airway is still open. This condition is commonly seen in post CVA dysphagic patients. These patients are frequently unable to segregate the oral bolus from the pharynx by apposition of their tongue base and soft palate, this condition results in premature spill and if pharyngeal sensation is deranged and swallowing is not initiated by entry of the bolus into the pharynx, it may result in predeglutitive aspiration. Deglutitive aspiration occurs due to incompetent or lack of closure of the glottis during swallowing sequence and the bolus invades the airway while being transported through the hypopharynx. Postdeglutitive aspiration develops when the bolus transport is incomplete and a large residue remains behind, in the pyriform sinus or valleculae at the end of the swallow sequence such as seen in Parkinsonism, post CVA, myasthenia gravis and multiple sclerosis. This large residue is either inhaled in or overflows into the trachea when the glottis opens and respiration is resumed.

Etiology of oropharyngeal dysphagia

Because of the variety of organs involved in oropharyngeal swallowing, dysphagia results from a large number of causes that may affect the muscular apparatus of the oropharynx and/or their related neuromuscular plate, peripheral, as well as central nervous systems [3, 21, 38, 42, 85]. These diseases may affect the oropharyngeal transport, deglutitive airway closure, or both. Table 3 lists a summary of the causes of oropharyngeal dysphagia. Neuromuscular diseases are responsible for approximately 80% of the cases while local structural lesions of the oropharynx account for the rest [25]. Oropharyngeal dysphagia has been reported in approximately 25% of adults following head injury, of which 94% have been reported to recover in about three months [96]. Oropharyngeal dysphagia also poses a significant clinical problem in post CVA patients. Abnormalities in this group include a variety of disturbances in the swallowing sequence such as: delay to initiate swallowing, diminished tongue control, and abnormalities of laryngeal closure [11, 94].

Malignancies of the head and neck account for approximately 10% of all the cancers in North America. The total number of newly diagnosed cases of head and neck cancer in the United States, excluding skin cancer, is estimated at 78,000. Relative frequencies of primary tumors at the anatomic sites are approximately as follows: 40% oral cavity, 25% larynx, 15% oro/hypopharynx, 27% major salivary gland, and 13% in the remaining sites. Age specific inci-

Table 3: *Causes of oral/pharyngeal dysphagia.*

Peripheral and central nervous system	Local structural lesions
Cerebrovascular accident	Surgical resection of oropharynx/larynx
Head injury	Oropharyngeal carcinoma
Parkinson's disease	Laryngeal carcinoma
Huntington's chorea	Zenker's diverticulum
Multiple sclerosis	Extrinsic compression:
Amyotrophic lateral sclerosis	Enlarged thyroid gland
CNS tumor	Senile ankylosing hyperostosis
Tabes dorsalis	of the cervical spine
Disorders of the central nervous system	Rheumatoid cricoarytenoid arthritis
(e. g., Alzheimer's disease)	Radiation injury
Bulbar poliomyelitis	Neuromuscular damage
Peripheral neuropathies	Salivary gland damage
Post traumatic	Cricopharyngeal abnormalities:
Friedreich spastic ataxia	Achalasia
Familial dysautonomia	Fibrosis
	Proximal esophageal webs and rings

Muscular/neuromuscular	Pharmacologic agents
Inflammatory muscle diseases	Antihistamines
Polymyositis	Anticholinergics
Dermatomyositis	Phenothiazines
Inclusion body myositis	
Muscular dystrophies (myotonic oculopharyngeal)	
Kearns-Sayre syndrome	
Metabolic myopathy (thyroid associated myopathy)	
Alcoholic myopathy	
Myasthenia gravis	

dence increases markedly after age 50 and male to female ratio is over 3 : 1 [71]. Surgical resection and/or radiation therapy in these patients results in considerable oropharyngeal dysphagia with significant management problems [30].

The cricopharyngeal muscle comprises the main component of the upper esophageal sphincter (UES) and its dysfunctions are becoming an increasingly recognized cause of dysphagia. In 1707, Valsalva proposed the designation cricopharyngeal (CP) muscle for the most distal muscle fibers of the pars cricopharyngea of the inferior pharyngeal constrictor, after he recognized its anatomical and functional identity [93].

Normal deglutitive UES opening is determined by 1) transient UES relaxation (i.e., loss of active cricopharyngeus tone), 2) persistence of minimal passive tension, namely, normal distensibility of the CP muscle, 3) active traction on the UES generated by anterior hyoid and laryngeal movement which, in turn, is induced by contraction of the suprahyoid muscles (i.e., geniohyoid and mylohyoid), and 4) pulsion forces imparted to the relaxed UES by oncoming pharyngeal bolus.

Abnormalities of either of these opening factors causes disordered UES opening which results in a compromised transsphincteric flow that comprises the pathophysiological basis for the majority of disorders of the UES.

Primary neurogenic cricopharyngeus muscle dysfunction includes cricopharyngeal achalasia and discoordination of UES relaxation and opening with pharyngeal peristalsis due to a variety of neurogenic causes such as: cerebrovascular hemorrhage, and Parkinson's disease. Primary myogenic cricopharyngeus dysfunction includes loss of elasticity as well as fibrotic changes of the UES that prevents its adequate opening during swallowing. A variety of causes, including gastroesophageal reflux and aging have been suggested to be responsible for these changes. Recently, a case of Crohn's disease involving the cricopharyngeus muscle, presenting as progressive dysphagia to solid food, has been reported [74]. In secondary cricopharyngeus dysfunction the pathology lies within the suprahyoid muscles, due to inflammatory change such as seen in myositis and inclusion body myositis. These patients are incapable of exerting adequate traction force to pull the UES open during swallowing. These patients typically lack normal laryngeal elevation. In this condition, excitatory impulses to the cricopharyngeal muscle are inhibited normally during swallowing and results in manometric relaxation of the UES, but the UES does not open adequately due to insufficient traction. Depending on the severity of the condition, patients suffering from UES dysfunction may present with aspiration pneumonia, swallow related cough, choking, repeated swallowing, food sticking in the throat, and weight loss.

Killian, in the early part of the century, suggested the discoordination between activities of the inferior pharyngeal constrictor and cricopharyngeus muscle as the cause of Zenker's diverticulum [50]. There is increasing evidence that inadequate opening or distensibility of the UES results in abnormally high intrabolus pressure (the pressure inside the bolus traveling ahead of the peristaltic wave). This increased intrabolus pressure seems to play a pathogenetic role in the development of Zenker's diverticulum. In a study of 14 patients with Zenker's diverticulum and dysphagia, Cook et al. reported a significant increase in intrabolus pressure along with a significant decrease in the area of the opening of the UES in patients compared to healthy controls [14]. The intrabolus pressure significantly decreased after cricopharyngeal myotomy [82]. Depending on the size of the symptomatic Zenker's diverticulum, the presenting symptom may range from pharyngeal dysphagia or gargling in the throat to regurgitation and aspiration [6]. It may result in halitosis, a trachael fistula, bleeding or it may harbor carcinomas.

Oropharyngeal dysphagia associated with the disruption of the normal laryngeal innervation ranges from minimal cough to severe frequent deglutitive aspiration with swallowing. These patients present with various degrees of hoarseness, aspiration pneumonia and weight loss. Etiology of the laryngeal paralysis includes insults to the recurrent and/or superior laryngeal nerve due to a variety of surgical procedures, inflammatory, and central nervous system diseases. An average of 10% of the laryngeal paralysis, however, is reported idiopathic [67].

Because of the proximity to the pharynx, symptomatic structural abnormalities of the most proximal portion of the esophagus may present with symptoms of cervical dysphagia.

These abnormalities include proximal esophageal rings that are usually reflux induced, but in rare instances they may be congenital. They may be complete or several incomplete rings arranged in a manner that result in luminal compromise. Dysphagia is usually for solid food. Cervical symptoms and choking develops when bolus impaction occurs. Diagnosis is confirmed with an esophagogram. Endoscopy and biopsy will determine the possible inflammatory nature of the ring as well as the status of the proximal esophagus. Reflux symptoms such as heartburn may be absent or minimal.

Proximal esophageal webs, as seen in Plummer−Vinson or Paterson, Brown, Kelly syndrome, occur in the upper 2−4 cm of the esophagus and are associated with iron deficiency anemia. Dysphagia is often associated with aspiration symptoms. There have been reports of an association between these webs and post cricoid carcinoma. Diagnosis is usually made by barium swallow study in lateral projection. Proximal esophageal webs may be associated with Zenker's diverticulum and graft versus host disease following bone marrow transplantation.

Proximal esophageal strictures may occur as the result of lye ingestion, nasogastric tube placement, and reflux disease. However, isolated involvement of the proximal esophagus is rare. If the proximal end of the stricture is close to the UES, patients may present with symptoms of cervical dysphagia.

Malignant strictures of the proximal esophagus induced by squamous cell carcinoma or adenocarcinoma in the setting of Barrett's esophagus will also present with symptoms of cervical dysphagia and need to be included in the differential diagnosis of any esophageal stricture.

Oral/pharyngeal dysphagia in degenerative neuronal diseases

A significant percent of patients with degenerative neuronal diseases experience difficulty swallowing. Although the exact prevalence of dysphagia in this group is not known, it has been reported to be between 18 and 89% in various diseases [9, 26, 32, 40, 41, 43, 45, 58, 59, 72, 89, 95]. Typically, dysphagia is more pronounced for liquid boluses than for solid food. They also experience difficulty swallowing crumbly material as well as boluses with high viscosity. Although the presenting symptoms are generally similar to dysphagic conditions caused by other pathologies, the objective finding on videofluoroscopic examination is mainly indicative of discoordination of lingual function, oral/pharyngeal bolus transit, inadequate pharyngeal constrictor function, discoordination between the transit and airway protective aspect of oral/pharyngeal phase of swallowing and abnormal upper esophageal sphincter opening (Table 4).

Initial evaluation

Oropharyngeal dysphagia (OPD) may result from a variety of abnormal conditions that extend across various disciplines. Diagnostic modalities, although in the majority of cases, will lead to the identification of a specific derangement in the oral or pharyngeal phases of swallowing, they rarely help in determination of the causative factors. Therefore, a multidisciplinary approach is needed, not only in identifying the cause or causes leading to OPD, but for its management. The approach to the OPD patient must be systematic. This starts with obtaining a detailed history of the problem, followed by a physical and neurological examination. Special attention has to be given to the concomitant disorders that may be responsible for oropharyngeal dysphagia such as thyroid disease, previous radiation therapy of the head and neck, neurologic disease or trauma, diabetes mellitus, Parkinson's disease, anemia, connective tissue diseases such as rheumatoid arthritis, scleroderma, Sicca syndrome, Raynaud's phenomenon, and rheumatologic diseases such as polymyositis, dermatomyositis, myotonia, and mysthenia gravis. History of recurrent pneumonia, weight loss, water and sour brash, regurgitation, and heartburn must be sought and a careful account of the use of medications including tranquilizers, ulcer, and cancer medications needs to be taken. Since some symptoms of oropharyngeal dysphagia, such as hoarseness, could be either due to unilateral paralysis of the cords or inflammation of the glottis due to frequent aspiration of food, correct diagnosis requires a thorough laryngologic examination. This, again, emphasizes the need for a multidisciplinary approach to the OPD patients. This team may consist of representatives from the following disciplines: 1) Gastroenterology, 2) Otolaryngology, 3) Radiology, 4) Dentistry, 5) Speech/Language Pathol-

Table 4: *Oral/pharyngeal dysphagia in neuronal diseases: videofluoroscopic findings.*

Parkinson's disease:
- abnormal lip control
- abnormal tongue control
- abnormal soft palate movement
- poor bolus manipulation/control
- abnormal triggering of pharyngeal phase
- incomplete pharyngeal clearance time
- tracheal aspiration

Dementia:
- lingual dysfunction
- abnormal bolus control
- discoordination of oral and pharyngeal phase
- epiglottal dysmotility
- pharyngeal constrictor paresis
- incomplete pharyngeal clearance
- incomplete UES opening
- aspiration

Closed head trauma:
- defective tongue control
- abnormal pharyngeal peristalsis
- abnormal laryngeal elevation/closure
- aspiration

Cerebrovascular accident:
- incomplete oral bolus clearance
- abnormal lingual function
- delayed pharyngeal phase
- pharyngeal residue
- aspiration

Multiple sclerosis:
- difficulty in mastication
- difficulty manipulating/control of bolus
- delay in pharyngeal phase
- impaired pharyngeal contraction/clearance
- aspiration

Post-polio syndrome:
- unilateral/bilateral tongue weakness
- pharyngeal paralysis (paresis)
- absent/incomplete epiglottic tilt
- poor laryngeal elevation
- poor laryngeal closure
- laryngeal penetration/aspiration
- incomplete UES opening

Huntington's disease:
- abnormal preparatory phase (mastication, bolus control)
- premature spill
- incomplete oral bolus clearance
- repetitive swallows
- lingual chorea
- tracheal aspiration
- discoordination of swallowing & breathing

Brainstem stroke:
- delayed initiation of swallow
- pharyngeal residue
- incomplete UES opening
- aspiration

Alzheimer's disease:
- abnormal preparatory phase
- abnormal initiation of pharyngeal phase
- defective pharyngeal clearance
- incomplete UES opening
- aspiration

Dysphagia is experienced more with:
- liquids (hot), than solids
- crumbly and high viscosity materials

ogy, and 6) Neurology. The role of individual members depends on the expertise available in respective institutions. However, the oropharyngeal dysphagia patient needs to be approached and cared for like any other patient by a single managing physician. Multidisciplinary working conferences to decide on diagnosis and management of unusual cases is most helpful.

Diagnostic modalities

The approach to the oropharyngeal dysphagia patient is evolving. Until recently, barium studies were the only modality available and used for evaluation of OPD patients. During the past decade, several other modalities such as: manometry, endoscopy, ultrasonography, and scintigraphy have been introduced to this field. Intense research via various disciplines is ongoing, making the approach to the oropharyngeal dysphagia patient a dynamic and improving phenomenon. Quantitative normalcy data are becoming available and study recordings and test substances are more standardized allowing interstudy comparison and better understanding of the results. With the advent of videorecorders and digitalization technology, endoscopic and fluoroscopic images are videotaped and analyzed later using the slow motion and frame-by-frame movements capability of the tape recorder. This technology allows the accurate timing of the events. Availability of specially designed timers allows synchronization of several investigative modalities. This synchronization allows determination of temporal relationship of various events such as bolus movement and airway closure during oropharyngeal swallowing. Since not all of the structures of the oropharynx during swallowing are adequately seen by one single modality, this multisystem recording is essential for studying the coordination of oropharyngeal swallowing events.

Modified barium swallow

Currently, videofluoroscopic recording of a modified barium swallow is the diagnostic modality of choice. During this study, recordings of a variety of boluses with different consistencies and volumes are made for subsequent analysis and these recordings are also used for future comparisons to evaluate progress. This technique not only provides adequate information about the movement of the barium bolus through the aerodigestive tract and documents misdirection of the bolus into the airway, it also provides vital information about the anatomy and function of the individual anatomical components of the aerodigestive tract and airway involved in swallowing [19, 62]. Additionally, this modality is used to evaluate the effect of various postural and breathing techniques on the efficiency, as well as safety, of swallowing [44, 60]. Normal and abnormal videofluoroscopic findings of swallowing (Table 5) have been published extensively [20, 29, 60]. On videofluoroscopy, abnormalities of the oral phase of swallowing manifest themselves as inadequate clearance of the barium bolus from the mouth leaving a barium residue behind, or piece-meal swallowing due to inadequate tongue function, or difficulty initiating the swallowing sequence due to impaired cognitive, or neural function [19, 60]. Patients with difficulty controlling the labial or facial muscles will not be able to hold the

Table 5: *Abnormalities of the oropharyngeal phase of swallowing (seen by videofluoroscopy).*

Oral phase	Pharyngeal phase
Anterior spill of the bolus from the mouth	Decreased or absent coupled anterocephalad movement of the hyoid bone and larynx
Inability to gather the bolus on the dorsum of the tongue	
Posterior spill into the pharynx	Lack of or abnormal epiglottal descent
Abnormal lingual palatal contact	Lack or incomplete palatal movement
Impaired tongue movement	Abnormal pharyngeal wall movement
● Repetitive	Laryngeal aspiration
● Disorganized	Abnormal unilateral/bilateral residue
Difficulty in initiating swallow	● Valleculae
Residue in the oral cavity	● Pyriform sinus
● Sublingual	Incomplete opening of the upper esophageal sphincter
● Sulci	

barium bolus in their anterior mouth and will end up drooling during swallow. Premature spill of the oral content into the pharynx before the pharyngeal phase is activated will catch the airway off guard and may result in predeglutitive aspiration. This abnormality commonly occurs with impaired palatal and/or lingual control.

Abnormalities of the pharyngeal phase of swallowing documented by videofluoroscopy include concomitant absent or diminished upward/forward movement of the larynx and hyoid bone, indicating inadequate suprahyoid muscle contraction. This abnormality may be accompanied by entry of the barium into the airway beyond the level of true vocal cords (aspiration). An incompetent velopharyngeal closure mechanism due to inadequate elevation and/or weak posterior movement of the palate and uvula may result in regurgitation of barium into the nasopharynx. This abnormality could develop after CVA or other neurogenic causes, inflammatory disorders of striated muscles, or following surgical excisions. Abnormalities of the oral phase of swallowing may or may not be accompanied with abnormalities of the pharyngeal phase of swallowing.

Abnormalities in the transport function during oropharyngeal swallowing results in hypopharyngeal residue. Abnormal lingual, pharyngeal or UES function, singularly or in combination, may be responsible. Unilateral involvement of the pharynx results in ipsilateral post deglutitive bulging of the pharyngeal wall and residue in the same side [15, 19].

Misdirection of the barium into the airway may be due to intrinsic abnormalities of the glottal adductor muscles resulting in ineffective glottal sphincteric mechanism or lack of coordination between glottal closure and transport function of the oropharynx commonly seen in neurologically impaired patients.

Abnormal opening of the upper esophageal sphincter during swallowing seen by videofluoroscopy, may be due to lack of or impairment of its relaxation, decreased UES compliance, or inadequate traction by the suprahyoid muscles. Correct diagnosis requires manometric evaluation of the UES for its resting pressure and its swallow-induced relaxation. Diagnosis of cricopharyngeal achalasia cannot be made solely by its radiographic appearance.

Videoendoscopy

The chronic nature of oropharyngeal dysphagia requires assessment of therapeutic results and progress with repeated videofluoroscopic studies. Because of the radiation exposure and also difficulty in moving some patients to the radiology suite, a videoendoscopic approach to the evaluation of oropharyngeal dysphagia has been developed [7, 8, 53, 54, 77, 81]. In this technique a small diameter endoscope, such as a laryngoscope or bronchoscope, is inserted

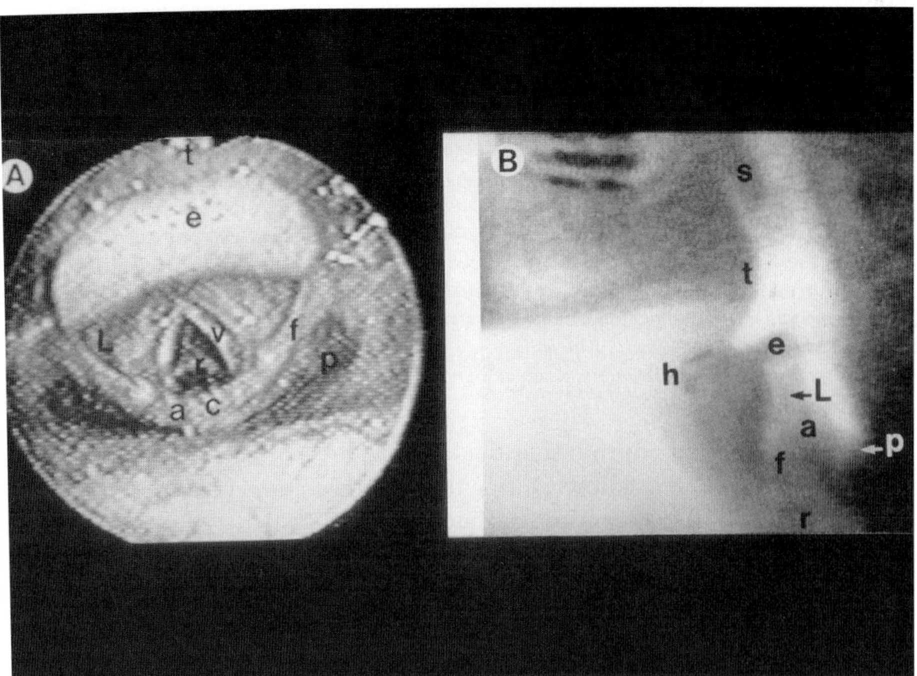

Fig. 5: Hypopharynx and glottis viewed by videoendoscopy (A) and videofluoroscopy (B). Although most of the anatomical structures involved in swallowing are visualized by both modalities, the hyoid bone is observed only by the x-ray technique, whereas vocal cords are visualized better by endoscopy. a, arytenoid; c, posterior commissure; e, epiglottis; f, aryepiglottic fold; h, hyoid bone; L, laryngeal vestibule; p, pyriform sinus; r, trachea; v, vocal cord.
Reproduced by permission from Shaker at al. Semin. Gastrointest. Dis. 3(3) (1992) 115−128.

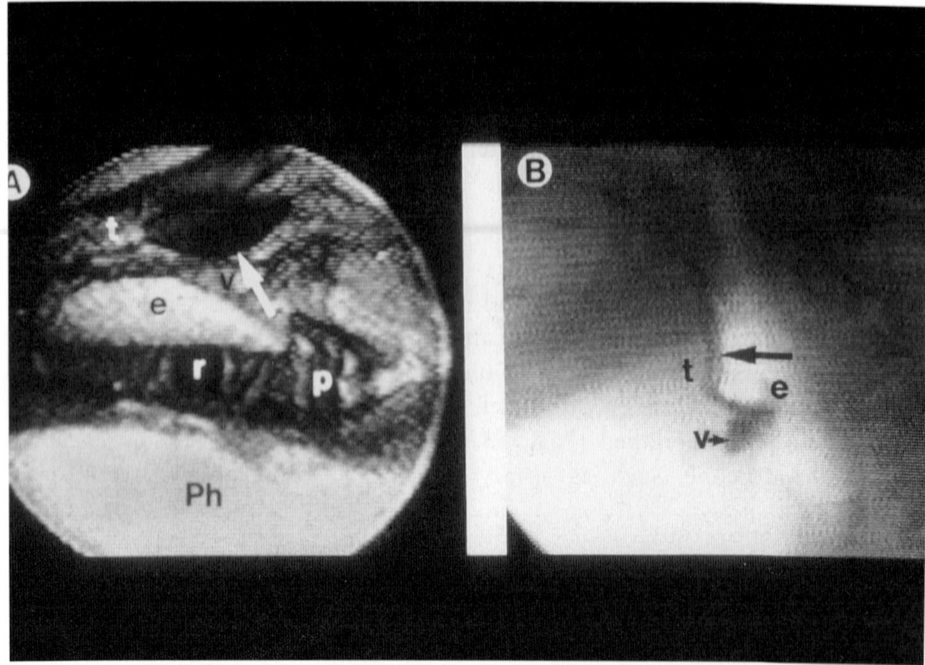

Fig. 6: *Still frames of videoendoscopic (A) and videofluoroscopic (B) views of premature spill (arrow) of oral bolus into the pharynx in the oropharyngeal dysphagic patient. On videofluoroscopy it is observed that the barium contrast spilled prematurely over the posterior aspect of the tongue and has filled the space between the posterior aspect of the tongue and anterior aspect of the free margin of the epiglottis (the valleculae). Similarly, on videoendoscopy it is observed that the blue-colored water has entered the pharynx prematurely and is over the posterior aspect of the tongue entering the valleculae. e, epiglottis; p, pyriform sinus; ph, posterior pharyngeal wall; r trachea; t, posterior aspect of the tongue; v, valleculae.*
Reproduced by permission from Shaker et al. Semin. Gastrointest. Dis. 3(3) (1992) 115−128.

through the nose and positioned at the level of posterior nares. In this position, the patient is asked to swallow. During this swallow, normal features of pharyngeal seal, namely the adduction of the superior constrictor and postero/orad elevation of palate seen as a bulging in the nasopharynx, is examined, then the scope is advanced to the level of free margin of the epiglottis. At this position the glottis is clearly seen (Figs. 5−7) and its adduction function is examined by having the patient produce different vowels. Following this, a 5−10 ml water bolus colored with blue food dye is given through the mouth and the patient is instructed to hold the bolus in the mouth for 20 seconds. During this time the back of the tongue is observed videoendoscopically for presence or absence of unilateral or bilateral spill or entry of colored water into the airway (predeglutitive aspiration). The presence of spill is seen in patients with abnormalities of the tongue and/or palate control. Following this stage, the scope is withdrawn

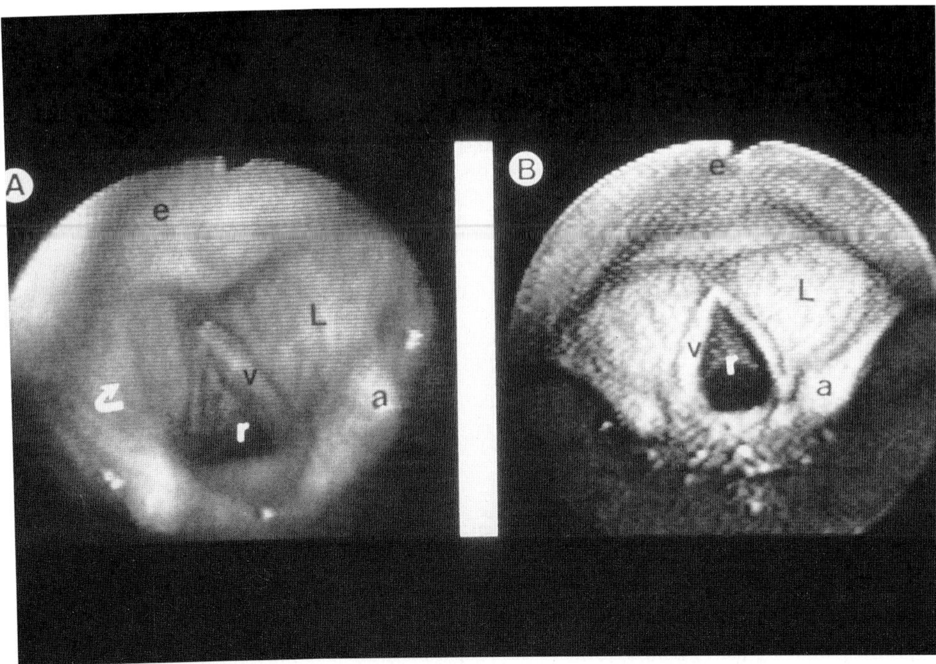

Fig. 7: *Endoscopic views of the glottis in a dysphagic patient (A) and a normal volunteer (B) after swallowing 5 ml of blue-colored water. As noted, the patient's vestibule is stained (arrow) after swallowing 5 ml of colored water, whereas, the healthy volunteer's vestibule is not, except for the staining edges. a, arytenoids; e, epiglottis; L, laryngeal vestibule; r, trachea; v, vocal cord. Reproduced by permission from Shaker et al. Semin. Gastrointest. Dis. 3(3) (1992) 115−128.*

to the level of the posterior nares and the patient is asked to swallow once. Then the scope is immediately advanced to the level of the epiglottis. On the way toward the epiglottis, attention is given to the presence or absence of blue staining of the retro palatal pharynx, indicative of nasal regurgitation due to abnormalities of the velopharyngeal closure mechanism. This abnormality may be caused by inadequate elevation and posterior movement of the soft palate and uvula. Then the inner aspect of the epiglottis, aryepiglottic fold, posterior commisure, and true vocal cords are examined for the presence or absence of staining. In a study of normal volunteers in our laboratory, only the outer edges of the epiglottis and aryepiglottic-fold were stained with blue dye. Endotracheal coloring with the blue dye is easily seen, proving aspiration. The patients are then asked to cough once and since, during cough the laryngeal vestibule remains open, expulsion of blue material from the trachea can be seen and is indicative of aspiration. Following this phase, the presence or absence of residue in the pyriform sinus and valleculae is determined and overflow of residue into the trachea through the posterior commisure is sought.

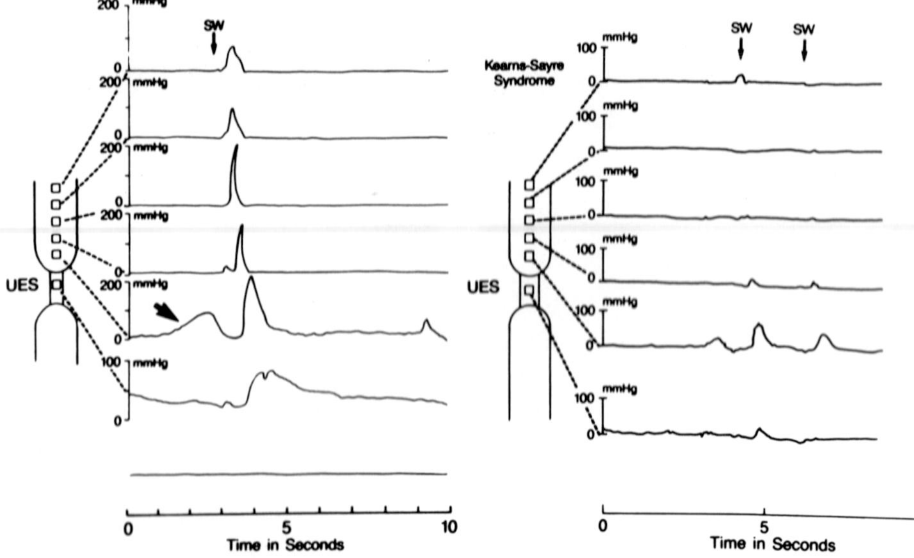

0   5   10   0   5

Time in Seconds   Time in Seconds

Fig. 8: *Pharyngeal peristalsis recorded using intraluminal strain-gauges in a patient with Kearns-Sayre syndrome and its comparison with age-matched control. The recording sites are 1.5 cm apart. During swallowing the bottom two sites record from the UES. The third from the bottom records the hypopharynx and the top three record from the proximal pharynx. As seen, the proximal pharyngeal pressure amplitude is significantly lower compared to the controls. However, the amplitude 1.5 cm above the UES (third from bottom) where the posterior tongue thrust is recorded, is similar to the control.*
Reproduced by permission from Shaker et al. Gastroenterology 103 (1992) 1328−1331.

Manometry

Although the use of intraluminal strain-gauges for pharyngeal manometry has resulted in a significant increase in our knowledge about the pharyngeal pressure phenomena, this modality still remains mainly a research tool and its clinical application is limited to the evaluation of dysphagia patients with primary muscle diseases. An example of these disorders is Kearns−Sayre syndrome, a mitochondrial disease which, in addition to external ophthalmoplegia and cardiac conduction defects and limb weakness [51, 64] may involve the pharyngeal constrictors, but dysphagic symptoms develop late in the disease. Significant diminution of the pharyngeal peristaltic pressure wave amplitude is the main finding (Fig. 8).

Because the pharynx is radially, as well as axially an asymmetric cavity, orientation of the pressure transducers needs to be ascertained and preferably similar in all studies in order to obtain meaningful data. In our laboratory, the posterior orientation has been used since it yields the most consistent results. Concurrent pharyngeal and UES manometry helps detect discoordination between the UES relaxation and arrival of pharyngeal peristalsis in the hyopharynx. Use of manometry to evaluate the oral phase in dysphagic patients has generally been unsuccessful and this modality continues to be used for research purposes.

Disordered deglutitive UES opening is a common clinical problem among the elderly and patients with neurological abnormalities. It may result in incomplete pharyngeal clearance and aspiration. It is commonly referred to as cricopharyngeal (CP) achalasia. Delayed or failure of cricopharyngeal muscle opening has been reported in 30–50% of brain stem lesions, central degenerative disorders, posterior cerebellar artery thrombosis, as well as in bulbar paralysis [10, 21, 34]. The term cricopharyngeal achalasia was originally used by radiologists upon observation of a prominent pharyngo-esophageal segment during swallowing causing inadequate opening of the pharyngo-esophageal junction in patients with cervical dysphagia (Fig. 9). However, comparing the mechanism of closure and opening of the CP (striated) muscle with that of the lower esophageal sphincter (smooth) muscle to which the term achalasia was first applied, as well as comparing the innervation and maintenance of basal tone by the two organs, the term cricopharyngeal achalasia needs to be viewed more critically.

As discussed above, normal uES opening basically requires the existence of normal cricopharyngeal relaxation and distensibility as well as normal contractile force of the suprahyoid muscles. Traditionally, UES resting tone and deglutitive relaxation have been studied by intraluminal manometry. Because of the orad displacement of the UES during swallowing and its to-and-fro movement during breathing, the use of a sleeve sensor has been advocated for this purpose. This 6 cm long sensor which acts similar to a Sterling resistor, provides continuous measurement of the UES pressure [46] and records the maximal squeeze pressure regardless of the axial sphincter movement along the length of the device. Shorter pressure sensors, either strain gauges or pneumohydraulic side holes, may remain within the sphincter at rest. However, during swallowing they will drop into the cervical esophagus, due to the upward movement of the sphincter, and yield intraesophageal pressure which may be misinterpreted as UES relaxation (Fig. 10).

Differentiating between deglutitive relaxation and opening of the CP muscle by intraluminal manometry is impossible. The sudden intraluminal UES pressure decline during swallowing, commonly referred to as UES relaxation, reflects the effect of (a) CP relaxation and (b) UES opening of various degrees. Concurrent manometry and fluoroscopy also provides information which is the summation of the two effects of relaxation and opening. For this reason concurrent manometry, electromyography (Fig. 11) and videofluoroscopy is essential to differentiate the effects of these phenomena.

A relatively common change in UES morphology observed during pharyngoeso-phageal barium studies is a prominent posterior indentation at the level of the UES; cricopharyngeal bar. Although rarely associated with dysphagia, its observation has been reported in 5% of patients older than 40 years who did

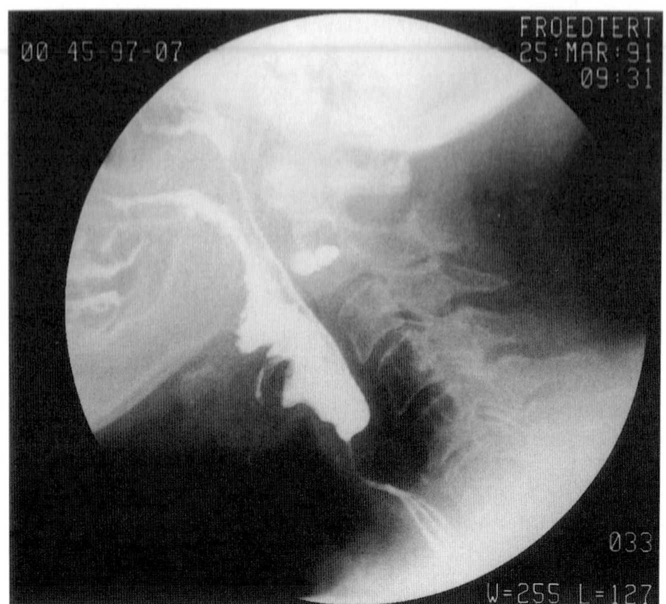

9a

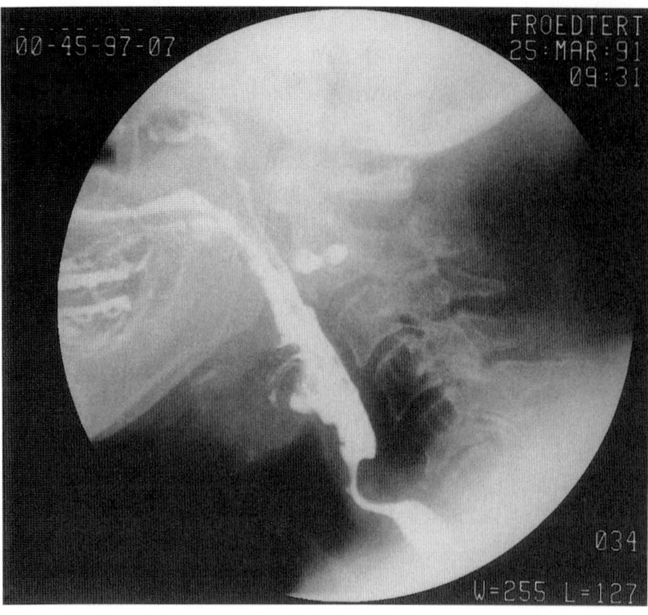

9b

not have symptoms [28, 75]. Despite the common notion of spasm or failed relaxation, the pathogenesis of cricopharyngeal bar is not fully known. A recent study by Dantas et al. [18] has shown a normal resting pressure, as well as normal deglutitive relaxation, in individuals with cricopharyngeal bar. However, the upstream (intrabolus) pressure was found to be higher than that of normal controls. Also found was reduced dimension of UES during passage of barium, suggestive of reduced compliance of the cricopharyngeal muscle.

Ultrasonography

Ultrasound for evaluation of the oral phase of swallowing has been successfully used [83, 87]. Since this modality is noninvasive and does not disturb the physiology of the oral phase of swallowing, it could be used in addition to videofluo-

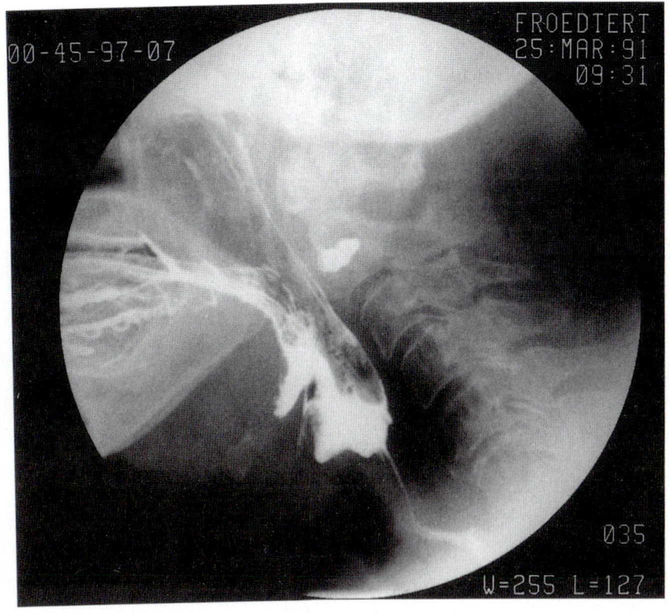

Fig. 9: *An example of a modified video barium swallow in a patient with cricopharyngeal achalasia resulting in a feeling of incomplete swallow, deglutitive cough and pharyngeal residue. A. Barium bolus is seen in the pharynx during the pharyngeal phase of swallowing immediately before the UES opens. A trace of barium from previous swallow is seen within the UES and proximal esophagus. Vestibular penetration and nasal regurgitation are also seen.*
B. Barium bolus is seen transversing the UES. Prominent indentation induced by incomplete opening of the CP muscle is seen. The result is severe narrowing of the UES lumen. However, barium bolus has filled the proximal esophagus. Also present is nasal regurgitation and vestibular penetration.
C. Pharyngeal phase swallowing is now ended. UES has closed, however, a large amount of barium is left behind in the hypopharynx.

roscopy to evaluate the dysphagic patients. Using this modality, Sonies et al. have described subtle, subclinical changes of the oral phase of swallowing in the aged [86].

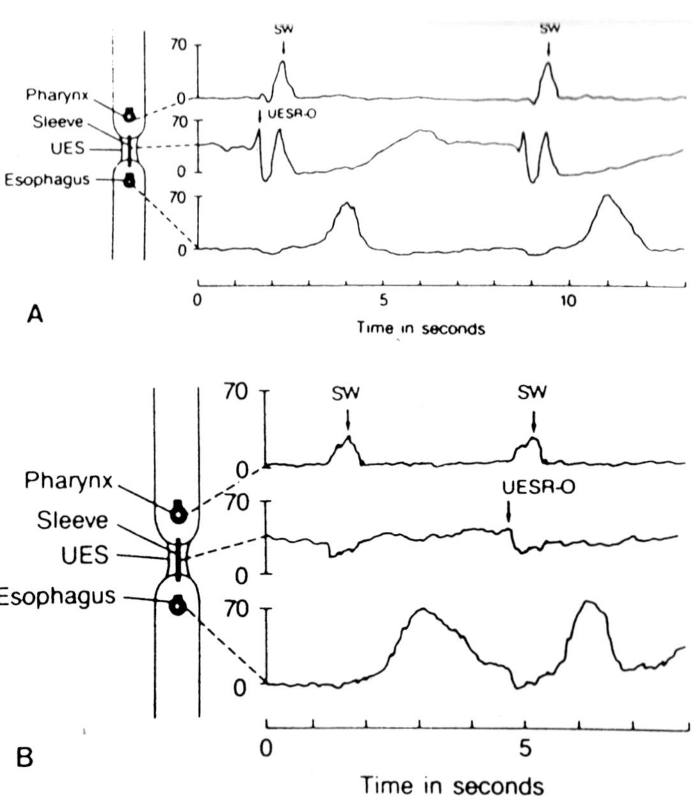

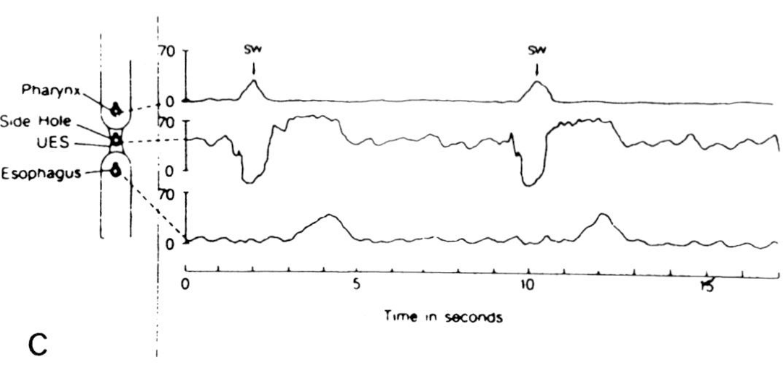

Management

Only a minority of the patients with oropharyngeal dysphagia are amenable to medical/surgical therapy. The majority, however, require patient retraining and use of various swallowing maneuvers and techniques to achieve an adequate and safe swallow.

Cricopharyngeal dilatation and myotomy has been performed for a variety of neurogenic and myogenic causes of oropharyngeal dysphagia with variable results. However, controlled clinical trials and outcome studies are lacking. In general, myotomy yields good results in CP achalasia due to primary CP muscle involvement. The results are less predictable for primary neurogenic causes if other parts of the swallowing apparatus are also involved. The role of myotomy in secondary CP achalasia is controversial since deglutitive relaxation and abolition resistance to flow is present in this group. The rationale for the cricopharyngeal myotomy, which usually is extended to the lower part of the inferior pharyngeal constrictor and upper part of the cervical esophagus, is to eliminate the resistance of the UES against the flow of the swallowed bolus. Under normal conditions this resistance is eliminated by timely relaxation, opening and closure of the UES. However, in a variety of conditions because of the discoordination of the UES and pharynx or because of ineffective pharyngeal function, the UES acts as a relative resistor to the bolus flow. It is in these conditions that cricopharyngeal myotomy may improve pharyngeal bolus transit and reduce aspiration. Recently, endoscopic transmucosal botulinum toxin injection into the CP muscle has been tried in patients with CP achalasia. However, close proximity of the injection area and the vocal cords raises special concern about possible respiratory complications. On the other hand, because of the temporary effect of the botulinum toxin, this new technique could potentially be used to select patients who will benefit from CP myotomy.

Fig. 10: *A. An example of complete manometric deglutitive UES relaxation in an elderly during UES manometry using a sleeve device. As seen, after the onset of UES relaxation (UESR-O), the UES pressure sharply declines to slightly below atmospheric pressure indicating complete UES relaxation.*
B. An example of UES manometry in a cricopharyngeal achalasia patient using a sleeve device. As seen with each swallow, contrary to the example in Section A, although the UES pressure reduces, it does not decline to the atmospheric pressure. The reduction in UES pressure during swallowing in this patient is felt to be due to anterocephalad displacement of cricoid cartilage as a result of suprahyoid muscle contraction.
C. An example of UES manometry using a pneumohydraulic side hole in the patient with cricopharyngeal achalasia. During swallowing, due to orad excursion of the UES, the side hole of the manometric catheter which was within the UES during resting was displaced into the proximal esophagus and recorded esophageal pressure, thus yielding a spurious UES relaxation. Reproduced by permission from Shaker et al. Gastroenterology 103 (1992) 1328–1331.

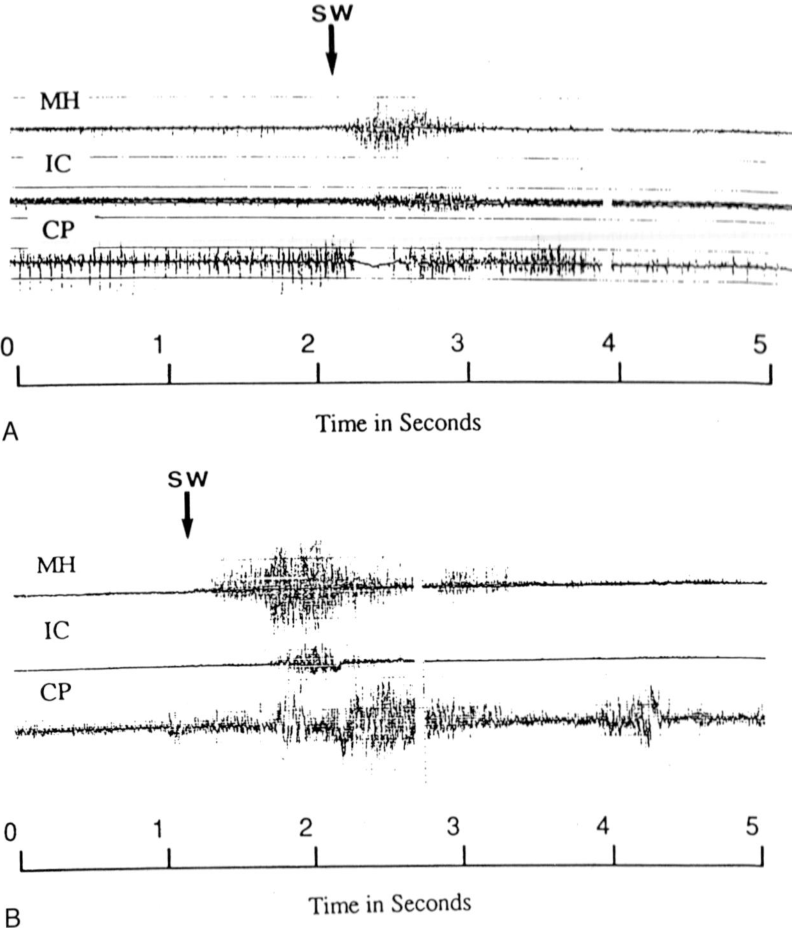

Fig. 11: *Examples of electromyographic recordings from the mylohyoid/geniohyoid muscle group (MH), inferior pharyngeal constrictor (IC) and cricopharyngeal muscle (CP) from a normal control (A) and a patient with CP achalasia (B) during dry swallow. As seen, the MH and IC do not exhibit any tone before swallow, whereas CP maintains a basal tone during resting. In the normal control subject, swallowing results in transient inhibition of CP tone, myoelectrical activity of the mylohyoid/geniohyoid group and the inferior constrictors. In the patient with CP achalasia, however, swallowing does not result in inhibition of the CP tone.*
Reproduced by permission from Shaker et al. Chapter 25 in: W. J. Snape (ed.): Consultations in Gastroenterology, pp. 177–186. W. B. Saunders, Co., Philadelphia, PA 1996.

Surgical treatment of Zenker's diverticulum has evolved with advances in the understanding of its pathophysiology. Treatment: Transcutaneous extra-mucosal cricopharyngeal myotomy with or without diverticulectomy [5] or diverticulopexy [33] traditionally have been the treatment of choice depending upon the size of the diverticulum and yield excellent results in over 90% of cases. However, the endoscopic transmucosal cricopharyngeal myotomy technique, proposed originally by Mosher and popularized by Dahlman and Mattsons, is reported to be relatively safe and yields excellent results. Vengensky et al. reported successful resolution of dysphagia after cricopharyngeal myotomy in a patient with acute cricopharyngeal obstruction due to dermatomyositis [95]. Gagic [34] reported excellent results of cricopharyngeal myotomy in patients with Zenker's diverticulum, and idiopathic hypertrophy of the cricopharyngeal muscle and marked improvement in patients with vagal injuries, amyotrophic lateral sclerosis and post CVA, however, no improvement was achieved in a patient with myotonia dystrophica. Two patients developed aspiration pneumonia and respiratory arrest. Logemann has reported [60] that the results of cricopharyngeal myotomy are superior when pathology is mainly in the UES, there are pharyngeal propulsive forces present and patients are able to close their airway voluntarily. Since the major barrier against pharyngeal regurgitation of gastric acid, namely the UES, is ablated by myotomy, pulmonary complications of gastroesophageal reflux postoperatively, remains a major concern in patients who undergo cricopharyngeal myotomy.

In patients with an inadequate deglutitive glottal closure mechanism such as patients after partial laryngectomy due to malignancy, Parkinson's disease, amyotrophic lateral sclerosis, the deglutitive airway closure could be improved by injection of nonabsorbable material such as teflon [4, 60, 76], into the post hemilaryngectomy pseudo cords or lateral thyroarytenoid muscle. Injection of teflon will result in bulk formation in the injection site and displaces the true cord or surgically constructed pseudo cord toward the midline. This new fixed position of the cord or the pseudo cord facilitates glottal closure during swallowing since the adduction of functioning cord will result in contact of the two cords and closure of introitus of the trachea. Teflon injection of the cords has also been successfully used to prevent aspiration in patients with various types of vocal cords paralysis due to lesion of recurrent laryngeal and/or superior laryngeal nerve as a result of various surgical, inflammatory or central nervous system disorders [52, 73].

The majority of oropharyngeal dysphagia patients, however, require specialized rehabilitation of their swallowing function. Maintaining an adequate nutrition during this period is essential [35, 36, 61, 68], otherwise the vicious cycle of malnutrition − oropharyngeal dysphagia/complications − malnutrition, will selfperpetuate.

Swallow therapy is done with the help of videofluoroscopy [60] and recently, videoendoscopy [7]. Swallowing studies using any modality are time consuming. In order to be helpful, it needs to be tailored to the specifications of each patient and when the pathology is determined, various techniques and maneuvers have to be tried until the efficient and safe swallow is produced.

Table 6: *Postural swallowing techniques.*

- Utilize gravity to move the bolus
- Hide away the airway from the bolus path
- Possibly reduce the laryngeal entrance
- Eliminate the weak side from bolus path
- Direct bolus to the stronger side

Table 7: *Swallow maneuvers.*

- Close the airway before and during swallow (supraglottic-swallow)
- Increase posterior tongue movement (effort-full swallow)
- Prolong UES opening and laryngeal elevation (Mendelsohn maneuver)

Several therapeutic maneuvers (Table 6) are used to improve the oropharyngeal bolus transport and airway safety. A change in bolus size and/or consistency is helpful in some patients, while in others swallowing with the head in a specific position may help safe passage of bolus through the hypopharynx. Flexion of the head by displacing the larynx under the epiglottis reduces the chance for aspiration, while rotating the head toward the weaker side will relatively close this side and improve pharyngeal transit. Similarly, tilting the head toward the weaker side will direct the bolus laterally, and may improve pharyngeal bolus transit and prevent aspiration.

Patients with predeglutitive and deglutitive aspiration may benefit from specific therapeutic maneuvers (Table 7) such as supraglottic swallow [51]. In this maneuver, patients take a deep breath and hold breathing, then swallow. Swallowing is followed by a voluntary cough before resumption of respiration which clears the larynx of aspirated material.

In patients with impaired pharyngeal transit and post deglutitive aspiration, Mendelsohn's [19, 60] maneuver may improve pharyngeal emptying and prevent aspiration. In this maneuver, patients are taught to generate a sustained laryngeal and hyoid bone elevation during swallowing in order to increase the UES traction and prolong its opening. This results in improved pharyngeal emptying. Observing the fluoroscopy monitor during this maneuver greatly enhances the patient's learning and compliance. In the elderly, with decreased opening of the upper esophageal sphincter, "Shaker's" exercise (isotonic and isometric head raising) has been shown to increase the cross sectional area of the UES [80]. This approach may potentially be helpful for dysphagic patients with disordered UES opening.

Summary

In summary oropharyngeal dysphagia develops as a result of dysfunction of transport and/or airway protective aspects of the oropharyngeal phase of swallowing. These dysfunctions occur due to a variety of muscular, peripheral and central nervous system disorders, malignancies of oropharyngeal cavity, surgical and radiation therapy of these malignancies. Symptoms of oropharyngeal dysphagia are highly specific and should be rarely considered psychogenic. Diagnosis and management of oropharyngeal dysphagia optimally requires a multidisciplinary team approach led by a managing physician.

References

1. Ardran, G. M., F. H. Kemp: The protection of the laryngeal airway during swallowing. Br. J. Radiol. 25 (1952) 406−416.
2. Ardran, G. M., F. H. Kemp: A radiographic study of movements of the tongue in swallowing. Dent. Practitioner 5 (1955) 252−261.
3. Ardran, G. M., F. H. Kemp, C. Wegelius: Swallowing defects after poliomyelitis. Br. J. Radiol. 30 (1957) 169−189.
4. Arnold, G.: Vocal rehabilitation of paralytic dysphonia: IX technique of intracordal injection. Arch. Otolaryngol. 76 (1962) 358−368.
5. Barclay, A. E.: The normal mechanism of swallowing. Laryngoscope 37 (1927) 235−262.
6. Barthlen, W., H. Feussner, C. Hannig et al.: Surgical therapy of Zenker's diverticulum: low risk and high efficiency. Dysphagia 5 (1990) 13−19.
7. Bastian, R. W.: Videoendoscopic evaluation of patients with dysphagia: an adjunct to the modified barium swallow. Otolaryngol. Head Neck Surg. 104 (1991) 339−350.
8. Bevan, K., M. V. Griffiths: Chronic aspiration and laryngeal competence. J. Laryngol. Otol. 103 (1989) 196−199.
9. Bird, M. R., M. C. Woodward, E. M. Gibson et al.: Asymptomatic swallowing disorders in elderly patients with Parkinson's disease: a description of findings on clinical examination and videofluoroscopy in sixteen patients. Age Ageing 23 (1994) 251−254.
10. Bonavena, L., N. A. Khan, T. R. DeMeester: Pharyngoesophageal dysfunctions: The role of cricopharyngeal myotomy. Arch. Surg. 120 (1985) 541−549.
11. Butcher, II, R. B.: Treatment of chronic aspiration as a complication of cerebrovascular accident. Laryngoscope 92 (1982) 681−685.
12. Clark, G.: Deglutition apnoea. J. Physiol. London 54 (1920) 59.
13. Cook. I. J., W. J. Dodds, R. O. Dantas et al.: Opening mechanism of the human upper esophageal sphincter. Am. J. Physiol. 20 (1989) G748−G759.
14. Cook, I. J., M. Gabb, V. Panagopoulos et al.: Zenker's diverticulum: a defect in upper esophageal sphincter compliance? Gastroenterology 96 (1989) A98.
15. Curtis, D. J., D. F. Cruess, M. Crain et al.: Lateral pharyngeal outpouchings: a comparison of dysphagic and asymptomatic patients. Dysphagia 2 (1988) 156−161.
16. Curtis, D. J., D. F. Cruess, A. H. Dachman et al.: Timing in the normal pharyngeal swallow. Invest. Radiol. 19 (1984) 523−529.
17. Curtis, D. J., G. U. Sepulveda: Epiglottic motion: video recording of muscular dysfunction. Radiology 148 (1983) 473−477.

18. Dantas, R. O., I. J. Cook, W. J. Dodds et al.: Biomechanics of cricopharyngeal bars. Gastroenterology 99 (1990) 1269−1274.
19. Dodds, W. J., J. A. Logemann, E. T. Stewart: Radiologic assessment of abnormal oral and pharyngeal phases of swallowing. A. J. R. 154 (1990) 965−974.
20. Dodds, W. J., E. T. Stewart, J. A. Logemann: Physiology and radiology of the normal oral and pharyngeal phases of swallowing. A. J. R. 154 (1990) 953−963.
21. Donner, M. W., M. L. Silbiger: Cinefluorographic analysis of pharyngeal swallowing in neuromuscular disorders. Am. J. Med. Sci. 251 (1966) 600−616.
22. Doty, R. W.: Influence of stimulus pattern on reflex deglutition. Am. J. Physiol. 166 (1951) 142−158.
23. Doty, R., J. F. Bosma: An electrophysiological analysis of reflex deglutition. J. Neurophysiol. 19 (1956) 44−60.
24. Doty, R., W. Richmond, A. Storey: Effect of medullary lesions on coordination of deglutition. Exp. Neurol. 17 (1967) 91−106.
25. Duranceau, A., E. R. Lafontaine, R. Taillefer et al.: Oropharyngeal dysphagia and operations on the upper esophageal sphincter. Surg. Annu. 19 (1987) 317−362.
26. Edwards, L. L., E. M. M. Quigley, R. F. Pfeiffer: Gastrointestinal dysfunction in Parkinson's disease: frequency and pathophysiology. Neurology 42 (1992) 726−732.
27. Ekberg, O.: Defective closure of the laryngeal vestibule during deglutition. Acta Otolaryngol. (Stockh.) 93 (1982) 309−317.
28. Ekberg, O.: Epiglottic dysfunction during deglutition in patients with dysphagia. Arch. Otolaryngol. 109 (1983) 376.
29. Ekberg, O., G. Nylander: Cineradiography of the pharyngeal stage of deglutition in 150 individuals without dysphagia. Br. J. Radiol. 55 (1982) 253−257.
30. Ekberg, O., G. Nylander: Pharyngeal dysfunction after treatment for pharyngeal cancer with radiotherapy. Gastrointest. Radiol. 8 (1983) 97−104.
31. Enomoto, S., G. Schwartz, J. P. Lund: The effects of cortical ablation on mastication in the rabbit. Neurosci. Lett. 82 (1987) 162−166.
32. Feinberg, M. J., O. Ekberg, L. Segall et al.: Deglutition in elderly patients with dementia: findings of videofluorographic evaluation and impact on staging and management. Radiology 183 (1992) 811−814.
33. Ferguson, M. K.: Evolution of therapy for pharyngoesophageal (Zenker's) diverticulum. Ann. Thorac. Surg. 51 (1991) 848−852.
34. Gagic, N. M.: Cricopharyngeal myotomy. Canad. J. Surg. 26 (1983) 47−49.
35. Ganger, D., R. M. Craig: Swallowing disorders and nutritional support. Dysphagia 4 (1990) 213−219.
36. Granieri, E.: Nutrition and the older adult. Dysphagia 4 (1990) 196−201.
37. Groher, M. E.: The prevalence of swallowing disorders in two teaching hospitals. Dysphagia 1 (1986) 3−6.
38. Hellemans, J., W. Pelemans, G. Vantrappen: Pharyngoesophageal swallowing disorders and the pharyngoesophageal sphincter. Med. Clin. North. Am. 65 (1981) 1149−1171.
39. Hockman, C. H., D. Bieger, A. Weerasuriya: Supranuclear pathways of swallowing. Prog. Neurobiol. 12 (1979) 15−32.
40. Horner, J., M. J. Alberts, D. V. Dawson et al.: Swallowing in Alzheimer's disease. Alzheimer Dis. Assoc. Disord. 8 (3) (1994) 177−189.
41. Horner, J., F. G. Buoyer, M. J. Alberts et al.: Dysphagia following brain-stem stroke: clinical correlates and outcome. Arch. Neurol. 48 (1991) 1170−1173.
42. Hurwitz, A. L., J. A. Nelson, J. K. Haddad: Oropharyngeal dysphagia. Dig. Dis. Sci. 20 (1975) 313−323.
43. Jones, B., D. W. Buchholz, W. J. Ravich et al.: Swallowing dysfunction in the postpolio syndrome: a cinefluorographic study. A. J. R. 158 (1992) 283−286.

44. Jones, B., M. W. Donner: How I do it: examination of the patient with dysphagia. Dysphagia 4 (1989) 162–172.
45. Kagel, M. C., N. A. Leopold: Dysphagia in Huntington's disease: a 16-year retrospective. Dysphagia 7 (1992) 106–114.
46. Kahrilas, P. J., W. J. Dodds, J. Dent et al.: A method for continuous monitoring of upper esophageal sphincter pressure. Dig. Dis. Sci. 32 (1987) 121–128.
47. Kahrilas, P. J., W. J. Dodds, J. Dent et al.: Upper esophageal sphincter function during deglutition. Gastroenterology 92 (1988) 52–62.
48. Kawasaki, M., J. Ogura: Interdependence of deglutition with respiration. Ann. Otol. Rhinol. Laryngol. 77 (1968) 906–913.
49. Kawasaki, M., J. Ogura, S. Takenouchi: Neurophysiologic observations of normal deglutition. I. Its relationship to the respiratory cycle. Laryngoscope 74 (1965) 1747–1765.
50. Killian, G.: The mouth of the esophagus. Laryngoscope 17 (1907) 421–480.
51. Kosmorsky, G., D. R. Johns: Neuro-ophthalmologic manifestations of mitochondrial DNA disorders: chronic progressive external ophthalmoplegia, Kearns–Sayre Syndrome and Leber's Hereditary Optic Neuropathy. Neurol. Clin. 9 (1991) 147–161.
52. Koufman, J. A., G. Isaacson: Laryngoplastic phonosurgery. Otolaryngol. Clin. North. Amer. 24 (1991) 1151–1177.
53. Langmore, S. E., K. I. Schatz, N. Olson: Endoscopic and videofluoroscopic evaluations of swallowing and aspiration. Ann. Otol. Rhinol. Laryngol. 100 (1991) 678–681.
54. Langmore, S. E., K. Schatz, N. Olsen: Fiberoptic endoscopic examination of swallowing safety: a new procedure. Dysphagia 2 (1988) 216–219.
55. Larson, C.: Neurophysiology of speech and swallowing. In: W. Perkins, J. Northern (Eds.): Seminars in Speech and Language (ed. 6), pp. 337–348, 1985.
56. Larson, C., K. Byrd, C. Garthwaite et al.: Alterations in the pattern of mastication after ablations of the lateral precentral cortex in rhesus macaques. Exp. Neurol. 70 (1980) 638–651.
57. Layne, K. A., D. S. Losinski, P. M. Zenner et al.: Using the Fleming Index of dysphagia to establish prevalence. Dysphagia 4 (1989) 39–42.
58. Lazarus, C., J. A. Logemann: Swallowing disorders in closed head trauma patients. Arch. Phys. Med. Rehabil. 68 (1987) 79–84.
59. Leighton, S. E. J., M. J. Burton, W. S. Lund: Swallowing in motor neurone disease. J. Royal Soc. Med. 87 (12) (1994) 801–805.
60. Logemann, J. A.: Evaluation and Treatment of Swallowing Disorders. College-Hill Press, Boston, Massachusetts 1983.
61. Logemann, J. A.: Factors affecting ability to resume oral nutrition in the oropharyngeal dysphagic individual. Dysphagia 4 (1990) 202–208.
62. Logemann, J. A.: Manual for the videofluorographic study of swallowing. College-Hill Press, San Diego 1986.
63. Logemann, J. A., Swallowing physiology and pathophysiology. Otolaryngol. Clin. North. Am. 21 (1988) 613–623.
64. McKelvie, P. A., J. B. Morley, E. Byrne et al.: Mitochondrial encephalomyopathies: a correlation between neuropathological findings and defects in mitochondrial DNA. J. Neurol. Sci. 102 (1991) 51–60.
65. Miller, A. J.: Characteristics of the swallowing reflex induced by peripheral nerve and brain stem stimulation. Exp. Neurol. 34 (1972) 210–222.
66. Miller, A. J.: Significance of sensory inflow to the swallowing reflex. Brain Res. 43 (1972) 147–159.
67. Montgomery, W. W. (Ed.): Laryngeal paralysis. In: Surgery of the Upper Respiratory System. Vol. II, 2nd Ed., pp. 607–676. Lea & Febiger, Philadelphia 1989.
68. O'Gara, J. A.: Dietary adjustments and nutritional therapy during treatment for oral-pharyngeal dysphagia. Dysphagia 4 (1990) 209–212.

69. Ramsey, G. H., J. S. Watson, R. Gramiak et al.: Cinefluorographic analysis of the mechanism of swallowing. Radiology 64 (1955) 498−518.

70. Ravich, W. J., R. S. Wilson, B. Jones et al.: Psychogenic dysphagia and globus: reevaluation of 23 patients. Dysphagia 4 (1989) 35−38.

71. Rice, D. H., R. H. Spiro (Eds.). In: General Management Guidelines. Current Concepts in Head and Neck Cancer, pp. 1−15. American Cancer Society, USA 1989.

72. Robbins, J., R. L. Levine: Swallowing after unilateral stroke of the cerebral cortex: preliminary experience. Dysphagia 3 (1988) 11−17.

73. Rontal, E., M. Rontal: Vocal cord injection techniques. Otolaryngol. Clin. North. Amer. 24 (1991) 1141−1149.

74. Rowe, P. H., P. R. Taylor, G. E. Sladen et al.: Cricopharyngeal Crohn's disease. Postgrad. Med. J. 63 (1987) 1101−1102.

75. Seaman, W. B.: Cineroentgenographic observations of the cricopharyngeus. Amer. J. Roentgenol. 96 (1966) 922.

76. Sessions, D., R. Zill, J. Schwartz: Deglutition after conservation surgery for cancer of the larynx and hypopharynx. Otolaryngol. Head Neck Surg. 87 (1979) 779−796.

77. Shaker, R., M. Bowser, W. J. Hogan et al.: Videoendoscopic characterization of abnormalities in pharyngeal phase of swallowing. Gastroenterology 100 (1991) A494.

78. Shaker, R., I. J. S. Cook, W. J. Dodds et al.: Pressure-flow dynamics of the oral phase of swallowing. Dysphagia 3 (1988) 79−84.

79. Shaker, R., W. J. Dodds, R. O. Dantas et al.: Coordination of deglutitive glottic closure with oropharyngeal swallowing. Gastroenterology 98 (1990) 1478−1484.

80. Shaker, R., M. Kern, R. C. Arndorfer et al.: Augmentation of deglutitive UES opening in the elderly by exercise. Gastroenterology 108 (4) (1995) A688.

81. Shaker, R., B. Martin, W. J. Dodds et al.: Comparison of videoendoscopic and videofluoroscopic evaluation of patients with cervical dysphagia. Gastrointest. Endosc. 37 (1991) 277.

82. Shaw, D. W., I. J. Cook, M. E. Simula et al.: Restoration of normal upper esophageal sphincter compliance following cricopharyngeal myotomy in patients with Zenker's diverticulum. Gastroenterology 98 (1990) A122.

83. Shawker, T. H., B. C. Sonies, M. Stone et al.: Real-time visualization of tongue movement during swallowing. J. C. U. 11 (1983) 485−490.

84. Shin, T., T. Maeyama, I. Morikawa et al.: Laryngeal reflex mechanism during deglutition − observation of subglottal pressure and afferent discharge. Otolaryngol. Head Neck Surg. 99 (1988) 465−471.

85. Silbiger, M. L., R. Pikielney, M. W. Donner: Neuromuscular disorders affecting the pharynx. Invest. Radiol. 2 (1967) 442−448.

86. Sonies, B. C., M. Stone, T. Shawker: Speech and swallowing in the elderly. Gerontology 3 (1984) 115−123.

87. Sonies, B. C., J. Weiffenbach, J. C. Atkinson et al.: Clinical examination of motor and sensory functions of the adult oral cavity. Dysphagia 1 (1987) 178−186.

88. Storey, A. T.: Interactions of alimentary and upper respiratory tract reflexes. In: B. J. Sessle, A. J. Hannam (Eds.): Mastication and Swallowing: Biological and Clinical Correlates, pp. 22−36. University of Toronto Press, Toronto, Canada 1976.

89. Stroudley, J., M. Walsh: Radiological assessment of dysphagia in Parkinson's disease. Br. J. Radiol. 64 (1991) 890−893.

90. Sumi, T.: The activity of brain-stem respiratory neurons and spinal respiratory motorneurons during swallowing. J. Neurophysiol. 26 (1963) 466−477.

91. Talley, N. J.: Onset and disappearance of gastrointestinal symptoms and functional gastrointestinal disorders. Am. J. Epidemiology 136 (1992) 165−177.

92. Trupe, E. H., H. Siebens, A. Siebens: Prevalence of feeding and swallowing disorders in a nursing home. Paper presented at the American Congress of Rehabilitation Medicine, Boston 1984.

93. Van Overbeek, J. J. M., H. C. Betlem: Cricopharyngeal myotomy in pharyngeal paralysis. Ann. Otol. 88 (1979) 596−602.
94. Veis, S. L., J. A. Logemann: Swallowing disorders in persons with cerebrovascular accident. Arch. Phys. Med. Rehabil. 66 (1985) 372−375.
95. Vencovsky, J., F. Rehák, P. Pafko et al.: Acute cricopharyngeal obstruction in dermatomyositis. J. Rheumatol. 15 (1988) 1016−1018.
96. Winstin, C. J.: Neurogenic dysphagia. Phys. Ther. 63 (1983) 1992−1996.
97. Yotsuya, H., K. Nonaka, Y. Ide: Studies on positional relationships of the movements of the pharyngeal organs during deglutition in relation to the cervical vertebrae by x-ray TV cinematography. Bull. Tokyo Dent. Coll. 22 (1981) 159−170.
98. Yotsuya, H., Y. Saito, Y. Ide: Studies on temporal correlations of the movements of the pharyngeal organs during deglutition by x-ray TV cinematography. Bull. Tokyo Dent. Coll. 22 (1981) 171−181.

Management of lower gastrointestinal alterations in degenerative nervous diseases

J. Weber

Does management depend on the neurological diagnosis?

The management of lower gastrointestinal tract disorders in nervous diseases depends mainly on the topographic level of the lesions but very little on the aetiologic diagnosis of the degenerative disease.

Topographic levels of gut control

Colonic motility

In our knowledge, nothing is known about colonic transit abnormalities in case of cortical injuries. In case of basal ganglia injury, Jost and Schimrigk [12] have found that transit time was globally increased in 25 patients with Parkinson's disease, when compared to 25 controls matched for age and sex.

The anterior and posterior parts of the brain stem are respectively involved in the control of the right and left colonic transit [18]. This study is confirmed by Staiano and Del Giudice [15], who found that left colonic transit was prolonged in 16 children with traumatic brain stem lesions. The thoraco lumbar sympathetic spinal cord centre and the sacral parasympathetic spinal cord centre control the distal colonic transit as shown by Beuret-Blanquart et al. [3]. Finally, the vagus nerve, the sympathetic peripheral nerves, and the pelvic nerves provide the peripheral pathways for the nervous control of the lower part of the gastrointestinal tract [11]. It has been shown by Werth et al. [21] that a peripheral neuropathy could be responsible for a right colonic transit increase.

Anorectal function

The frontal cortical area and basal ganglia are involved in the voluntary control of rectoanal motility [1, 19]. A defecation centre is present in the anterior part of the pons as shown by Weber et al. in adults [18] and confirmed by Staiano and Del Giudice in children [15]. The thoracolumbar sympathetic spinal cord centre and the sacral parasympathetic spinal cord centre control the anorectal reflexes [3]. Patients with a peripheral neuropathy also present with anorectal disturbances, such as a decreased anal resting pressure and an increased sensory threshold for rectal distension [20].

Role of the etiologic diagnosis in the management of gastrointestinal disturbances

Diseases of the central nervous system
There is no difference in the management of gastrointestinal dysfunctions in vascular cortical diseases and in Alzheimer's or Parkinson's diseases, because in all these nervous pathologies the main lower GI tract dysfunction is due to a loss of voluntary control of the rectoanal reflexes themselves, responsible for the impaired defecation.

The management of colonic constipation and of faecal incontinence follows the same rules in the Shy-Drager syndrome and in a brain stem vascular stroke.

There is no difference between the gastrointestinal symptoms of a patient with a traumatic spinal cord lesion, multiple sclerosis, or Strümpell's disease.

Diseases of the peripheral nervous system
Finally, there is no major difference in the management of the lower GI tract symptoms in a patient with diabetic, alcoholic or degenerative neuropathy.

Whatever the degenerative disease, the main complaint of these patients is an association of transit constipation, with or without straining at stools, and faecal incontinence.

Management of transit constipation

We have seen that transit constipation, in case of a lesion of either central or peripheral nervous system, is secondary to an increased total and segmental colonic transit time. The occurrence of colonic constipation must be assessed with a radiopaque colonic transit time as described by Bouchoucha et al. [7].

Only the left colonic transit time is increased

In our experience, the conventional treatment of constipation with non-irritant laxatives is most often sufficient to improve the distal colonic transit [20].

Parasympathomimetic drugs such as cisapride could be useful. In patients with Parkinson's disease, Jost and Schimrigk have shown that cisapride therapy was always associated with a significant acceleration of the left colonic transit [12]. When the topographic level of the neurological lesion is the spinal cord, the efficacy of cisapride seems less clear. de Groot and de Pagter [9], Binnie et al. [4], and Etienne et al. [10], claimed that cisapride can improve the colonic transit in case of spinal cord injury. Conversely, in a placebo-controlled randomized double-blind study, de Both et al. [8] and Badiali et al. [2] failed to show any improvement of colonic transit with cisapride in case of spinal cord lesion. It could be hypothesised that cisapride could have had a major effect on colonic transit in case of sacral spinal cord injury as in the study of Etienne et al. [10], and that it has no major effect in case of suprasacral spinal cord injuries as reported by de Both [8], and Badiali [2].

The stimulation of sacral anterior roots can improve left colonic motility as shown by Varma et al. [16] and Binnie et al. [5, 6]. The increased motility induced by this stimulation could be responsible for an increased colonic transit because the patients treated with this method had a clinical improvement of constipation and defaecation frequency were clinically improved in patients treated with this method, as shown by Mc Donagh et al. [14], and Binnie et al. [6].

In case of increased right colonic transit time

The treatment of constipation is much more difficult. Conventional laxatives are most often ineffective, and it becomes necessary to try irritant laxatives. In case of failure, a surgical treatment must be considered.

Right or left colostomy, or caecostomy improve colonic transit in case of resistant colonic constipation. Recently, Koyle et al. [13] have used a surgical procedure resulting in a continent catheterizable appendicocecostomy in 22 patients with neurological diseases. With this procedure it was possible to administer daily a large volume enema via the appendicocecostomy. Sixteen patients reported total continence 4 months or longer after surgery. The use of the Malone antegrade continence enema could be an interesting option for neurogenic patients with proximal colonic transit constipation.

Defaecation disorders

Defaecation disorders such as straining at stools or impaired voluntary control of the defaecation reflex, may be managed by the use of daily suppositories or manual manoeuvres when they can be made by the patient himself.

Electrical stimulation of the sacral anterior roots have been successfully used for initiating the defaecation reflex [14]. In a prospective study of 12 patients with complete supraconal spinal cord lesions, Mc Donagh et al. have shown that in 6 cases, a complete daily defaecation could be obtained using the implant, without manual help for defaecation. In all but one of the patients, the total time taken to complete defaecation was reduced, and all were free from constipation. This technique could be particularly useful in case of degenerative lesions in which patients cannot use their hands to manually help defaecation.

Faecal incontinence

Treatment of faecaloma

Almost all neurologic patients have faecal incontinence due to faecaloma. This incontinence for solid or liquid stools may be dramatically improved by treatment and also by avoiding the recurrence of a reappearance of the rectal faecaloma. The best way is to empty the rectum every day and as completely as possible, using the manoeuvres and various treatments previously described.

Gas incontinence

Gas incontinence is due to the loss of the reflex and voluntary contraction of the striated anal sphincter at the moment of the defaecation reflex. This incontinence cannot be improved in case of a complete absence of voluntary control of the anal sphincter, but when a voluntary contraction still exists, this contraction may be improved by biofeedback therapy, as shown by Whitehead et al. [22] and Wald [17] in congenital neurologic lesions. Anorectal manometry is very useful in such cases to quantify the level of voluntary anal contraction that is still possible.

References

1. Ashraf, W., R. F. Pfeiffer, M. M. Quigley: Anorectal manometry in the assessment of anorectal function in Parkinson's Disease: a comparison with chronic idiopathic constipation. Movement Disorders 9 (1994) 655–663.
2. Badiali, D., E. Corazziari, F. I. Habib et al.: A double-blind controlled trial on the effect of cisapride in the treatment of constipation in paraplegic patients. J. Gastrointest. Motil. 3 (1991) 263–267.
3. Beuret-Blanquart, F., J. Weber, J. P. Gouverneur et al.: Colonic transit and anorectal manometric anomalies in 19 patients with complete transection of the spinal cord. J. Auton. Nerv. Syst. 30 (1990) 199–208.
4. Binnie, N. R., G. H. Creasey, P. Edmond et al.: The action of cisapride on the chronic constipation of paraplegia. Paraplegia 26 (1988) 151–158.
5. Binnie, N. R., A. N. Smith, G. H. Creasey et al.: Motility effects of electrical anterior sacral nerve stimulation of the parasympathetic supply of the left colon and anorectum in paraplegic subjects. J. Gastrointest. Mot. 2 (1990) 12–17.
6. Binnie, N. R., A. N. Smith, G. H. Creasey et al.: Constipation associated with chronic spinal cord injury: the effect of pelvic parasympathetic stimulation by the Brindley stimulator. Paraplegia 29 (1991) 463–469.
7. Bouchoucha, M., G. Devroede, P. Arhan et al.: What is the meaning of colorectal transit time measurement? Dis. Colon Rectum 35 (1992) 773–782.
8. de Both, P. S. M., G. H. de Groot, H. R. Slootman: Effects of cisapride on constipation in paraplegic patients: a placebo-controlled randomized double-blind cross-over study. Europ. J. Gastroenterol. Hepatol. 4 (1992) 1013–1017.

9. de Groot, G. H., G. F. de Pagter: Effects of cisapride on constipation due to a neurological lesion. Paraplegia 26 (1988) 159−161.

10. Etienne, M., M. Verlinden, A. Brassinne: Treatment with cisapride of the gastrointestinal and urological sequelae of spinal cord transection: case report. Paraplegia 26 (1988) 162−164.

11. Gonella, J., M. Bouvier, F. Blanquet: Extrinsic nervous control of motility of small and large intestines and related sphincters. Physiol. Rev. 67 (1987) 902−961.

12. Jost, W. H., K. Schimrigk: Cisapride treatment of constipation in Parkinson's disease. Movement disorders 8 (1993) 339−343.

13. Koyle, M. A., D. V. Kaji, M. Dusque et al.: The malone antegrade continence enema for neurogenic and structural fecal incontinence and constipation. J. Urol. 154 (1995) 759−761.

14. Mc Donagh, R. P., W. M. Sun, R. Smallwood et al.: Control of defecation in patients with spinal injuries by stimulation of sacral anterior nerve roots. Br. Med. J. 300 (1990) 1494−1497.

15. Staiano, A., E. Del Giudice: Colonic transit and anorectal manometry in children with severe brain damage. Pediatrics 94 (1994) 169−173.

16. Varma, J. S., N. Binnie, A. N. Smith et al.: Differential effects of sacral anterior root stimulation on anal sphincter and colorectal motility in spinally injured man. Br. J. Surg. 73 (1986) 478−482.

17. Wald, A.: Use of biofeedback in treatment of fecal incontinence in patients with myelomeningocele. Pediatrics 68 (1981) 45−49.

18. Weber, J., P. Denis, B. Mihout et al.: Effect of brain stem lesion on colonic and anorectal motility. Study of three patients. Dig. Dis. Sci. 30 (1985) 419−425.

19. Weber, J., T. Delangre, D. Hannequin et al.: Anorectal manometric anomalies in seven patients with frontal lobe brain damage. Dig. Dis. Sci. 35 (1990) 225−230.

20. Weber, J.: Constipation in spinal cord lesions, multiple sclerosis and diabetes mellitus. In: M. A. Kamm, J. E. Lennard-Jones (Eds.): Constipation, pp. 273−277. Wrightson Biomedical Publishing Ltd., Petersfield, UK 1994.

21. Werth, B., B. Meyer-Wyss, B. Spinas et al.: Non-invasive assessment of gastrointestinal motility disorders in diabetic patients with and without cardiovascular signs of autonomic neuropathy. Gut 33 (1992) 1199−1203.

22. Whitehead, W. E., L. S. Bosmajian, E. D. Morill-Corbin et al.: Treatment of faecal incontinence in children with spina bifida: comparison of biofeedback and behaviour modification. Arch. Phys. Med. Rehabil. 67 (1986) 218−224.

Visceral manifestations in spinal cord lesions

D. De Grandis, V. Tugnoli

Introduction

In higher animals, particularly in mammals, the upper regions of the central nervous system (CNS) have progressively assumed the control of the spinal cord functions. Therefore the spinal cord, isolated from the CNS, is capable of carrying out only few regulatory functions at the segmental or plurisegmental level.

After a damage of the long myelinated fibers, the conscious sensations of affected dermatomes are completely lost and this is clinically fundamental, in order to define the level of the lesion. An objective test in low cooperative patients may be the evoked potentials and especially the dermatomeric ones.

Sudomotor and cutaneous vasomotor activity may be used to test the level of vegetative involvement in dorsal spinal lesions, in absence of diffuse hypothermia. A practical method to monitor the area of sympathetic involvement may be the exploration of the sudomotor activity through the sympathetic skin response (SSR), applicable to every segment.

An exact clinical evaluation of the level and extension of the lesions may be fundamental, but sometimes it may be hard, in critical phase, to differentiate between complete and incomplete lesion and to determine the cranio-caudal width of the segmental damage.

In a man an acute transection of spinal cord results in immediate and permanent paralysis of all voluntary movements and at the same time all reflexes, evoked below the lesion, are temporarily extinguished. Provided that the patients receive fundamental care after 2−6 weeks, depending on the level of injury, the reflexes reappear, often with a pathological profile. This reversible neurological areflexia, which is manifest after acute global spinal lesions, is typically defined as spinal shock. This transitory absolute absence of reflexes may be referred not only to the striated muscle response following stretch or cutaneous stimulation, but also to the different vegetative reactions leading to an abnormal control of bladder, bowel, cardiovascular and thermoregulatory functions.

There are several similarities in the pattern of motor and vegetative responses in acute and chronic phases after a spinal damage. Therefore, in order to better understand the pathogenesis, we have compared some motor symptoms to the vegetative ones. Particularly the sympathetic regulation of temperature and the cardiovascular activity will be taken into consideration, both involved in the upper segments damage of the spinal cord.

The upper motoneuron syndrome has both "negative" and "positive" symptoms. The negative features are weakness, loss of dexterity and shock. The positive signs are abnormal posture and tonus, exaggeration of proprioceptive reflexes producing "spasticity" and an abnormal pattern of some exteroceptive responses of the limbs producing flexor withdrawal spasms, extension reaction and the classical Babinsky response [3].

The same approach may be applied to the interpretation of visceral reactions, with the presence of decreased reflex activity and reduced modulation (negative symptoms), and abnormal reaction with global activation of both cutaneous and muscular portions of sympathetic system (positive features).

Negative features

The acute responses to the crash of pyramidal tract fibers are paralysis and profound hyporeflexia for the innervated musculature, a condition referred to as "shock". The clinical findings will be those of a deep flaccid paralysis involving all muscle groups and of a complete stretch and cutaneous areflexia. With traumatic spinal cord lesions, the onset of spinal shock is said to be immediate and it may last typically from 2 to 6 weeks. The less abrupt is the onset of pathology, the more likely is the patient to bypass the shock phase. Some reflexes are later recovered to a limited extent and some of them become even stronger than before.

A minority of patients never develop hyperreflexia, even if some reflex activities usually appear. The reasons for persistence of hypotonia in a few are unclear. Severe spinal trauma may be accompanied by wide motor neuron damage or plurisegmentary gray matter involvement, secondary to ischemia or traction with secondary root damage. This happens frequently at the lumbar enlargement. It may be difficult to recognize in the acute phase the presence of a plurisegmental anterior and posterior horns involvement. Only combined neurophysiological testings, as evoked potentials and electrical or magnetic direct root stimulation are able to demonstrate, 6−7 days after the trauma, the peripheral damage and the degeneration of the lower motor neuron.

We possess a very incomplete and unsatisfactory knowledge of the causes of spinal shock and the mechanisms which bring about the recovery of reflexes.

By testing the excitability of lower motoneuron through antidromic excitation, the recurrent response, we can observe its complete disappearance lasting few weeks, with a progressive reappearance, at the same time with the cutaneous-plantar and other flexor responses.

As in the motor system, acute interruption of the tonic and phasic excitatory influences from the higher centers, particularly the brainstem nuclei, produces a complete abolition in both tonic and reflex autonomic activity, probably due to an hypoexcitability of preganglionic autonomic neurons. This "vegetative shock" causes hypothermia, hypotension and in presence of high level lesion above the fifth dorsal, bradycardia. All these symptoms are due to a loss of sympathetic tone below the lesion [5]. Deep hypothermia is particularly liable to develop soon after the acute spinal cord section [7], due to the paralytic cutaneous vasodilatation of acute phase.

Blood pressure will be mainly regulated by blood volume and posture and stimulation below the lesion will not produce any change in arterial pressure. The paraplegic patients present hypotension soon after the injury without tachycardia. The reason is presumably the abolition of sympathetic nerve activity and perhaps a little contribution is brought by muscular flaccid paralysis [5].

Mechanically ventilated patients with acute lesions above C5 are prone to severe bradycardia and cardiac arrest during trachael suction or other maneuvers activating vagal reflexes [5].

In patients with incomplete pyramidal involvement, other negative signs are weakness and loss of dexterity in fine movements, particularly of the fingers.

Chronic tetraplegic subjects have basal systolic and diastolic arterial pressure about 15–20 mm Hg below normal values, due probably to a reduction of sympathetic activity [9]. They experience both orthostatic hypotension with tilt and overshoot of arterial pressure when returned to the horizontal position [5].

This is referable to the lack of the sympathetic components of the baroreflex with their influences on muscle sympathetic activity.

After several weeks blood pressure can be maintained in most patients, generally without symptoms, in the sitting position. Local reflexes and change in blood circulating volume are the cause of the compensatory mechanisms.

In subjects with thoracic cord lesions, sweating is present in the area connected to the neurons above the lesions level. Sweating may also be present below the lesions in absence of gray matter damage. This is the result of spinal local reflex following warming or other stimuli [8]. These subjects present a large oscillation in temperature, since the central fine regulation is lost, as a consequence of the interruption of the pathways to the glands and smooth muscles organs.

Positive features

As reported above, signs of hyperactivity of motor system appear few weeks after acute spinal section. These may be summarized in three points: abnormal muscular tonus and posture, increased proprioceptive reflexes and anomalous cutaneous responses. Several muscles, joints and skin afferents are able to evoke a flexion withdrawal response of the lower limb, with a triple flexion (dorsiflexion of the ankle, flexion of the knee and of the hip). These afferents involve a common polysynaptic reflex pathway. Following complete spinal section syndrome, flexion reflexes are disinhibited, and the patient emerging from spinal shock passes through a phase of minimal reflex activity into one of flexor spasms. After a month the flexor reflexes can become extraordinarily strong and their occurrence is often accompanied by powerful vegetative reflexes, such as outbreaks of sweating, bladder and rectal contractions. The Mass Reflex of Riddoch is the sum of extremely strong flexor response and vegetative hyperreflexia.

Extensor reflexes develop more slowly than the flexor and are usually not very pronounced.

Deviations from this clinical picture, particularly strong extensor reflexes and increased muscle tone, shortly after the injury, are usually a sign of incomplete section of the spinal cord, with correspondent better prognosis.

If we test neurophysiologically the flexor reflex, we can observe together with the prolongation and exaggeration of the response two other aspects: an increased threshold and a stimulus-related change of latency, shape and duration. These stimulus-dependent changes regard both the intensity and the rate of repetition of the train.

In chronic tetraplegia with cervical or high thoracic level of lesion, deep, repetitive stimulation of the skin, muscle or viscera below the level may elicit massive reflex activation of the sympathetic and sacral parasympathetic activity, known as autonomic hyperreflexia or dysreflexia [5]. This abnormal pattern is due to a simultaneous activation of primary cutaneo-visceral and muscle sympathetic reflexes in an atypical and uncontrolled fashion [5].

Abnormal bursts of sympathetic activity preceding the sudomotor activity or vasoconstriction have been recorded in cutaneous or muscular nerves by microneurography. This contrasts with the reduction of spontaneous sympathetic activity to the same organs [9]. Compensatory symptoms may be present above the lesion level, like sweating, vasodilatation with flashing and bradycardia.

The abnormal balance of the autonomic nervous system and the impairment of vascular and cardiac control represent a life threatening factor which can precipitate the spinal damage itself or can lead to throbbing headache, ischemic or hemorrhagic neurologic deficit and seizures. These may represent the first manifestation of autonomic disorders [10].

Nociceptive stimulations, bladder distension, stimuli from muscles, joints and skin may be the evoking causes.

When the spinal cord injury determines the interruption of adequate supraspinal controls, the reciprocal influence between nociceptive and autonomic systems becomes abnormal. Painful stimuli are associated with exaggerated activation of both cutaneous and muscular part of sympathetic system and a prolonged vasoconstrictor response in superficial and deep segments is observed. This aspect, when widespread over large segments, can determine dangerous hypertensive crises, and can worsen the spontaneous painful crisis described by many patients with both complete and incomplete lesions.

Conclusions

The role of the CNS in the control of the visceral functions appears in all its evidence after spinal lesions. To compare the motor function with the vegetative regulation is not only a useful didactic approach, but may be relevant in clinical practice. A precise relation between motor and vegetative system is present not only in mass reaction, but also in all physiological responses.

Summary

The spinal cord lesion syndromes are clinical entities with their own features and prognosis strictly related to the level and rapidity of the onset, independently of the causes which play a minor role.

The motor and sensor symptoms are evident and help the clinician to establish the level of the lesion and is also important to assess the visceral manifestations. Particularly the analysis of the cardiovascular system and temperature regulation may be relevant to monitor the level and the type of lesion as well as to prevent some severe crisis and late complications. Similarity in the reflex activity has been found between somatic and visceral manifestations both in acute and chronic phases. After the initial shock, the hyperreflexia may assume a particular clinical relevance not only inside the somatic and visceral functions, but also within their reciprocal relationships.

Among visceral complications of spinal cord lesions, cardiac arrhythmias and acute hypertension are frequent occurrences [1, 2]. These symptoms have been always considered as the consequence of the autonomic hyperreflexia and they are found in upper cervical and dorsal lesions. Clinically they represent severe complications and can determine sudden deaths.

References

1. Arieff, A. J., E. L. Tigay, S. W. Pyzik: Acute hypertension induced by urinary bladder distension. Arch. Neurol. 6 (1962) 88–96.
2. Bors, E., J. D. French: Management of paroxysmal hypertension following injuries to cervical and upper thoracic segments of the spinal cord. A.M.A. Arch. Surg. 64 (1952) 803–812.
3. Burke, D.: Spasticity as an adaptation to pyramidal tract injury. In: S. G. Waxman (Ed.): Advances in Neurology, pp. 401–423. Raven Press, New York 1988.
4. Evans, D. E., A. I. Kobrine, H. V. Rizzoli: Cardiac arrhythmias accompanying acute compression of the spinal cord. J. Neurosurg. 52 (1980) 52–59.
5. Mathias, C. J., H. L. Frankel: Carciovascular control in spinal man. Annu. Rev. Physiol. 50 (1988) 477–492.
6. Meinecke, F. W., K. A. Rosenkranz, C. M. Kurek: Regulation of cardiovascular system in patients with fresh injury to the spinal cord: preliminary report. Paraplegia 9 (1971) 109–113.
7. Pledger, H. G.: Disorders of temperature regulation in acute traumatic tetraplegia. J. Bone Jt. Surg. 44 (1962) 110–113.
8. Silver, J. R., W. C. Randall, L. Guttmann: Spinal mediation of thermally induced sweating. J. Neurol. Neurosurg. Psychiatry 54 (1991) 297–304.
9. Stjernberg, L., H. Blumberg, B. G. Wallin: Sympathetic activity in man after spinal cord injury. Outflow to muscle below the lesion. Brain 109 (1986) 695–715.
10. Yarkony, G. M., R. T. Katz, Y. C. Wu: Seizures secondary to autonomic dysreflexia. Arch. Phys. Med. Rehabil. 67 (1986) 834–835.

Lower urinary tract dysfunction in spinal cord injury

Ph. E. V. Van Kerrebroeck

Introduction

In the majority of patients with spinal cord injury, a traumatic event is the cause of the lesion. A traumatic spinal cord injury therefore is the classical form of spinal cord injury. Spinal cord injuries can be the consequence of injury by a high velocity missile, fracture or fracture dislocation of the spinal column, or the consequence of sudden or severe hyperextension. With compression and shearing of the spinal cord, there is destruction of neurons and white matter with haemorrhage, particularly in the grey matter. Healing after the period of hematomyelia may produce a cystic cavity or syrinx. However frequently no lesion of the spinal cord is evident on macroscopic examination or at exploratory laminectomy or autopsy.

After the spinal cord injury there is sudden partial or complete loss of voluntary movement below the level of the lesion. Sensation loss often goes together with the motor deficit and can also be partial or complete and eventually at a different level. The level of the lesion will be decisive for the resulting type of lower urinary tract function. However the bony segments are numbered by the vertebral level but have a different relationship to spinal segmental levels at different locations. The spinal cord terminates at the level of vertebrae L_1-L_2 in the adult, the conus medullaris being located approximately at the level of vertebrae $Th_{12}-L_1$, indicating the discrepancy between vertebral and spinal segment level of injury in low thoracic, lumbar and sacral lesions. Most lesions occur where the mobility of the vertebral column is most pronounced, notable in the cervical spine and at the thoracolumbar transition. The neurological deficit will indicate the level of the spinal cord injury.

The first phase immediately after the trauma is called spinal shock phase and is associated with loss of all reflexes below the level of the lesion. In the spinal shock phase the detrusor presents areflexia, whereas the tonus in the periurethral striated muscle seems to return early, often within hours of the injury [10]. This period can persist for weeks to months and is followed by a period of increased reflex activity [12]. This occurrence of increased reflex activity is associated with hyperreflexia on examination of the deep tendon reflexes and the presence of extensor plantar responses. However when the injury damages the conus medullaris or the cauda equina, there is persistent absence of reflexes in the segments involved. There is laxity of the anal sphincter and a varying degree of flaccid paralysis of the lower extremities in conjunction with depressed or absent deep tendon reflexes. The bulbocavernosus reflex is absent or depressed. Often this deficit is accompanied by complete or partial sensory loss in the same segments.

In the phase of spinal shock urinary retention is the common symptom of bladder dysfunction followed by recovery of detrusor reflex function if the lesion is above the level of the conus medullaris. The recovery of detrusor reflexes is associated with impaired or complete loss of voluntary control. Autonomic dysreflexia may be present in the lesions above Th_6 [6]. In the case of a conus medullaris or cauda equina lesion, reflex contractions will be absent or partially present.

Classification of neurogenic lower urinary tract function

Classification of neurogenic lower urinary tract function in spinal cord injury is necessary not only for clarification but also to guide the therapeutic approach and to give an indication of the prognosis. Classifications of neuro-urological disorders including spinal cord injuries can be based on a description of the anatomic location of the neurologic lesion or on the detrusor and urethral dysfunction.

The neuro-anatomic or neurotopographic classification is more a neurological approach based on the site of the damage in the neuro-urological axis.

The classical classification of this type was created by Bors and Commarr [3]. In order to bring the lower urinary tract dysfunction on a comparable basis with the paralysis of skeletal muscle, they introduced the terms "upper motor neuron lesion" (lesions above the sacral micturition center) and "lower motor neuron lesion" (lesions below the sacral micturition center). They devote considerable attention to the completeness of the lesion and the degree of residual urine volume (balanced versus unbalanced).

They divided all spinal cord lesions in three different types (sensory neuron lesions, motor neuron lesions, combined sensory−motor neuron lesions).

This classification is very elaborate and therefore a simple classification based on the previous one has been introduced by T. Hald [11]. In this classification five categories are introduced on a neurotopographical basis (supraspinal lesions, suprasacral spinal lesions, infrasacral or sacral lesions, peripheral autonomous neuropathy, muscular lesions).

Another simple classification was proposed by Gibbon [9]. He divides the lesions in three categories: suprasacral lesions, sacral lesions, mixed lesions.

However since there is not always a fixed relationship between the type of disturbance in the somatic skeletal and the visceral innervation, these classifications have their limits. Another objection to this kind of classification is the fact that the terms upper and lower motor neuron do not make sense when applied to the parasympathetic nervous system. In a classical upper motor neuron lesion such as a spinal cord injury, it is not the upper neuron in the parasympathetic system which is damaged, nor is it the lower motor neuron of the parasympathetic system which is interrupted in a typical lower motor neuron lesion such as a cauda equina injury.

Furthermore these classifications take into account only the parasympathetic and somatic lower urinary tract innervation and not the sympathetic system.

Because of all these limitations functional or urological classifications were introduced. These classifications have the advantage that the disorders of the lower urinary tract can be classified on the basis of the type of function or dysfunction. This is an accurate method that can be performed in a standardized way, using urodynamic and neurophysiological methods. Based on this information an adequate treatment can be proposed.

Originally the type of bladder dysfunction was indicated as autonomous in case of a neurologic lesion resulting in a functional separation of the bladder from the sacral cord. On the other hand the reflex bladder resulted from a lesion above the sacral micturition center thus separating the bladder segmental reflexes from the higher control. Many subclassifications of these basic types were introduced since the term autonomous bladder and reflex bladder might include different neuro-anatomical entities. Indeed, further experience with the urodynamic evaluation of neurogenic bladder function showed that a fixed correlation of a neuro-anatomical lesion with a certain type of bladder dysfunction is not always true [5]. Another problem with many of the classifications was the fact that they did not take into account the dynamic and often pathologic interaction between the detrusor and the smooth and striated muscles of the urethra.

Since these three functional components were taken into account, different neurophysiologic classifications with therapeutic implications were developed. The first attempt to classify neurogenic bladder dysfunction according to this criteria was the classification of Bradley. This classification is based on his neuro-anatomical system of four loops. Disorders can be localised in one of the four loops (central nervous system pathology) or at the level of the peripheral innervation of the lower urinary tract (pathology of the peripheral motor or sensory nerves).

Another problem in the classification of lower urinary tract dysfunction in spinal cord injury is the lack of correlation between the symptoms and the physiopathological mechanisms as shown by urodynamic techniques. Therefore the functional status of the lower urinary tract as evaluated by urodynamic techniques is the most important information in view of the different treatment options.

Different forms of functional behaviour of the detrusor can be distinguished. The detrusor behaviour in spinal cord injury can be described as detrusor hyperreflexia, detrusor hyporeflexia or areflexia.

Detrusor hyperreflexia

Detrusor hyperreflexia is the most common form of detrusor dysfunction in spinal cord injury. It is characterized by involuntary detrusor contractions during bladder filling that cannot consciously be suppressed and that produce an increase in intravesical pressure of more than 15 cm H_2O [2]. In spinal cord injury this entity is almost always associated with a lesion cephalad to the sacral cord outflow. Several theories have been presented to explain the neurophysiologic basis of detrusor hyperreflexia following suprasacral neuologic lesions. The normal micturition reflex is not a simple segmental process but involves synapsing of long spinal cord tracts, presumably in the region of the pontine reticular formation. Following suprasacral spinal cord transection, the nature of the micturitional reflex changes from a long tract reflex to a segmental reflex. Whether this segmental pathway is normally present in humans and is unmasked by a suprasacral lesion, or whether it represents a new reflex pathway formed by collateral sprouting is not sure [17]. In any case, the end result is a new micturitional reflex center localised in the sacral cord [7]. The threshold of this center is decreased and therefore it is responsible for involuntary detrusor contractions at low intravesical volume.

Detrusor hyporeflexia or areflexia

Detrusor hyporeflexia or areflexia may be defined as the absence of a detrusor reflex at appropriately high intravesical volumes. However, the inability to elicit a detrusor reflex during cystometry does not mean the presence of a neurologic lesion, since a certain percentage of normals will have bladder areflexia under these circumstances. This disorder is usually caused by a lesion involving the sacral cord, the cauda equina or the pelvic nerves.

However detrusor behaviour cannot be described without taking into account the behaviour of the smooth and striated urethral musculature.

The striated musculature

In detrusor hyperreflexia, reflex interactions between the detrusor and the external striated sphincter are present. Bladder filling will result in increased activity of the external urethral sphincter. On the other hand bladder contraction will normally be associated with reflex inhibition of all activity in the external urethral sphincter [8]. In the intact individual, this reflex coordination is probably organised at a suprasacral level [1]. Spinal cord lesions between the sacral cord and the pons may therefore result in detrusor hyperreflexia and lack of appropriate coordination between the detrusor and the external sphincter (detrusor-sphincter dyssynergia). Detrusor hyperreflexia with sphincter dyssynergia may represent the unmasking of a facilitative reflex between the detrusor and the external sphincter or rather the formation of a new reflex by neural reorganisation. This can explain why dyssynergia rarely occurs in lesions other than those of the suprasacral spinal cord.

In patients with detrusor areflexia the striated sphincter may or may not be similarly affected. If the spinal lesion involves the innervation of the external sphincter, denervation will be present and relaxation will occur. This implies a lesion of the pudendal nucleus in the sacral cord or a pudendal nerve injury. In other patients the external sphincter retains its innervation and will not relax appropriately during attempts of voiding. Another explanation for nonrelaxation of the striated sphincter in complete lesions of the parasympathetic afferents is the continued input to the spinal cord via the intact sympathetic pathway thus constituting a stimulus for continuous striated sphincter activity. This phenomenon in the absence of detrusor contraction may not be called dyssynergia but nonrelaxation of the striated sphincter.

The smooth musculature

Rarely detrusor hyperreflexia is associated with an obstruction at the level of the smooth muscle sphincter [21]. A normal detrusor contraction is accompanied by synchronous neurogenic relaxation of the smooth muscle sphincter. A lesion situated above the sympathetic spinal cord outflow (Th_6) may result in loss of this appropriate inhibition of sympathetic discharge to the smooth muscle sphincter. This has most frequently been described in patients with clinical evidence of autonomic dysreflexia. This may be a manifestation of release of the sympathetic neurons in the thoracolumbar spinal cord from higher inhibitory centers.

Detrusor areflexia may also be associated with neurogenically mediated outlet obstruction at the level of the proximal smooth muscle sphincter [13], since opening of the proximal urethra is neurologically mediated and not the result of detrusor contraction. The coordination of this event occurs via the spinal reflexes. A decreased parasympathetic influence may thus result in detrusor areflexia combined with neurogenically mediated smooth muscle sphincteric obstruction.

The first classification based on urodynamic parameters was introduced by McClellan [18] and popularized by Lapides [16]. It consists of five categories of neurogenic bladder dysfunction: uninhibited neurogenic bladder, reflex neurogenic bladder, autonomous neurogenic bladder, sensory paralytic bladder, motor paralytic bladder.

The first two categories are secondary to upper motor neuron lesions and the last three secondary to interruptions in the sacral micturition reflex. However this classification is solely based on cystometry and does not take into account urethral pathology.

Therefore Krane and Siroky developed a practical classification with a therapeutical orientation [14]. They combine the uninhibited and reflex bladder under the heading of detrusor hyperreflexia since they do not differ with respect to therapy. For the same reason the sensory paralytic, motor paralytic and autonomous bladder are consolidated under the heading of detrusor areflexia. Both types of bladder dysfunction are subdivided with respect to their interaction with the striated and smooth muscle sphincters.

Their classification consists finally of seven categories:

I. Detrusor hyperreflexia
   with coordinated sphincters
   with striated sphincter dyssynergia
   with smooth muscle sphincter dyssynergia

II. Detrusor areflexia
   with coordinated sphincters
   with non-relaxing striated sphincter
   with denervated striated sphincter
   with non-relaxing smooth muscle sphincter

This classification is very easy to use in a specific patient, however other factors such as age, prognosis and symptoms must also be taken into account.

Pathophysiology of lower urinary tract dysfunction in spinal cord injury

Based on the classification of Krane and Siroky seven specific categories of neurogenic dysfunction of the lower urinary tract can be discriminated. The same categories can be found in patients with spinal cord injury. Each of these categories has its own pathophysiological mechanisms that are responsible for the urological pathology and symptomatology.

Detrusor hyperreflexia with coordinated sphincters is caused by a lesion of the suprasacral cord (or the higher centers). It must be presumed that there is some preservation of long tracts from the pontine region to sacral spinal center referring to an incomplete suprasacral spinal cord lesion. However the same pattern has been reported in cases of complete spinal cord lesion. The urodynamic evaluation in these patients will show involuntary detrusor contractions associated with periods of appropriate relaxation of the urethral closure mechanism due to suppression of the electrical activity in the external urethral sphincter. Since these patients cannot counteract the involuntary contractions by increasing the urethral resistance the major symptom is urgency and urge incontinence. These patients often void with high intravesical pressures [19]. However upper urinary tract deterioration will mostly only occur by intercurrent infection or an organic intravesical obstruction.

Detrusor hyperreflexia with dyssynergia of the striated urethral sphincter is often indicated as detrusor−sphincter dyssynergia. It is almost always present in patients with a complete spinal cord injury. During cystometry, the involuntary detrusor contractions are accompanied by concomitant bursts of electrical activity in the external urethral sphincter. This can be explained by the loss of coordinating reflexes involving higher central nervous centers. Several variants of abnormal striated sphincter responses in patients with a spinal cord injury are described. The striated sphincter can present a continuous hyperactivity or even a clonic activity. This activity is not related to detrusor activity but is the result of stimuli in the S_2 to S_4 afferent nerves regions (e. g. urinary tract infections, infected decubitus). These patients will also have a neurogenically mediated obstruction at the level of the external sphincter and therefore will be, from a functional point of view, similar to patients with true detrusor−sphincter dyssynergia.

Patients in this category will present all the symptoms of outflow obstruction with large residual volumes and a higher incidence of urinary tract infections. On cystometry high intravesical pressures are present during micturition with a poor flow and large residual urine. The detrusor contraction is often of short duration and ineffective [22]. However most of these patients will have some degree of incontinence caused by the detrusor hyperreflexia or by overflow.

There will be progressive detrusor hyperthrophy and obstruction at the level of the intramural segment. In other patients vesico-ureteral reflux will appear. Both are responsible for the high incidence of upper urinary tract disorders in this category of spinal cord injured patients.

Detrusor hyperreflexia and dyssynergia at the level of the smooth urethral sphincter is mostly seen in spinal cord injured patients with a lesion in the upper cord above the thoracolumbar sympathetic outflow at Th_6 to Th_{12}. This condition is always associated with autonomic dysreflexia. Due to the increased sympathetic outflow from the thoracolumbar spinal cord the proximal smooth sphincter is stimulated. During cystometry detrusor hyperreflexia is present with or without striated sphincter dyssynergia.

Detrusor areflexia with coordinated sphincters is the result of a sacral cord or more peripheral lesion without any obstruction at the level of the smooth or striated sphincter. During urodynamic examination complete detrusor areflexia is present and voiding is performed by straining using abdominal pressure increase to expel urine. During micturition a decrease in electrical activity of the striated sphincter is detected. This situation can be encountered in partial lesions.

Detrusor areflexia with a non-relaxing striated sphincter is found in the same categories of patients as the previous entity. During straining in an attempt to void there will be continued or even increased electrical activity of the striated sphincter. This is not a real detrusor-sphincter dyssynergia since no detrusor contraction is present. As these patients have large amounts of residual urine they are at risk for fibrotic changes in the bladder wall due to overdistension.

Detrusor areflexia with striated sphincter denervation will be present in case of lesions involving the parasympathetic and pudendal nervous system. This situation is present in severe cauda equina lesions. Urodynamics will reveal detrusor areflexia together with evidence of pudendal neuropathy (polyphasic potentials and/or positive giant waves on electromyography of the striated sphincter).

Detrusor areflexia with non-relaxation of the smooth sphincter is the result of the loss of parasympathetic influence on the sympathetic input to the proximal urethra at the peripheral level [23]. Every lesion of the parasympathetic system can be responsible through this mechanism for the loss of appropriate smooth sphincter relaxation.

Since a few years we try to classify the patients in our neuro-urological unit following this classification and found it very useful. Furthermore based on this classification a more rational treatment can be established.

Investigations of neurogenic lower urinary tract dysfunction

Radiological exploration

The upper urinary tract can be visualised with an intravenous urography or an ultrasound of the kidneys. These investigations permit to describe the anatomical situation and are the basis for further control. Dilatation of the upper urinary tract, due to obstruction or reflux can be detected as well as the presence of nefrolithiasis.

The diagnosis of vesico-ureteral reflux necessitates a (video-)miction-cystography eventually in combination with a urodynamic investigation.

Urodynamic examinations

Urodynamic examinations inform on the functional behavior of the lower urinary tract and can permit to predict the influence of lower urinary dysfunction on the upper urinary tract. This test permits also to detect the cause of incontinence and to classify the lower urinary tract dysfunction. Therefore urodynamic tests are the basis for further therapeutic decisions. The filling phase of the micturition cycle will be studied with a filling cystometry. Important parameters are the compliance of the bladder (pressure increase correlated with the filling volume, $\Delta V/\Delta P$) and the activity of the detrusor. The compliance of the bladder must be high (more than 10 for volumes up to 100 cc, more than 25 for volumes up to 500 cc). A low compliance is a bad prognostic sign for upper tract problems [19]. During the filling cystometry hyperreflexic detrusor activity can be present with a high intravesical starting pressure ($>$ 10 cm H_2O), increasing pressure with filling and intermittent detrusor contractions with high intravesical pressure ($>$ 100 cm H_2O).

If the motor innervation of the detrusor is damaged, detrusor acontractility may be present with a low starting pressure and slow pressure increase with filling. However a limited compliance can occur at some point of filling.

To distinguish real acontractility from unmasked reflex activity a rapid fill cystometry (flow $>$ 100 cc) or an icewater test can be performed [4]. For this test the bladder is filled at 25 cc/min with water at 4° Celsius and the bladder pressure registered. A positive test means an evident detrusor contraction with expulsion of the bladder content. This indicates the integrity of the sacral reflex arc and normal contractile capacity of the detrusor. However a negative icewater test is caused by hypo-activity of the detrusor in 30% of the patients [4].

During the evacuation phase of a urodynamic investigation detrusor−sphincter dyssynergia can be detected with electromyographic registration of the activity of the striated muscle of the external sphincter and the pelvic floor. Moreover the intravesical pressure necessary for evacuation of urine can be registered.

Neurophysiological tests

Neurophysiological tests can help to distinguish complete from incomplete spinal cord lesions since the clinical examination alone is not always sufficient.

The absence of somatosensory evoked potentials at the level of the cerebral cortex after stimulation below the level of the spinal cord injury, indicates a complete spinal cord injury. The evokability of potentials at the level of the detrusor after magnetic stimulation of the cauda equina permits to detect the integrity of the sacral motor nerves.

Kidney function evaluation

It is difficult to follow the exact kidney function in patients with spinal cord injury based on the serum creatinine level alone. Because of the reduced muscle mass in these patients, the serum creatinine level will only decrease when the kidney function is below 60% of the normal value [15].

The best test for kidney function evaluation is the determination of the creatinine clearance based on a 24-hour collection of urine. These values do not depend on the total muscle mass and are a better measure of the real kidney function. However the collection of the urine in patients with a spinal cord lesion and incontinence can be difficult.

Scintigraphic examinations can be helpful for the determination of the kidney function. These tests permit also to detect the flow of urine through the upper urinary tract and give an idea of the degree of obstruction [20].

References

1. Barrington, F. J. F.: The nervous mechanism of micturition. Q. J. Exp. Physiol. 8 (1914) 33−52.
2. Bates, P., W. E. Bradley, E. Glen et al.: Standardization of terminology of lower urinary tract function. Urology 9(2) (1977) 237−244.
3. Bors, E., A. E. Commarr: Classification. In: E. Bors, A. E. Commarr: Neurological Urology, pp. 129−135. Karger, New York 1971.
4. Bors, E., A. E. Commarr: Neurological disturbances of sexual function with special reference to 529 patients with spinal cord injury. Urol. Surv. 10 (1960) 191−201.
5. Bradley, W. E., S. Chou, C. Markland: Classifying neurologic dysfunction of the urinary bladder. In: S. Boyarsky: The neurogenic bladder, pp. 136−146. Williams and Wilkins, Baltimore 1967.
6. Commarr, A. E.: Autonomic dysreflexia. J. Am. Paraplegia Soc. 7 (1984) 4−11.
7. DeGroat, W. C.: Nervous control of the urinary bladder of the cat. Brain Res. 87 (1975) 201−207.
8. Diokno, A. C., S. A. Koff, L. F. Bender: Periurethral striated muscle activity in neurogenic bladder dysfunction. J. Urol. 112 (1974) 743−749.
9. Gibbon, N. O. K.: Nomenclature of neurogenic bladder. Urology 8(5) (1976) 423−432.
10. Guttmann, L., D. Whitteridge: Effect of bladder distention on autonomic mechanisms after spinal cord injuries. Brain 70 (1947) 361−405.
11. Hald, T., W. E. Bradley: Classification of neuromuscular disorders. In: T. Hald, W.E. Bradley: The urinary bladder. Neurology and dynamics, pp. 151−155. Williams and Wilkins, Baltimore 1982.
12. Hoppenfeld, S.: Aandoeningen van ruggemerg en zenuwwortels. Bohn, Scheltema & Holkema, Utrecht 1984.
13. Krane, R. J., C. A. Olsson: Phenoxybenzamine in neurogenic bladder dysfunction: clinical considerations. J. Urol. 110 (1973) 653−659.
14. Krane, R. J., M. B. Siroky: Classification of neuro-urologic disorders. In: R. J. Krane, M. B. Siroky: Clinical neuro-urology, pp. 143−158. Little Brown, Boston 1979.

15. Lange, S., R. Nagel, K. Winkel et al.: Classification of impaired renal evacuation by sequential scintigraphy. In: K. Winkel, D. Blaufox, L. Funck-Brentano: Radionuclides in Nephrology, pp. 97–101. Thieme, Stuttgart 1975.
16. Lapides, J.: Neuromuscular vesical and ureteral dysfunction. In: M. F. Campbell, J. H. Harrison: Textbook of Urology, pp. 616–627. Saunders, Philadelphia 1976.
17. Liu, C. N., W. W. Chambers: Intraspinal sprouting of dorsel root axons. Arch. Neurol. Psychiatr. 79 (1958) 46–52.
18. McClellan, F. C.: The neurogenic bladder. Thomas, Springfield 1939.
19. McGuire, E. J., J. R. Woodside, T. A. Borden: Upper urinary tract deterioration in patients with myelodysplasia and detrusor hypertonia: a follow-up study. J. Urol. 129 (1983) 823–826.
20. O'Reilly, P. H., H. J. Testa, R. S. Lauson: Diuresis renography in equivocal urinary tract obstruction. Br. J. Urol. 50 (1978) 76–79.
21. Scott, F. B., E. M. Quesada, D. Cardus: The use of combined uroflowmetry, cystometry and electomyography in evaluation of neurogenic bladder. In: S. Boyarsky: The neurogenic bladder, pp. 106–114. Williams and Wilkins, Baltimore 1967.
22. Thomas, D. G.: Spinal cord injury. In: A. R. Mundy, T. P. Stephenson, A. J. Wein: Urodynamics: principles, practice and application, pp. 260–272. Churchill-Livingstone, London 1984.
23. Torrens, M. J. Urethral sphincteric responses to stimulation of the sacral nerves in the human female. Urol. Int. 33 (1978) 22–29.

Gastrointestinal manifestations in spinal cord lesions

J. Weber

Three principal extrinsic vegetative nervous systems provide its extrinsic supply to the gut: the vagus nerves originating from the brain stem, the mesenteric nerves emanating from the prevertebral ganglia, and the pelvic nerves coming from the sacral segments of the spinal cord [15].

Upper part of the gut

The upper part of the gut (oesophagus, stomach, small bowel, proximal colon) receives a parasympathetic innervation from the brain stem via the vagus nerve, and a sympathetic innervation from the spinal cord (from C8 through T9) via the mesenteric nerves. In these conditions, there is little evidence that spinal cord lesions could produce any dysfunction in the upper part of the gut because only disturbances from the sympathetic supply of the extrinsic innervation could be involved in gastrointestinal manifestations. However, some disturbances of the upper gut motility related to a spinal cord dysfunction have been described.

Oesophagus

Thoren et al. [17] studied in 1988 the effects of thoracic epidural analgesia on lower oesophageal motility. Oesophageal manometric recordings were performed in twenty healthy volunteers before and after an epidural analgesia (T4 level). During epidural morphine oesophageal peristalsis, resting lower oesophageal sphincter (LOS) pressure and contraction of LOS after swallowing did not change, but the degree of LOS relaxation in response to swallowing decreased significantly. It has been concluded by the authors that if the sympathetic innervation of the oesophagus originating in the thoracic spinal cord is not involved in the control of the oesophageal peristalsis, it could be involved in the LOS relaxation after swallowing.

Stomach, small bowel and gallbladder

Five patients with complete high-cord transection (neurologic level above T1), and three patients with complete low-cord transections (neurologic level T10 or below) were studied in comparison with a healthy control group by Fealey et al. in 1984 [11]. Gastric emptying and antroduodenal motility was studied in all subjects. The duration of the phases and the cycle length of the interdigestive motor complex were similar in the three groups. However, the percentage of phases III of the interdigestive motor complex originating in the antrum and propagated to the duodenum was significantly decreased but only in patients with a high-cord transection, contrary to controls. Moreover, only patients with high-cord transection had a reduced cumulative gastric emptying at 60 min postprandially when compared with healthy controls. The authors concluded that the interruption of the cervical cord above the level of the sympathetic outflow to the gastrointestinal tract disturbs normal interdigestive antra-duodenal motor coordination and may delay the postprandial gastric emptying of liquid meals.

In 1987 Apstein and Dalecki-Chipperfield [2] reported that gallstone disease was significantly more prevalent in patients with spinal cord injury when compared with the control population. For these authors a possible explanation for this threshold increase in risk of gallstone disease among patients with spinal cord injury includes an abnormal gallbladder motility resulting in stasis, decreased intestinal transit leading to an abnormal enterohepatic circulation, and metabolic changes responsible for an abnormal biliary lipid secretion.

Finally, in normal subjects, Iovino et al. [13] found that an activation of the sympathetic nervous system selectively increases visceral but not somatic sensitivity and enhances in the gut both vagally and sympathetically driven reflexes.

Lower part of the gut

The lower part of gut (distal part of the colon and anorectal apparatus) receives a parasympathetic innervation from S2 through S4 via the pelvic nerves, and a sympathetic innervation from T9 through L2 via the hypogastric nerves. It is of clinical evidence that spinal cord injuries have major consequences on the colorectal function. Constipation and/or faecal incontinence are always found in patients with a spinal cord disease.

Constipation

Constipation may be explained by, at least, three pathophysiological mechanisms:

Slow colonic transit
In paraplegic subjects, a dramatic increase in total colonic transit time is always reported by authors studying colonic transit [3, 4, 5, 6, 9, 10] to explain the complaint of constipation. This increase in colonic time is only secondary to an increase in the distal colon transit time compared with the proximal colon

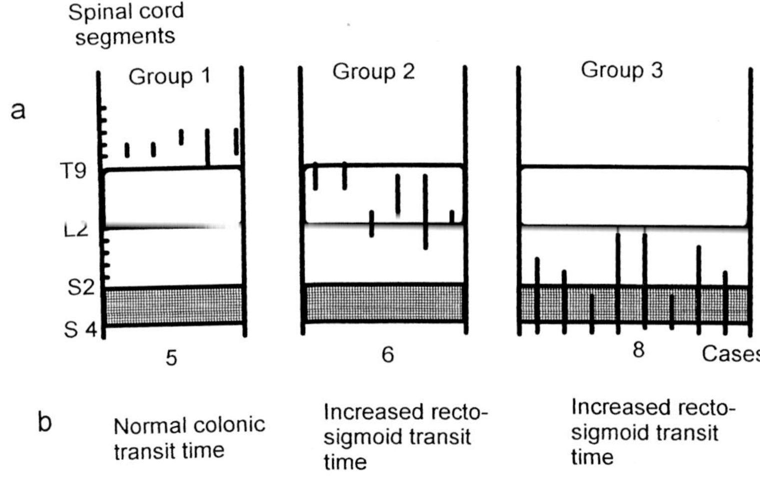

Fig. 1: *a) Level and number of injured spinal cord segments (the extent of the lesion is represented by black vertical lines) in three groups of patients with complete spinal transection. The white rectangles show the metameric location of the sympathetic centre (between T9 and L2), and the shaded rectangles show the metameric location of the parasympathetic centre (between S2 and S4). b) When the spinal lesion is above the sympathetic and parasympathetic centres, the colonic transit time is not different from that of control subjects. When the sympathetic or the parasympathetic centres are injured, the right and left colonic transit times are not different from those of controls, but the rectosigmoid transit time is increased (from Weber [20]).*

transit time. Indeed, it has been shown that only the distal part of colon is modified by a spinal cord lesion, whatever the spinal cord transection level [4]. In 19 patients with a complete spinal cord transection at different levels (above T9, between T9 and L2, and below L2) it has been shown that the right colonic transit was not different from that of controls, whatever the spinal cord transection level, and that transit time was increased only in the rectosigmoid colon (Fig. 1). Depending on the spinal cord injury level, two kinds of motility disturbances may be suggested: an increase in the nonperistaltic sympathetic controlled motility of the sigmoid colon in the case of a lesion of the thoracolumbar spinal cord (due to a lesion of the T9−L2 sympathetic centre), or a decrease of the peristaltic parasympathetic controlled motility of the sigmoid colon in case of a lesion of the sacral spinal cord (due to a lesion of the S2−S4 parasympathetic sacral centre). To confirm this last hypothesis, Varma et al. [18] and Binnie et al. [6], have shown that electrical stimulations of the anterior sacral roots (S2, S3 and S4) provoked colorectal peristaltic contractions associated with an increased colonic and rectal tone.

Knowing the pathophysiological mechanisms of slow transit in paraplegics could have a major impact on the choice of an appropriate treatment of constipation, since the electrical stimulation of sacral nerves has already been tried with a successful stimulation of the peristaltic parasympathetic motility. Conversely, to the best of our knowledge, no one has used beta-sympathomimetic drugs to restore the inhibitory control of non-peristaltic motility.

Gastro-colonic reflex

Recording colonic myoelectric activity, in the fasting state and after stimulation by a standard meal, Aaronson et al. [1] and Glick et al. [12] failed to show any increase in spike activity in spinal cord-injured subjects while it did in controls. Moreover, Aaronson et al. [1] found that those with a spinal cord injury had significantly more spike wave activity in the basal state than the controls. Finally, neostigmine significantly increased spike activity in both groups, with and without spinal cord injury. Conversely, Glick et al. [12] have shown that basal colonic motor and myoelectrical activity was normal. The difference between these two types may result from the difference between spinal cord injury levels. Aaronson's study [1] included 6 paraplegic subjects with different levels of spinal cord transection (between C5 and T12), and the other study [12] included 9 subjects with a thoracic level of transection (between T6 and T12). Another explanation could be the use of a different method of recording myoelectrical activity. Nevertheless, these two studies demonstrate clearly that the gastrocolonic reflex is always absent in spinal cord injury, suggesting that this reflex is mediated through the spinal cord.

Impaired defaecation

Defaecation depends on the integrity of the spinal reflexes controlling the motor activity of the anorectum and their modulation by conscious mechanisms.

It has been shown that a rectoanal dyssynergia exists in case of spinal cord lesion. Indeed, the rectoanal inhibitory reflex (RAIR) is still present in case of spinal lesion whatever the transection level, indicating that RAIR occurrence is independent of the spinal nerve control [4, 10, 19]. Nevertheless, RAIR is abnormal in patients with spinal cord lesion. Amplitude and/or duration of the reflex are not always correlated with the volume of rectal distention. Figure 2 shows that these abnormalities depend on the transection level. RAIR anomalies are more severe in patients with a sacral cord injury, suggesting the importance of the parasympathetic spinal centre in RAIR modulation [4, 16]. The external anal sphincter does not seem to play any role in RAIR anomalies because there is no tonic activity in paraplegic patients at rest, as we have shown previously [19]. Nevertheless, in these patients, the striated anal sphincter may play the same negative role during reflex defaecation that the striated urethral sphincter plays in the micturition reflex [19]. Thus, the distal constipation found in paraplegic patients, with incomplete voiding of the rectal ampulla during the defaecation reflex, could be explained by two types of rectoanal disorders: RAIR anomalies and striated anal sphincter dyssynergia.

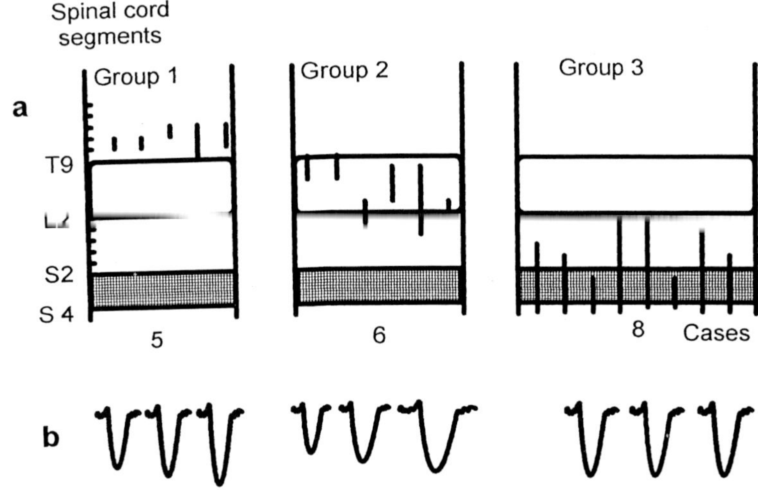

Fig. 2: *a) see Fig. 1.*
b) Three schematic RAIR responses obtained for increased rectal distending volumes, in each group. Group 1: when the rectal distending volume is increased, the RAIR amplitude, but not the RAIR duration is increased; group 2: when the rectal distending volume is increased, both the RAIR amplitude and duration are increased as seen in control subjects; group 3: when the rectal distending volume is increased, neither the RAIR amplitude nor the RAIR duration is increased (from Weber [20]).

Faecal incontinence

Faecal incontinence is a very common symptom in paraplegic patients. This may also be explained by at least three pathophysiological mechanisms:

Sigmoid and rectal faecaloma

The main consequences of both slow colonic transit and rectoanal dyssynergia is the occurrence of a rectosigmoid faecaloma. In our experience, a faecaloma is always found in the clinical examination of paraplegic patients. Very often faecal incontinence for solid and liquid stools is induced by a faecaloma [4]. Treatment and avoiding the recurrence of a faecaloma are the main principles of the therapeutic management of faecal incontinence in paraplegic subjects.

Impairment or decrease of conscious sensations

The lack of sensation coming from the anorectal apparatus is the main cause of faecal incontinence as shown by Caruana et al. [8]. It is well known that in case of injuries above the sacral spinal cord, sensations coming from the anorectal apparatus are always impaired. In these conditions, paraplegic patients lack all voluntary control of the defaecation reflex.

Absence of automatic and voluntary contractions in the external anal sphincter
Those are probably the most important pathophysiological factors explaining the compelling urge to defaecate as well as the faecal incontinence observed in paraplegic patients; in particular, gas incontinence is always present in paraplegics.

References

1. Aaronson, M. J., M. M. Freed, R. Burakoff: Colonic myoelectric activity in persons with spinal cord injury. Dig. Dis. Sci. 30 (1985) 295–300.
2. Apstein, M. D., K. Dalecki-Chipperfield: Spinal cord injury is a risk factor for gallstone disease. Gastroenterology 92 (1987) 966–968.
3. Badiali, D., E. Corazziari, F. I. Habib et al.: A double-blind controlled trial on the effect of cisapride in the treatment of constipation in paraplegic patients. J. Gastrointest. Motil. 3 (1991) 263–267.
4. Beuret-Blanquart, F., J. Weber, J. P. Gouverneur et al.: Colonic transit time and anorectal manometric anomalies in 19 patients with complete transection of the spinal cord. J. Auton. Nerv. Syst. 30 (1990) 199–208.
5. Binnie, N. R., G. H. Creasey, P. Edmond et al.: The action of cisapride on the chronic constipation of paraplegia. Paraplegia 26 (1988) 151–158.
6. Binnie, N. R., A. N. Smith, G. H. Creasey et al.: Motility effects of electrical anterior sacral nerve root stimulation of the parasympathetic supply of the left colon and anorectum in paraplegic subjects. J. Gastrointest. Motil. 2 (1990) 12–17.
7. Binnie, N. R., A. N. Smith, G. H. Creasey et al.: Constipation associated with chronic spinal cord injury: the effect of pelvic parasympathetic stimulation by the Brindley stimulator. Paraplegia 29 (1991) 463–469.
8. Caruana, B. J., A. Wald, J. P. Hinds et al.: Anorectal sensory and motor function in neurogenic fecal incontinence. Gastroenterology 100 (1991) 465–470.
9. de Both, P. S. M., G. H. de Groot, H. R. Slootman: Effect of cisapride on constipation in paraplegic patients: a placebo-controlled randomized double-blind cross-over study. Eur. J. Gastroenterol. Hepatol. 4 (1992) 1013–1017.
10. Devroede, G., P. Arhan, C. Duguay et al.: Traumatic constipation. Gastroenterology 77 (1979) 1258–1267.
11. Fealey, R. D., J. H. Szurszewski, J. L. Merritt et al.: Effect of traumatic spinal cord transection on human upper gastrointestinal motility and gastric emptying. Gastroenterology 87 (1984) 69–75.
12. Glick, M. E., S. Haldeman, H. Meshkinpour: The neurovisceral and electrodiagnostic evaluation of patients with thoracic spinal cord injury. Paraplegia 24 (1986) 129–137.
13. Iovino, P., F. Azpiroz, E. Domingo et al.: The sympathetic nervous system modulates perception and reflex responses to gut distention in humans. Gastroenterology 108 (1995) 680–686.
14. Read, N. W., L. Abouzekry: Why do patients with faecal impaction have faecal incontinence? Gut 27 (1986) 283–287.
15. Roman, C., J. Gonella: Extrinsic control of digestive tract motility. In: L. R. Johnson (Ed.): Physiology of the gastrointestinal tract (2nd ed.), pp. 507–553. Raven Press, New York 1987.
16. Shepherd, J. J., P. G. Wright: The response of the internal anal sphincter in man to stimulation of the presacral nerve. Am. J. Dig. Dis. 13 (1968) 421–427.

17. Thoren, T., E. Carlsson, S. Sandmark et al.: Effects of thoracic epidural analgesia with morphine or bupivacaine on lower oesophageal motility — an experimental study in man. Acta Anaesthesiol. Scand. 32 (1988) 391−394.
18. Varma, J. S., N. Binnie, A. N. Smith et al.: Differential effects of sacral anterior root stimulation on anal sphincter and colorectal motility in spinally injured man. Br. J. Surg. 73 (1986) 478−482.
19. Weber, J., F. Beuret-Blanquart, P. Ducrotté et al.: External anal sphincter function in spinal patients. Electromyographic and manometric study. Dis. Colon Rectum 34 (1991) 405−415.
20. Weber, J.: Constipation in spinal cord lesions, multiple sclerosis and diabetes mellitus. In: M. A. Kamm, J. E. Lennard-Jones (Eds.): Constipation, pp. 273−277. Wrightson Biomedical Publishing Ltd, Petersfield, UK 1994.

Management of lower gastrointestinal tract dysfunctions in patients with spinal cord injury

D. Badiali, M. Inghilleri, E. Corazziari

Introduction

Motor abnormalities of the gastrointestinal and biliary tract, as well as an increased prevalence of gallstone disease, esophagitis, chronic constipation and anal incontinence, have been reported in subjects with transection of the spinal cord.

A reduced pressure of the lower esophageal sphincter and a decreased velocity of the propagating motor activity were observed in paraplegic patients reporting esophageal symptoms such as heartburn, chest pain, intermittent dysphagia and the endoscopic-histologic evidence of esophagitis [20]. An autoptic study with no clinical information reported an increased prevalence of gallstones [2]. The transection of the cervical cord above the level of the sympathetic outflow to the gastrointestinal tracts may alter the normal interdigestive antro-duodenal motor coordination and delay gastric emptying [13]. Reduced bowel frequency and defaecatory dysfunctions are the most frequent and severe gastrointestinal complaints after cord injury.

With the exception of investigations of large bowel and anorectal motor functions most of these studies investigated epidemiological and physiopathological aspects and made little attempts to assess the relationship between the abnormal motor functions and symptoms, as well as the effect of the former on the clinical conditions.

Measurement of the large bowel transit, by means of radioopaque markers [18], showed a prolonged oro-anal transit time in paraplegic patients with spinal lesion located above the sacral level.

The evaluation of the large bowel segmental transit, expressed as transit index identified an abnormally slow transit mainly at level of the left colon and the rectum. These data indicate that after complete lesion of the spinal cord above the autonomic sacral nuclei, constipation is caused by slow transit through the left colon as well as by an altered defaecation. The former condition can be due to the increase of the intracolonic pressure by non-propagated contractions, and the lack of the gastrocolonic reflex, which may both impair transit through the colon and induce chronic constipation.

Manometric and electromyographic recording of the distal colon in paraplegics with suprasacral lesions have in fact reported an increased myoelectrical activity in basal fasting condition [1], and the absence of any postprandial propagated motor activity [15].

At the level of the rectoanal segment the lack of any conscious control of the pelvic and anal muscles predisposes to faecal incontinence, and on the other side, the impairment of the recto-anal inhibitory reflex [14, 26] or the persistence of external anal sphincter contraction during the attempts to evacuate [11, 22] is an obstacle to defaecation, which, in the presence of paralysis of abdominal and pelvic muscles, is not facilitated by the insufficient intrabdominal pressure increment during straining.

Patients with sacral or lower cord injury complain of faecal incontinence since the gastrocolonic reflex is preserved, anal tone and contractility is reduced and the conscious control of anal and pelvic muscles is lost [11, 21].

Constipation

Chronic constipation is the major gastrointestinal complaint after spinal cord injury which hardly responds to the usual conservative treatment and, not infrequently, leads to colo-rectal impaction and overflow faecal incontinence. In the management of chronic constipation, and in the attempt to prevent colo-rectal impaction, paraplegic subjects often use remedies which are unsuitable, scarcely effective, and unpredictable in their outcome. Thus constipation itself, the management of constipation and its side effects may, either alone or in variable conditions, reduce the wellbeing and the overall autonomy of paraplegic patients.

The ideal treatment of constipation in paraplegic patients should accelerate colonic transit, and evoke the defaecatory reflex at regular time intervals leading to predictable, effective, painless defaecations, and ultimately enhance patients' autonomy. The usual therapeutic measures, however, are less than optimal. Enemas and suppositories are not well accepted and, in patients with high cord lesion, they can not be used autonomously, and abdominal percussion and ano-rectal digitation can not be performed; laxatives can cause abdominal pain and their effect is not predictable since their use may be followed by episodes of faecal incontinence.

An attempt to optimize bowel movements and enhance patients' autonomy can be made, in addition to a high residue and adequately hydrated diet (15 g/die in dietary fibres and 1500 ml/die of water), with a sequential schedule of evacuating stimuli, aimed to identify, among several defaecatory stimuli, the one which, being equally effective, maximizes patient's control on his/her bowel.

A sequential progression of defaecatory stimuli may include the following steps: 1) abdominal massage and/or percussion; 2) perianal digitation; 3) anorectal digitation; 4) administration of glycerin suppository; 5) administration of laxative suppository; 6) enema and/or oral laxative. If patients are on daily laxatives and/or enemas, they are initially asked to refrain from them and to delay non spontaneous evacuations. Attempts to open the bowel according to the schedule should then be made, starting from the first step, and progressing to the successive step only if unsuccessful with the previous one.

In some paraplegic patients simple physical stimuli such as abdominal massage and perianal or anal digitation can induce inhibition of the anal sphincters (Fig. 1) and evacuation. The possible benefit of these maneuvers to initiate defaecation should be tested in each patient. It has been reported [4] that after a 4-week period of the previously described sequential treatment, the large bowel transit is accelerated, the weekly bowel evacuations are increased, and the use of oral laxatives is decreased (Fig. 2).

However in some patients the physical and/or pharmacological stimulation of the anorectal area may not be sufficient, and it is necessary to prescribe oral laxatives alone or in combination with one or more of the above mentioned anorectal stimuli. In prescribing laxatives some factors should be taken into account. Frequency of laxative assumption must be planned in order to avoid rectal impaction and overflow incontinence: daily administration is not necessary and usually three or less administrations per week are sufficient. Laxatives must be administered at the lowest effective dose and chosen among those with fewer side effects. It may be suggested to make an initial trial with the osmotic laxatives or PEG solutions; alternative approaches could take into consideration contact laxatives which, like bisacodyl, are scarcely absorbed from the intestine.

In 1988 three reports suggested that cisapride, at the dose of 40 mg per diem, may be of benefit in the management of chronic constipation in paraplegic patients. These papers, two case reports [10, 12] and one short term uncontrolled study [5] suggested that the use of cisapride does not trigger bowel opening, but it accelerates colonic transit and partially affects modality and frequency of defaecation.

In contrast, two double blind controlled trials [3, 9] did not confirm these favourable effects since neither the oro-anal transit time nor bowel habits differed significantly during cisapride and placebo administration (Fig. 3). However, it is still possible that cisapride might have therapeutic effects in patients who differ from those investigated in controlled clinical trials for the degree and/or the level of cord lesion.

To prevent reflex contraction of the bladder which may lead to urinary incontinence and vesico-pielic reflux, paraplegic patients with neurological bladder

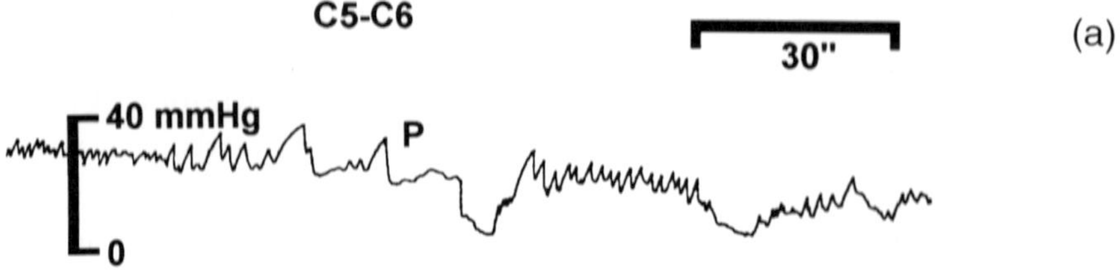

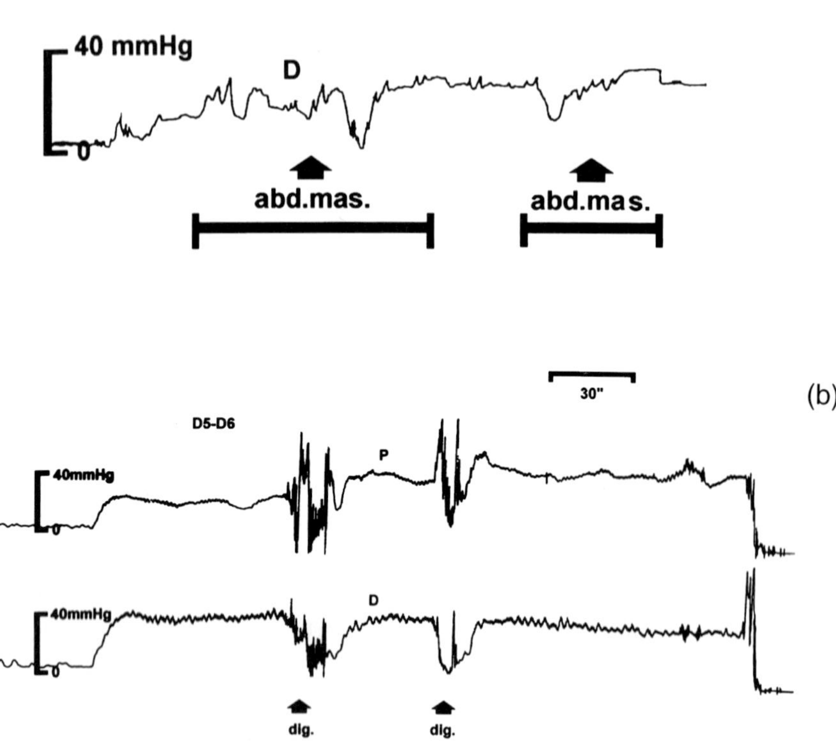

Fig. 1: *Two manometric tracings recorded from the the proximal (P) and distal (D) tract of the anal canal; (a) the anal canal pressure decreases during abdominal massage (abd. mas) and (b) during and following ano-rectal digitation (dig). Paraplegic patients can induce the relaxation of the anal canal and thus trigger defaecation by means of such maneuvers.*

can be submitted to rhizotomy, consisting in the surgical bisection of the posterior nerve roots of S2, S3, S4, with the implant of an electrostimulator capable to activate the process of micturition by stimulating the anterior sacral roots [7].

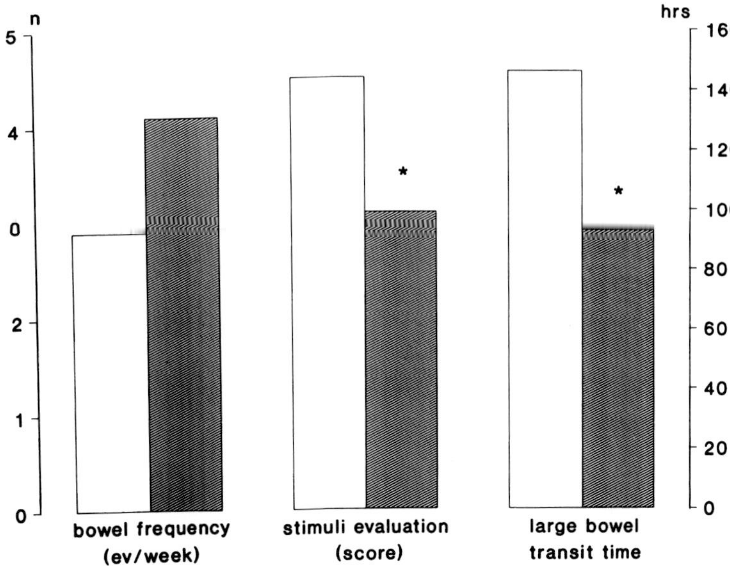

Fig. 2: *Comparison of bowel frequency, use of defaecatory stimuli and large bowel transit time in basal condition, before treatment (empty columns) and after a 4-week period of sequential treatment (striped columns). After treatment there is significant (*p < 0.05) improvement of the score evaluating the stimuli to defaecate and of the large bowel transit, but not of the bowel frequency (Badiali et al. [4]).*

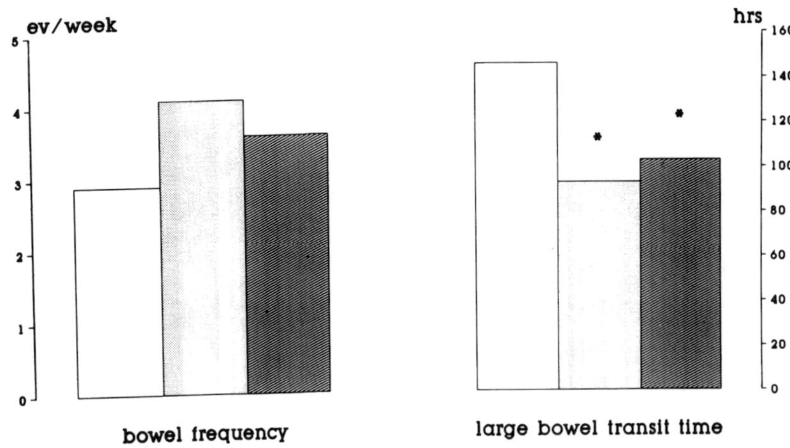

Fig. 3: *Comparison of bowel frequency and large bowel transit time in basal condition, before treatment (empty columns), during placebo (dotted columns) and cisapride treatment (striped columns). Bowel frequency did not differ during the three study periods; large bowel transit accelerated during placebo and cisapride treatment (*p < 0.02), but did not differ significantly between placebo and cisapride treatment (Badiali et al. [3]).*

Rhizotomy of S2–S4 affects also the motor function of the distal bowel and, in paraplegic patients, it may prevent the spinal excitatory reflexes, which in response to the increase of intra-abdominal pressure such as during straining, induce prolonged repetitive contractions of the rectosigmoid region (clusters of giant non-propagating contractions) and/or of the anal sphincter [22]. After rhizotomy, the act of defaecation, once triggered, is facilitated and becomes easier and more predictable because faeces find less resistance to enter into the rectum, and expulsion of faeces is not impaired by the paradoxical anal contraction during straining.

Since the distal colon and the anorectum are innervated by the parasympathetic and somatic nerve fiber outflow via the same sacral spinal roots used for electromicturition, the electro-stimulation has been proposed [8, 23] to induce defaecation in paraplegic patients by coordinating colorectal contraction and anal relaxation.

The electrostimulation of the individual sacral nerve roots induces different motor activity in the distal part of the gastrointestinal tract [17, 23]; it was observed that the electrostimulation of S3 induced contraction of the left and sigmoid colon, but no motor activity of the rectum; on the contrary the electro-stimulation of S4 induced a rectal contraction accompanied by anal relaxation, and no colonic activity. Rectosigmoid contraction coordinated with anal inhibition [17] was best achieved with the simultaneous electrostimulation of the 3 pairs of anterior sacral nerve roots (S2–S4). However the responses to root stimulation show wide intra-individual variability, and manometry of the colon and ano-rectum has been advocated to identify root level, pulse frequency and strength, which optimize the act of defaecation in the individual patient [17]. Complete unassisted defaecation is obtained in about 50% of the subjects with properly programmed sacral anterior root stimulator [17]. Autonomy of these patients is greatly improved since they achieve a normal bowel frequency while saving time spent to defaecate. Another study reported that in patients with electrostimulator there was an acceleration of the bowel transit and an increase of bowel frequency [6].

As expected the spontaneous defaecatory reflex is definitively lost after rhizotomy [18] and thus patients unresponsive to electrostimulation must permanently rely on digital maneuvers to defaecate. It would therefore appear that, despite some positive results, constipation (and/or faecal incontinence) can not be the only indications for rhizotomy and implantation of electrostimulators. On the other hand in patients who have already an implanted sacral electrostimulator to regulate micturition it is worthwhile to use the same technique to stimulate defaecation by programming it upon the indications of colorectoanal manometry.

Faecal incontinence

Faecal incontinence may be the consequence of rectal impaction and faecal overflow, an exaggerated rectal contraction in response to distension, the impairment of the conscious control of the anal contraction (lack of squeezing) [11, 14, 21, 22, 27]. The simple most important means to prevent faecal incontinence is to avoid prolonged rectal faecal stasis by maintaining a regular frequency of bowel evacuation.

The measures aimed to regulate stool consistency are also important. To obtain soft stools, and prevent faecaloma, it is important to balance the intake of fibers and water; patients should decrease, or even abolish, foods which can cause liquid stools (e. g. milk) and avoid or control the dose of oral laxatives. The administration of loperamide to increase the anal pressure [19] is not useful and it may worsen constipation.

Rhizotomy, which may potentially prevent faecal incontinence because it eliminates the reflex contraction of the rectum in response to its distension when filling with faeces [22] does not seem to be sufficiently reliable as a therapeutic means.

In patients with sacral or lower cord lesion, faecal incontinence is also caused by the reduced resting anal tone [21]. Bowel training is indicated in these subjects; a toilet training program using the less disturbing rectal maneuver or medication which triggers a satisfactory defaecatory stimulus, within thirty minutes after a meal (to take advantage of the gastrocolonic reflex), has been reported to be successful in managing faecal incontinence in 23/24 cooperative children with spina bifida [16]. The achievement of this goal required 6−12 weeks and the successful outcome correlated with the presence of the anocutaneous reflex [16]. A reduced compliance to the training program has been observed in young adult people, while inadequate technique in suppository insertion or in performing digital stimulation is the most frequent cause of therapeutic failure [16].

In those patients with very low or incomplete lesions, with residual control of the external anal sphincter, and preserved rectal sensitivity [25], the degree of continence can be improved with biofeedback and/or physiotherapy [24, 28].

Conclusions

In conclusion, chronic constipation, and related overflow faecal incontinence, represents the major gastrointestinal complaint in paraplegic patients.

A sequential schedule of evacuatory stimuli, combined with a high fiber diet enables to identify the therapeutic measures which, in the individual patient, optimize frequency and modality of evacuation obtaining the best result to defaecate with the minimal side effects.

In patients with sacral electrostimulator implanted to regulate micturition, the same technique can be programmed, on the indication of colorectoanal manometry, to induce unassisted and effective defaecation.

The best treatment for faecal incontinence is the management of bowel habit.

References

1. Aaronson, M. J., M. M. Freed, R. Burakoff: Colonic myoelectric activity in persons with spinal cord injury. Dig. Dis. Sci. 30 (1985) 295–300.
2. Apstein, M. D., K. Dalecki-Chipperfield: Spinal cord injury is a risk factor for gallstone disease. Gastroenterology 92 (1987) 966–968.
3. Badiali, D., E. Corazziari, F. I. Habib et al.: A double-blind controlled trial on the effect of cisapride in the treatment of constipation in paraplegic patients. J. Gastroint. Motility 3 (1991) 263–267.
4. Badiali, D. et al.: Sequential treatment of chronic constipation in paraplegic subjects. Spinal Cord, in press.
5. Binnie, N. R., G. H. Creasey, P. Edmond et al.: The action of cisapride on the chronic constipation of paraplegia. Paraplegia 26 (1988) 151–158.
6. Binnie, N. R., A. N. Smith, G. H. Creasey et al.: Constipation associated with chronic spinal cord injury: the effect of pelvic parasympathetic stimulation by the Brindley stimulator. Paraplegia 29 (1991) 463–469.
7. Brindley, G. S., C. E. Polkey, D. N. Rushton: Sacral anterior root stimulation for bladder control in paraplegia. Paraplegia 20 (1982) 365–381.
8. Brindley, G. S., C. E. Polkey, D. N. Rushton: Sacral anterior root stimulation for bladder control in paraplegia: the first 50 cases. J. Neurol. Neurosurg. Psychiatry 49 (1986) 1104–1114.
9. de Both, P. S. M., G. H. de Groot, H. R. Slootman: Effects of cisapride on constipation in paraplegic patients: a placebo-controlled randomized double blind cross-over study. Eur. J. Gastroenterol. Hepatol. 4 (1992) 1013–1017.
10. de Groot, G. H., G. F. de Pagter: Effects of cisapride on constipation due to a neurological lesion. Paraplegia 26 (1988) 159–161.
11. Devroede, G., P. Arhan, C. Duguay et al.: Traumatic Constipation. Gastroenterology 77 (1979) 1258–1267.
12. Etienne, M., M. Verlinden, A. Brassinne: Treatment with cisapride of the gastrointestinal and urological sequelae of spinal cord transection: case report. Paraplegia 26 (1988) 162–164.
13. Fealey, R. D., J. H. Szurszewski, J. L. Merritt et al.: Effect of traumatic spinal cord transection on human upper gastrointestinal motility and gastric emptying. Gastroenterology 87 (1984) 69–75.
14. Frenckner, B.: Function of the anal sphincters in spinal man. Gut 16 (1975) 638–644.
15. Glick, M. E., H. Meshkinpour, S. Haldeman et al.: Colonic dysfunction in patients with thoracic spinal cord injury. Gastroenterology 86 (1984) 287–294.
16. King, J. C., D. M. Currie, E. Wright: Bowel training in spina bifida: importance of education, patient compliance, age, and anal reflexes. Arch Phys Med Rehabil 75 (1994) 243–247.
17. MacDonagh, R. P., W. M. Sun, R. Smallwood et al.: Control of defecation in patients with spinal injuries by stimulation of sacral anterior nerve roots. Br. Med. J. 300 (1990) 1494–1497.

18. Menardo, G., G. Bausano, E. Corazziari et al.: Large-bowel transit in paraplegic patients. Dis. Colon Rectum 30 (1987) 924−928.
19. Read, M., N. W. Read, D. C. Barber et al.: Effects of loperamide on anal sphincter function in patients complaining of chronic diarrhea with fecal incontinence and urgency. Dig. Dis. Sci. 27 (1982) 807−814.
20. Stinneford, J. G. et al.: Esophagitis and esophageal motor abnormality in patients with chronic spinal cord injury. Paraplegia 131 (1993) 384−392.
21. Sun, W. M., N. W. Read, T. C. Donnelly: Anorectal function in incontinent patients with cerebral disease. Gastroenterology 99 (1990) 1372−1379.
22. Sun, W. M., R. MacDonagh, D. Forster et al.: Anorectal function in patients with complete spinal transection before and after sacral posterior rhizotomy. Gastroenterology 108 (1995) 990−998.
23. Varma, J. S., N. Binnie, A. N Smith et al.: Differential effects of sacral anterior root stimulation on anal sphincter and colorectal motility in spinally injured man. Br. J. Surg. 73 (1986) 478−482.
24. Wald, A.: Use of biofeedback in treatment of fecal incontinence in patients with myelomeningocele. Pediatrics 68 (1981) 45−49.
25. Wald, A.: Biofeedback for neurogenic fecal incontinence: rectal sensation is a determinant of outcome. J. Ped. Gastroenterol. Nutrition 2 (1983) 302−306.
26. Weber, J., F. Beuret-Blanquart, P. Ducrotte et al.: External anal sphincter function in spinal patients. Dis. Colon Rectum 34 (1991) 409−415.
27. Whearley, I. C., K. J. Hardy, J. Dent: Anal pressure studies in spinal patients. Gut 18 (1977) 488−490.
28. Whitehead, W. E., E. Parker, L. Basmajian et al.: Treatment of faecal incontinence in children with spina bifida: comparison of biofeedback and behaviour modification. Arch. Phys. Med. Rehabil. 67 (1986) 218−224.

Gastrointestinal disorders in neuromuscular and neurological diseases in childhood

P. J. Milla

Neuromuscular disease of the gut and disorder of the extrinsic innervation and central nervous system may result in alteration of gastrointestinal motor activity which is clinically significant and interfere with its normal propulsive function in the absence of anatomic abnormality. Whilst such disorders may be acute due to transient inflammatory or metabolic changes in this review we will only be concerned with chronic changes. Motor dysfunction of the gut may be regional or diffuse but not uncommonly although the clinical presentation is regional careful physiological studies will reveal dysfunction in other areas of the gut. Neuromuscular disease and extrinsic nerve disorder causes abnormalities of motor activity by disturbing different levels of control; either the smooth muscle end organ, intermediate regulatory pathways, the intrinsic innervation of the gut or higher centres involving the extrinsic innervation.

Smooth muscle

Damage to smooth muscle cells would result in reduced contractile activity of the gut with reduced intra-luminal pressure generated in the intestine and delayed transit of luminal contents. Motility recordings might be expected to show contractions of reduced amplitude with or without a normal pattern of contraction. The delayed transit might result in bacterial overgrowth and malabsorption.

Nerve

Enteric nervous system

Disease may be primarily of the intrinsic enteric nerves with or without involvement of the extrinsic autonomic nerves or of the central nervous system. Damage or disorder of the intrinsic enteric innervation may be restricted to one or other of the major nerve plexuses, the submucosal or myenteric plexus or to both. The myenteric plexus may be thought of as the motor division of the enteric nervous system and the submucosal plexus the sensory and secreto-motor division. Thus damage to the myenteric plexus would result in disruption of normally observed patterns of contractile activity and disorder of the sub-mucosal plexus perhaps visceral hyperalgesia or increased intestinal secretion. Whilst denervation might be expected to release the smooth muscle from its customary inhibition resulting in increased contractility, it is unlikely that this will result in consistent patterns of abnormality which are functionally effective. Some processes will be restricted to one type of neuron whereas others will be completely unselective resulting in damage to both inhibitory and excitatory networks. Myenteric plexus disease may be due to a wide variety of disorders including developmental disorders typified by Hirschsprung's disease, ingestion of environmental toxins, toxins from intestinal bacterial pathogens, viral infec-tions such as cytomegalovirus infection, inflammatory infiltrative and parasitic disorders such as amyloidosis, Chagas' disease. Lymphoma and vasculitic and ischaemic disorders are extremely rare in childhood and occur with much greater frequency in adult life.

Central and autonomic nervous system

There is increasing evidence to suggest that disease outside the gut disrupts normal patterns of activity varying with the level of nervous involvement. The central nervous system might disturb normal patterns of activity through the autonomic nervous system. In general, parasympathetic stimulation stimulates motor activity and sympathetic activity suppresses it. Increased sympathetic activity is well recognised in stress which has been shown to disturb small intestinal motility. This may be an important factor in some functional bowel disorders. Autonomic abnormalities may co-exist with myenteric plexus disease and may cause pupillary disorders, abnormalities of sweating and of cardiovas-cular control. Familiar forms of autonomic dysfunction (the Riley-Day Syn-drome) are well known to the paediatrician.

That the central nervous system may be responsible for patterns of the activity is common every day experience either as a strong emotional reaction or as an expression of underlying psycho-pathology. Increasing numbers of studies of the effects of stress and sleeping [25] disturbing fasting small intestinal motility provides support for the more every day observations. It is however also clear that central nervous system disease may be associated with disturbed gastroin-testinal motor activity and this is best exemplified by the gastro-oesophageal reflux associated with severe cerebral palsy. Indeed where central nervous sys-tem disease exists disturbance of motor function in the gut occurs where there is the greatest density of afferent and efferent fibres connecting gut and brain. Thus, fore gut disorders such as gastro-oesophageal reflux are very common in association with central nervous system disease.

Clinical disorders

Disorders of swallowing

In children swallowing disorders rarely present as isolated problems and most often occur in infants and children with multiple handicaps. A number of conditions pre-dispose to impaired swallowing and include central and peripheral nervous system dysfunction, diseases of muscle and structural anomalies of the

Table 1: *Swallowing disorders in children.*

1 Prematurity
2 Upper airway and pharyngeal anomalies
  a nasal and naso-pharyngeal disorders
     — choanal atresia and stenosis
     — septal deflections
     — tumours
  b oral cavity and oro-pharynx
     — defects of lip
     — cleft lip and/or cleft palate
     — craniofacial syndromes eg Pierre Robin Syndrome
  c Laryngeal
     — laryngeal stenosis and webs
     — laryngomalacia
     — laryngeal cleft
3 Congenital defects of trachea and oesophagus
  a Tracheo-oesophageal fistula/atresia
  b Oesophageal strictures and webs
  c Vascular anomalies eg double aortic arch
4 Neurological disorders
  a Central nervous system disease
     — hypoxic brain damage eg cerebral palsy
     — cortical atrophy, microcephaly
     — infections
     — myelomeningocele
     — trauma
  b Peripheral nervous system disease
     — traumatic
     — congenital
     — inflammatory eg Guillain-Barre Syndrome
     — poliomyelitis
  c Neuromuscular disease
     — myotonic muscular dystrophy
     — myasthenia gravis
  d Miscellaneous
     — cricopharyngeal achalasia
     — dysautonomia
     — aberrant cervical thymus

oral cavity and pharynx. Other groups at risk of developing dysfunctional swallowing and its complications include preterm infants with poor co-ordination of breathing and swallowing and infants with chronic pulmonary disease. The spectrum of swallowing disorders will not be reviewed in detail and is provided in Table 1 [26].

Table 2: *Oesophageal motor disorders.*

1   Disorders that effect the striated muscle oesophagus
   a Cricopharyngeal dysfunction
   b Myopathic disease
      − myotonic muscular dystrophy
      − oculo pharyngeal dystrophy
   c Inflammatory myopathies eg dermatomyositis
   d Neurological disorders
      − motor neurone disease
      − bulbar palsy eg Moebius Syndrome
      − myasthenia gravis
      − infection eg poliomyelitis, botulism
2   Disorders that effect the smooth muscle oesophagus
   a Primary oesophageal motor disorders eg achalasia
   b Secondary eosophageal motor disorders
      − congenital malformation
      − collagenosis
      − neuromuscular disorders
      − infections eg Chagas Disease

Oesophageal disorders

Abnormalities of oesophageal function occur frequently and may be primarily confined to the oesophagus or secondary to systemic illness. The disorders can be divided into two groups depending upon whether the upper third striated muscle portion of the oesophagus is predominantly effected or the lower two thirds of the smooth muscle oesophagus. Conditions effecting the latter are much commoner than the former. The former will tend to present with disorders of swallowing and these will be caused by a variety of systemic muscular disease or neurological conditions. These are shown in Table 2.

Disorders of the smooth muscle portion of the oesophagus

Achalasia

Achalasia is a motor disorder of the oesophagus that presents as functional obstruction at the oesophago-gastric junction [3]. It is characterised by abnormalities of function of the lower oesophageal sphincter and of the body of the oesophagus. The lower oesophageal sphincter does not relax normally in association with swallowing and the pressure of the sphincter is increased. In the body of the oesophagus peristalsis is abnormal and there may be episodes of oesophageal spasm. The illness is uncommon with an incidence in the United Kingdom of between 0.11 and 0.31 cases per 10^5 children per year [13]. Whilst in the past numerous theories have existed regarding the pathogenesis of the condition the consensus of the body of information now available would suggest that this is a neuropathic condition effecting the myenteric plexus of the lower oesophagus. In the majority of cases there is ganglion cell degeneration with progression to aganglionosis resulting in loss of inhibition to the oesophageal smooth muscle [23]. In only one circumstance is the etiology of the neuro degenerative disorder known and that is in Chagas' disease [12].

The condition presents more commonly in adults than in children but the youngest patient reported is a 900 g fourteen day old premature infant [18]. The mean age at diagnosis is however 8.8 years and the duration of symptoms prior to diagnosis twenty three months. The most prominent symptoms on presentation are dysphagia and vomiting. The dysphagia occurs initially with solids but progresses to liquids. Patients often describe the sensation of food getting caught in the middle to lower chest and as a consequence of the symptoms the children are usually very slow eaters.

At the present time oesophageal motility remains the diagnostic method of choice though scintiscanning and radiography are useful screening tests [23]. Endoscopy provides useful information regarding the oesophageal mucosa prior to treatment being started.

Treatment

The goal of therapy is to relieve the functional obstruction at the level of the lower oesophageal sphincter either by pharmacological means using calcium channel blockers such as nifedipine or isosorbide dinitrate. Non-pharmacological treatments consist of dilatation by bougienage or balloon, or surgery. The most common surgical treatment being a Heller's myotomy. In the author's unit a long or extended myotomy is used together with an anti-reflux procedure and this has resulted in excellent control of the dysphagia and of the obstructive symptoms [5].

Gastro-oesophageal reflux disease

It is common for infants to have recurrent problems with vomiting during the first year of life. In the majority this does not cause serious symptoms, but in some, results in a variety of associated disorders including failure to thrive due to loss of calories from vomiting or refusal to feed, irritability, iron deficiency anaemia, haematemesis and stricture as a consequence of oesophagitis and apnoeic episodes, wheezing and aspiration pneumonia [14]. It is important to realise that gastro-oesophageal reflux in infancy may occur secondary to any process that interrupts normal gastrointestinal motility but in particular with a hiatus hernia, gastric outlet obstruction, a malrotation, intrinsic neuromuscular disease of the oesophagus and severe neurological disease such as cerebral palsy. Up to two thirds of patients with severe cerebral palsy suffer from gastro-oesophageal reflux.

The commonest mechanism for gastro-oesophageal reflux is inappropriate relaxation of the sphincter occurring independently of swallow induced peristalsis. Whether an individual patient develops other symptoms such as oesophagitis or aspiration pneumonia may however be determined by the effectiveness of secondary peristalsis in clearing refluxed material [11].

Investigations of gastro-oesophageal reflux related disease fall into three groups. Investigations to detect its presence and define its severity; determination of complicating disease such as a stricture or aspiration pneumonia and lastly an investigation of the potential underlying causes. In order to manage the conditions a 24 hour intra-oesophageal pH study to determine the presence and severity of reflux together with an upper gastrointestinal contrast study to detect the presence of anatomical abnormality and an endoscopy for oesophagitis are required [14]. Oesophageal manometry is extremely useful in determining the underlying physiological mechanism of the disorder but clinically is of little value. Treatment is in three phases and consists of positioning and thickening of feeds for those who are thriving but spitting up, the addition of prokinetic agents such as domperidone and cisapride together with antacid or H2 blockade to reduce acid secretion. Lastly those, particularly with oesophagitis, that fail medical treatment, those who have respiratory symptoms and those who have a stricture will require surgical treatment with a fundoplication.

Disorders of the stomach

Gastric outlet obstruction

Gastric outlet obstruction is mostly commonly present as hypertrophic pyloric stenosis in which the grossly thickened pylorus results in a well recognised clinical presentation of projectile vomiting and failure to thrive. The nature of the pathological process which causes the condition is not clear though most evidence suggests that it is a neuropathy [6] and that it may particularly effect nitrergic nerves [15]. Hypertrophic pyloric stenosis perhaps should be thought of as extremely isolated pseudo-obstructive lesion in the majority of cases.

Other forms of functional gastric outlet obstruction may be associated with dysrhythmia of the gastric antral smooth muscle, particularly in the situation where there is a persistent tachygastria.

Small intestinal and colonic disease

Chronic idiopathic intestinal pseudo-obstruction

Intestinal pseudo-obstruction is a clinical syndrome characterised by signs of intestinal obstruction but without demonstrable organic occlusion. As a result bacterial overgrowth and diarrhoea is a very common problem in these patients. The condition is due to disease of the smooth muscle coats, the extrinsic or intrinsic nerves or alteration of their neuroendocrine environment. Disorder of the humoral and endocrine environment will not be considered further here.

Enteric nervous system disease

Disease of the enteric nervous system may be familial and limited entirely to the gut as in congenital absence of argyrophil nerves [24] (which is inherited as an X-linked or perhaps in some an autosomal recessive trait) and familial megaduodenum [9] or as part of a familial peripheral and autonomic neuropathy such as familial visceral neuropathy [21]. In isolated conditions of the enteric nerves other than achalasia and pyloric stenosis, short small intestine and malrotation there are no specific clinical features. The disorder of the enteric nervous system may be due to either primary or secondary disease and in children it is nearly always primary. Over 90% of cases present during the first year of life, mostly commonly at or around birth [16]. It seems likely that those that present at or shortly after birth are due to defects of development or intra-uterine catastrophes such as might occur with neurotropic viruses. Defective development may occur at any point in the complex process of colonisation of the gut by migrating neural crest cells and this process may be held up at any point. At the present time a number of genetic factors are known which appear to control different aspects of this process including the ret gene [20], the endothelin B receptor [19], the endothelin 3 ligand [1], possibly the trk gene [8] and some of the homeobox genes. The ret gene is also associated with multiple endocrine neoplasia in which giant submucosal ganglia and myenteric plexus hyperplasia are observed together with obstructive symptoms [7].

The etiology of enteric nervous damage occurring after birth is similarly poorly understood; in many cases in older children enteric neuropathy may be due to one of a number of secondary conditions such as collagenosis. Mention should also be made of a ten year old child which we have recently studied who presented with acute severe constipation proven to be associated with an inflammatory denervating process effecting the intrinsic enteric nerves. An IgG circulating myenteric antibody was found in her peripheral circulation similar to that described in the paraneoplastic syndrome associated with oat cell carcinoma of the lung [10].

Disorders affecting intestinal smooth muscle

In adult life intestinal muscle disease usually occurs secondary to a number of different conditions including dystrophia myotonica, systemic sclerosis, Ehlers-Danlos syndrome, dermatomyositis and systemic lupus erythematosus. In only a minority is there smooth muscle disease restricted to the gut. The reverse is true in children and smooth muscle disease as part of a systemic disease occurs extremely rarely. The majority of children suffer from two syndromes the pathogenesis of which is not understood.

Hollow visceral myopathy syndrome

This condition may occur sporadically or familially and when in families appears to be inherited as an autosomal dominant or an X-linked dominant trait [22]. The disease process is not restricted to any particular regions of the gut and may effect the oesophagus, stomach, small or large intestine. In the author's experience the urinary tract is nearly always effected with a hydro-ureter and megacystis [17].

Megacystis microcolon hypoperistalsis syndrome

A similar but different disease occurring sporadically is the megacystis microcolon hypoperistalsis syndrome described in neonates by Berdon et al. [2].

Diagnostic techniques

In order to understand the pseudo-obstructive disorder and plan rational treatment the involved areas must be defined and at least the physiology of the effected areas studied. Such studies may involve radiology and transit studies using either radioopaque pellets or scintiscanning. Manometry is helpful in delineating both the extent of the disease and the nature of the disease process causing the disorder [27]. We have shown particularly in the small intestine that measurement of fasting motor activity is a useful diagnostic procedure as phase 3 activity can be used as a probe of the integrity of the enteric neuromusculature. In neuropathic processes contractions are of normal amplitude but are bizarre in wave form, abnormally propagated and phase 3 activity is ill formed. Whereas in muscle disease contractile activity is of low amplitude and poorly propagated with phase 3 often being apparently not present [4].

Latterly we have used surface electrogastrography as a screening test and find this an excellent method for determining the nature of the underlying disease where there is diffuse disorder of the bowel (Fig. 1).

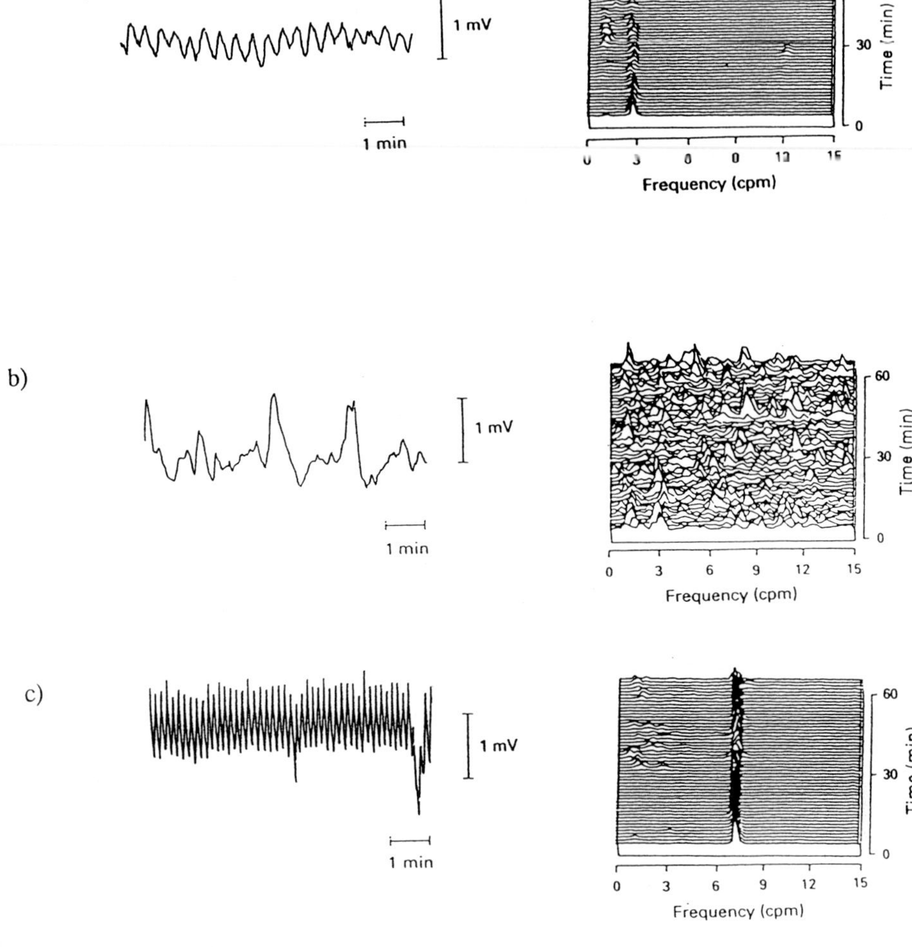

Fig. 1: *Surface electrogastrography. a) control subject. b) smooth muscle myopathy. c) visceral neuropathy.*

The mortality of these conditions is high, as much as 40% in muscle disease, but with careful treatment of infection, particularly of the urinary tract and of bacterial overgrowth, the use of decompression surgery, a terminal ileostomy, and judicious use of parenteral nutrition allow survival to adult life.

Idiopathic megarectum and megacolon in children

A very large majority, probably in excess of 90% of children who present with chronic constipation do not have neurological disease or neuromuscular disease of the gut. But it should be remembered that constipation is extremely common in children with central nervous system disease, particularly where this results in mental retardation and is presumably due to the loss of central inhibition to the gastrointestinal tract.

However it is clear that neuromuscular disease may present simply as chronic constipation and some 5% of children with Hirschsprung's disease may present in this way. So called pseudo-Hirschsprung's disease may be due to a wide variety of conditions most of which have been described in the section on intestinal pseudo-obstruction but which also importantly includes the so called condition of intestinal neuronal dysplasia. Whether this is an intrinsic developmental disorder of the enteric nervous system of the hind gut is at this time controversial but the condition clearly does occur in association with Hirschsprung's disease. Lastly, very unusually some children with smooth muscle disease isolated to the lower part of the hind gut may present with constipation.

References

1. Baynash, A. G., K. Hosoda, A. Giaid et al.: Interaction of endothelin-3 with endothelin-B receptor is essential for development of epidermal melanocytes and enteric neurons. Cell 79 (1994) 1277−1285.
2. Berdon, W. E., D. H. Baker, W. A. Blane et al.: Megacystis-microcolon-intestinal hypoperistalsis syndrome: a new cause of intestinal obstruction in the new born. Am. J. Roentgenol. 126 (1976) 957−964.
3. Berquist, W. E., W. J. Byrne, M. E. Ament et al.: Achalasia: diagnosis, management and clinical course in 16 children. Pediatrics 71 (1983) 798−805.
4. Devane, S. P., A. M. Ravelli, W. M. Bisset et al.: Gastric antral dysrhythmias in children with chronic idiopathic intestinal pseudoobstruction. Gut 33 (1992) 1477−1481.
5. Emblem, R., M. D. Stringer, C. M. Hall et al.: Current results of surgery for achalasia of the cardia. Arch. Dis. Childh. 68 (1993) 749−751.
6. Friesen, S. R., A. S. E. Pearse: Pathogenesis of congenital pyloric stenosis: histochemical analyses of pyloric ganglion cells. Surgery 53 (1963) 604−607.
7. Hofstra, R. M. W., R. M. Landsvater, I. Ceccherini et al.: A mutation in the RET proto-oncogene associated with multiple endocrine neoplasia type 2B and sporadic medullary thyroid carcinoma. Nature 367 (1994) 375−376.
8. Kapur, R., B. Doggett, E. Olsen: Colonisation of the murine large intestine by ganglion cell precursors is blocked by an inhibitor of trk-family receptor tyrosine kinases. Pediatric Pathology Laboratories and Medicine 15 (1995) 345.
9. Law, D. H., E. A. Ten Eyck: Familial megaduodenum and megacystis. Am. J. Med. 33 (1962) 911−922.
10. Lennon, V. A., D. F. Sas, M. F. Busk et al.: Enteric neuronal auto-antibodies in pseudoobstruction with small cell lung carcinoma. Gastroenterology 100 (1991) 137−142.
11. Mahony, M. J., M. Migliavacca, L. Spitz et al.: Motor disorders of the oesophagus in gastro-oesophageal reflux. Arch. Dis. Childh. 63 (1988) 1333−1338.
12. Martin, S., J. V. Campos, W. I. Tafuri: Chagas enteropathy. Gut 14 (1973) 910−919.
13. Mayberry, J. B., M. J. Mayell: Epidemiological study of achalasia in children. Gut 29 (1988) 90−93.

14. Milla, P. J.: Reflux vomiting. Arch. Dis. Child. 65 (1990) 996−999.
15. Milla, P. J.: Gastric outlet obstruction in children. New England Journal of Medicine 327 (1992) 558−559.
16. Milla, P. J.: Intestinal pseudo-obstruction in children. In: M. A. Kamm, J. E. Lennard-Jones (Eds.): Constipation, pp. 251−258. Wrightson Biomedical Publishing Ltd., Petersfield, UK 1994.
17. Milla, P. J., B. D. Lake, L. Spitz et al.: Chronic idiopathic intestinal pseudo-obstruction in infancy: smooth muscle disease. In: G. Labo, M. Bortolotti (Eds.): Gastrointestinal Motility, pp. 125−131. Cortina International, Verona 1984.
18. Polk, H. C., T. H. Burford: Disorders of the distal esophagus in infancy and childhood. American Journal of Diseases of Children 108 (1964) 243−251.
19. Puffenberger, E. G., K. Hosoda, S. S. Washington et al.: A missense mutation of the endothelin-B receptor gene in multigenic Hirschsprung's disease. Cell 79 (1994) 1257−1266.
20. Romeo, G., P. Ronchetto, Y. Luo et al.: Point mutations affecting the tyrosine kinase domain of the RET proto-oncogene in Hirschsprung's disease. Nature 367 (1994) 377−378.
21. Schuffler, M. D., T. D. Bird, S. M. Sumi et al.: A familial neuronal disease presenting as intestinal pseudo-obstruction. Gastroenterology 75 (1978) 889−898.
22. Schuffler, M. D., M. C. Lowe, A. H. Bill: Chronic idiopathic intestinal pseudo-obstruction. 1. Hereditary hollow visceral myopathy. Clinical and pathological studies. Gastroenterology 73 (1977) 339−344.
23. Sendes, A., F. Smok, I. Braghetto et al.: Gastro-oesophageal sphincter pressure and histological changes of the distal esophagus in patients with achalasia of the oesophagus. Digestive Disease Sciences 30 (1985) 941−945.
24. Tanner, M. S., B. Smith, J. K. Lloyd: Functional intestinal obstruction due to deficiency of argyrophil neurones in the myenteric plexus. Arch. Dis. Childh. 51 (1978) 837−841.
25. Thompson, D. J., E. Richelson, J. R. Malagelada: Perturbation of upper gastrointestinal function by cold stress. Gut 24 (1983) 277−283.
26. Weiss, M. H.: Dysphagia in infants and children. Otolaryngology Clinics of North America 21 (1988) 727−735.
27. Wozniak, E. R., T. R. Fenton, P. J. Milla, : Fasting small intestinal motor activity in chronic idiopathic intestinal pseudo-obstruction. Pediatr. Res. 18 (1984) 1060.

Genetic aspects of myopathies

E. Gussoni, C. G. Bönnemann, E. M. McNally, L. M. Kunkel

Muscular dystrophies are a heterogeneous group of disorders affecting predominantly skeletal muscle. The severity of their phenotype is broad and varies among different disorders as well as within a given type of dystrophy. The most common and most severe type of muscular dystrophy is the X-linked Duchenne muscular dystrophy (DMD), but other non X-linked dystrophies have also been identified in various populations, and are generally referred to as autosomal muscular dystrophies [15]. Duchenne muscular dystrophy is an ultimately lethal disorder affecting 1 in 3,500 newborn males. It is characterized by progressive skeletal muscle weakness due to necrosis of muscle cells and substitution of connective tissue for skeletal muscle, and eventual cardiac and respiratory failure [15]. Patients affected by DMD may also manifest gastrointestinal complications, including gastric hypomotility and intestinal pseudo-obstruction [3, 12].

The understanding of the molecular pathogenesis of muscular dystrophies began with the identification and cloning of the gene that causes Duchenne muscular dystrophy. The DMD gene, the largest known human gene, is located on Xp21 and its size spans 2.5 million base pairs. The full length transcript from this gene is 14 Kb and contains about 79 exons that, when translated, yield a high molecular weight protein, named dystrophin [9]. At least 7 different promoters have been discovered in the dystrophin gene. Some of these promoters regulate the expression of tissue specific isoforms of dystrophin in skeletal muscle, brain, retina, kidney and peripheral nerve, for review, see Ahn 1993 [2]. Since the different promoters are located within introns throughout the dystrophin gene, some of these dystrophin isoforms may have smaller sizes than the full length protein. For example, the peripheral nerve promoter encodes for a protein of 116 kD [6] and the general promoter for a 71 kD isoform [11].

Dystrophin is expressed at its highest levels in skeletal and cardiac muscle, where it constitutes 0.001% of total cellular protein and is expressed at much lower levels in brain and smooth muscle. Immunohistochemical studies on normal skeletal muscle tissue sections using anti-dystrophin antibodies have localized this protein at the level of the sarcolemma as a continuous staining along the membrane. In contrast, dystrophin is absent or severely reduced in muscle of DMD patients.

Clinical studies have shown that DMD patients have a delayed gastric emtpying time compared to normal controls [3]. This abnormality has been attributed to the lack of dystrophin in the smooth muscle layers of the gastrointestinal tract

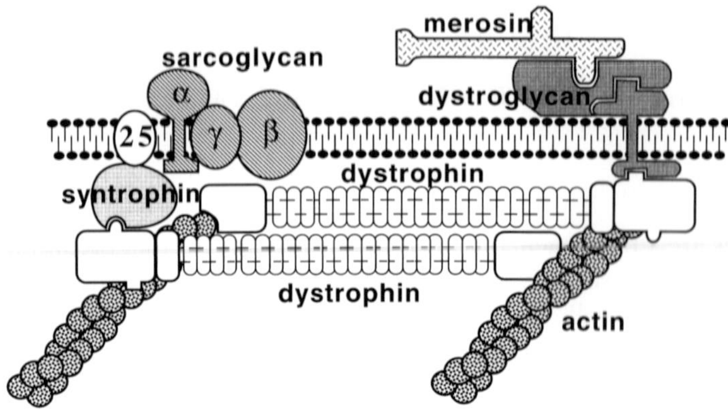

Fig. 1: *Dystrophin glycoprotein complex (DGC).*

[3]. Histological findings have shown that the longitudinal muscle layer is more affected than the circular layer in DMD patients [3, 12].

By western blot analysis on normal smooth muscle extract, dystrophin can be detected as a single band of about 400 kD, a slightly lower molecular weight than full length dystrophin in skeletal muscle [5]. Immunohistochemical studies using anti-dystrophin antibodies on intestine tissue sections have shown immunoreactivity at the level of the sarcolemma of smooth muscle cells.

In contrast to striated muscle, dystrophin appears as a discontinuous labeling of the surface of the cell membrane. In transverse sections the labeling appears punctate, while in longitudinal view it forms a stripe-like pattern [5]. A similar pattern of expression can be detected by immunohistochemistry on smooth muscle tissue sections using antibodies against vinculin. Vinculin is a protein highly expressed in the adherens junctions, areas of the smooth muscle cell membrane which appear dense by electron microscopy studies. In contrast, dystrophin is not expressed in the adherens junctions, thus implying that vinculin and dystrophin are present in different domains of the smooth muscle cell membrane. Vinculin is thought to play a role in connecting F-actin to the sarcolemma of the smooth muscle cell.

Biochemical studies on skeletal muscle cell extracts have elucidated some of the interactions between dystrophin and other proteins (Fig. 1). Dystrophin is composed of four domains which may play different functional roles in skeletal muscle as well as other tissues. The amino-terminus of dystrophin links the cell cytoskeletal protein filamentous actin (F-actin) (Fig. 1), followed by a long central portion of spectrin-like repeats (rod domain). Loss of portions of the amino-terminus of dystrophin results in the severe DMD phenotype, while in-frame alterations in the rod domain usually give rise to the allelic milder form of DMD, Becker muscular dystrophy (BMD). The carboxyl-terminus of dystrophin contains a cysteine-rich domain which is associated with a complex of proteins named dystrophin-associated proteins (DAPs) (Fig. 1). This complex of proteins has been shown to biochemically copurify with dystrophin in skeletal muscle membrane extracts, suggesting a tight association between these proteins and dystrophin [7, 8, 10, 17, 20]. Loss of the dystrophin domain that binds this complex of proteins usually results in the severe DMD phenotype, suggesting that this portion of dystrophin plays an important functional role. The dystrophin-associated proteins can be divided into at least three subgroups. The first, dystroglycan, is composed of two glycosylated proteins, α and β dystroglycan which link dystrophin to the extracellular matrix protein component laminin 2, thus completing a bridge between cell cytoskeleton and extracellular matrix (Fig. 1). The second subgroup of proteins, sarcoglycan, is composed of at least three proteins, named α, β, γ sarcoglycan whose functional role remains unknown and an as yet uncharacterized 25 kD protein (Fig. 1). The third subgroup of proteins associated with dystrophin include at least two intracellular proteins: a 59 kD component named syntrophin and a 94 kD component named A_0 (Fig. 1).

Immunohistochemical studies using antibodies against members of the dystrophin-associated proteins have shown that muscle of DMD patients has reduction or absence of several components of the complex. In DMD this reduction is a secondary event to the absence of dystrophin, suggesting that these proteins interact with each other and thus also disintegrate as a complex. Two intriguing possibilities can be raised by these findings: one that mutations in any of the genes encoding for these proteins may result in a series of pathogenic events common to the dystrophic phenotype, the second that some of the dystrophin-associated proteins may be the primary deficiency in forms of autosomal muscular dystrophies.

Findings from our as well as other laboratories recently reported the cloning of genes encoding for components of the sarcoglycan complex and their identification as the primary cause of three types of autosomal recessive muscular dystrophy [4, 13, 16] (Table 1).

α-sarcoglycan previously referred to as adhalin is a 50 kD integral membrane glycoprotein associated with dystrophin. Immunohistochemical studies of α-sarcoglycan revealed its deficiency in muscle of patients with severe childhood autosomal muscular dystrophy (SCARMD). The human α-sarcoglycan gene was cloned and its chromosomal localization subsequently identified on 17q21 [14, 19]. Further studies have shown that a subset of autosomal muscular dystrophy patients carry mutations in the α-sarcoglycan gene with variable severity in their clinical phenotype [18, 19], although a substantial number of patients did not have mutations in this gene, making the absence of α-sarcoglycan a secondary deficiency in these disorders.

Table 1: *Muscular dystrophies.*

Type	Recessive/dominant	Gene	Chromosome
Duchenne MD	recessive	dystrophin	Xp
Becker MD	recessive	dystrophin	Xp
Limb Girdle MD, type 1	dominant	unknown	5q
Limb Girdle MD, type 2A	recessive	calpain	15q
Limb Girdle MD, type 2B	recessive	unknown	2q
Limb Girdle MD, type 2C	recessive	γ-sarcoglycan	13q
Limb Girdle MD, type 2D	recessive	α-sarcoglycan	17q
Limb Girdle MD, type 2E	recessive	β-sarcoglycan	4q
Congenital MD	recessive	merosin	6q

More recently, we showed that mutations in the γ-sarcoglycan gene are the primary deficiency in the chromosome 13-linked SCARMD [16] (Tab. 1).

Our laboratory also isolated and characterized the rabbit and human cDNAs encoding for β-sarcoglycan, a 43 kD transmembrane dystrophin-associated protein [4]. The β-sarcoglycan gene was localized on human chromosome 4q12 [4, 13]. Subsequently, 64 patients with presumed autosomal muscular dystrophy were screened for mutations in the β-sarcoglycan gene. In one patient with a Duchenne-like severe muscular dystrophy we found mutations in this gene on both alleles [4].

With the cloning and identification of the genes encoding for the members of the sarcoglycan complex associated with dystrophin, it is now possible to identify in the population patients with different types of muscular dystrophies that carry mutations in these genes (Table 1).

Other proteins associated with dystrophin have been characterized, but these proteins have not yet been associated to be involved in neuromuscular disorders. Syntrophin is a 59 kD cytoplasmic protein associated with dystrophin. At least 3 different types of syntrophins have been characterized in humans, one acidic and two basic syntrophins, according to their respective biochemical properties. These proteins are encoded by 3 separate genes located on different chromosomes in humans [1]. They show different patterns of tissue expression, suggesting that complexes of variable composition may exist in different tissues [1].

The discovery and characterization of several isoforms of dystrophin as well as of the dystrophin-associated proteins hints at the potential complexity of interactions among these proteins, and raises interesting questions about possible functions in skeletal muscle as well as in other tissues. In smooth muscle many questions concerning dystrophin and its associated proteins still need to be addressed. Very little is known about the expression of different dystrophin isoforms in smooth muscle as well as the members of the DAG complex. It will be important to understand the interactions between dystrophin and the associated proteins specifically in smooth muscle. This might allow a better understanding of disorders characterized by abnormalities in smooth muscle including muscular disorders restricted to the gastrointestinal tract.

Finally, a deeper understanding of the pathogenic aspects underlying some severe forms of muscular dystrophy may lead to the design of a therapeutic approach applicable to more than one form of muscular dystrophy.

References

1. Ahn, A. H., C. A. Feener, E. Gussoni et al.: The three human syntrophin genes are expressed in diverse tissues, have distinct chromosomal location and each bind to dystrophin and its relatives. J. Biol. Chem. 271 (1996) 2724−2730.
2. Ahn, A. H., L. M. Kunkel: The structural and functional diversity of dystrophin. Nature Genet. 3 (1993) 283−291.
3. Barohn, R. J., E. J. Levine, J. O. Olson et al.: Gastric hypomotility in Duchenne's muscular dystrophy. N. Engl. J. Med. 319 (1988) 15−18.
4. Bönnemann, C. G., R. Modi, S. Noguchi et al.: Mutations in the dystrophin-associated glycoprotein β-sarcoglycan cause autosomal recessive muscular dystrophy with disintegration of the sarcoglycan complex. Nature Genet. 11 (1995) 266−273.
5. Byers, T. J., L. M. Kunkel, S. C. Watkins: The subcellular distribution of dystrophin in mouse skeletal, cardiac and smooth muscle. J. Cell Biol. 115 (1991) 411−421.
6. Byers, T. J., H. G. W. Lidov, L. M. Kunkel: An alternative dystrophin transcript specific to the peripheral nerve. Nature Genet. 4 (1993) 77−80.
7. Campbell, K. P.: Three muscular dystrophies: loss of cytoskeleton-extracellular matrix linkage. Cell 80 (1995) 675−679.
8. Ervasti, J. M., K. P. Campbell: Membrane organization of the dystrophin-glycoprotein complex. Cell 66 (1991) 1121−1131.
9. Hoffman, E. P., R. H. J. Brown, L. M. Kunkel: Dystrophin: the protein product of the Duchenne muscular dystrophy locus. Cell 51 (1987) 919−928.
10. Ibraghimov-Beskrovnaya, O., J. M. Ervasti, C. J. Leveille et al.: Primary structure of dystrophin-associated glycoproteins linking dystrophin to the extracellular matrix. Nature 355 (1992) 696−702.
11. Lederfein, D., Z. Levy, N. Augier et al.: A 71-Kilodalton protein is a major product of the Duchenne muscular dystrophy gene in brain and other nonmuscle tissues. Proc. Natl. Acad. Sci. USA 89 (1992) 5346−5350.
12. Leon, S. H., M. D. Schuffler, M. Kettler et al.: Chronic intestinal pseudoobstruction as a complication of Duchenne's muscular dystrophy. Gastroenterology 90 (1986) 455−459.
13. Lim, L. E., F. Duclos, O. Broux et al.: β-sarcoglycan: characterization and role in limb-girdle muscular dystrophy linked to 4q12. Nature Genet. 11 (1995) 257−265.
14. McNally, E. M., M. Yoshida, Y. Mizuno et al.: Human adhalin is alternatively spliced and the gene is located on chromosome 17q21. Proc. Natl. Acad. Sci. USA 91 (1994) 9690−9694.
15. Morgan Hughes, J. A.: Diseases of striated muscle. In: A. Ashbury, G. M. McKhann, W. I. McDonald (Eds.): Diseases of the Nervous System, pp. 164−196. Saunders, Philadelphia 1992.
16. Noguchi, S., E. M. McNally, K. Ben Othmane et al.: Mutations in the dystrophin-associated protein γ-sarcoglycan in chromosome 13 muscular dystrophy. Science 270 (1995) 819−822.

17. Ohlendieck, K., K. P. Campbell: Dystrophin-associated proteins are greatly reduced in skeletal muscle from mdx mice. J. Cell. Biol. 115 (1991) 1685−1694.
18. Piccolo, F.: Primary adhalinopathy: a common cause of autosomal recessive muscular dystrophy of variable severity. Nature Genet. 10 (1995) 243−245.
19. Roberds, S. L., Leturcq, F., Allamand, V. et al.: Adhalin mRNA and cDNA sequence are normal in the cardiomyopathic hamster. Cell 78 (1994) 625−633.
20. Yoshida, M., E. Ozawa: Glycoprotein complex anchoring dystrophin to sarcolemma. J. Biochem. 108 (1990) 748−752.

Genetics of Hirschsprung's disease

S. Lyonnet, T. Attié, P. Edery, J. Amiel, A. Pelet,
C. Nihoul-Fékété, A. Munnich

Genetics of Hirschsprung's disease (HSCR)

HSCR is a congenital disorder characterized by the absence of the parasympathetic intrinsic ganglion cells in the submucosal and myenteric plexuses of the hindgut [17]. This frequent condition (1/5,000 live births) results in intestinal obstruction in neonates and in severe constipation in infants and adults. HSCR is regarded as a neurocristopathy [10] related to the premature arrest of the craniocaudal migration of neural crest cells toward the anal end of the rectum, between the 5th and the 12th week of gestation [20]. The earlier the cessation of migration, the larger the aganglionic segment. In the majority of cases (80%), the aganglionic tract involves the rectum and the sigmoid colon only (short-segment HSCR), while in 20% of cases, it extends toward the proximal end of the colon (long-segment HSCR).

A genetic etiology for HSCR was indicated by several observations [8, 11, 12]:

1) the increased risk of recurrence for sibs of affected individuals (4%);
2) the unbalanced sex-ratio (Male : Female 4 : 1);
3) the association of HSCR with other genetic diseases, malformation syndromes and/or chromosomal anomalies such as Multiple Endocrine Neoplasia type 2 (MEN 2), Waardenburg syndrome, trisomy 21, interstitial deletion of either chromosome 10 or chromosome 13;
4) the existence of large HSCR families (10%) likely to indicate an autosomal dominant mode of inheritance with variable expression and low penetrance;
5) and several animal models of colonic aganglionosis segregating as mendelian traits.

The high frequency of sporadic cases (80−90%), the variable expressivity (different extent of the aganglionic tract among related patients) and the incomplete, sex dependent penetrance were considered for a long time as an indication that both a complex pattern of inheritance (sex-modified multifactorial disease) and more than one major gene (genetic heterogeneity) were possibly involved in HSCR. Segregation analyses performed on different sets of patients and families suggested various models of inheritance depending on the length of the aganglionic tract [8]. In particular, they supported an autosomal dominant mode of inheritance with incomplete penetrance in long-segment HSCR and an autosomal recessive or multifactorial modes of inheritance in short-segment HSCR.

Localisation of a major disease gene for HSCR to chromosome 10

The observation of a patient with total colonic aganglionosis associated with a *de novo* interstitial deletion of chromosome 10 (10q11.2−21.2, [23]) was followed by linkage analyses with subsets of highly informative microsatellite DNA markers previously mapped to that candidate region (examination of the segregation of the disease allele with respect to the segregation of alleles at known marker loci). Consequently, a dominant gene for HSCR was indeed mapped to the proximal long arm of chromosome 10 [2, 22].

Independently, linkage analyses combined with physical mapping, allowed the mapping of a gene for MEN 2 to the same chromosomal region. The *RET* proto-oncogene, encoding a receptor tyrosine kinase expressed in neural crest-derived tissues, physically mapped in the HSCR-MEN2 genetic region was therefore considered as a candidate gene for both disorders. Indeed, no recombinant was observed with the *RET* proto-oncogene locus demonstrating its close vicinity with the HSCR locus. Furthermore, other patients presenting with HSCR and an interstitial deletion of chromosome 10q encompassing the *RET* gene were reported.

The RET proto-oncogene

RET, a receptor tyrosine kinase

On the basis of structural homologies, *RET* encodes a receptor tyrosine kinase (RTK, [34]). RTKs are cell-surface proteins which possess an extracellular ligand binding domain, a single hydrophobic transmembrane region and a cytoplasmic domain with an intrinsic tyrosine kinase (TK) activity (Fig. 1). Receptor dimerization is followed by autophosphorylation which takes place with tyrosine residue phosphorylation of one receptor molecule by the other in the dimer. The *RET* ligand is still unknown, but one may hypothesize that *RET* engages homophilic binding to a second *RET* molecule, or perhaps heterophilic binding to another cadherin molecule, which could trigger its tyrosine kinase activity.

The *RET* gene is composed of 21 exons spanning more than 60 Kb of genomic DNA. The *RET* promoter and the first exon are separated from the remaining coding exons by a large intron of more than 20 Kb. The *RET* gene produces 5 mRNA species ranging in size from 3.9 to 7 Kb. These transcripts are predicted to encode two *RET* protein isoforms with alternative 9 or 51 carboxy-terminal aminoacids. More recently, alternative splicing of the *RET* gene involving the 5′ exons of the extracellular domain have been identified. The role of these alternative 5′ splicing variants in normal developmental processes and their respective significance in neoplastic growth remain to be elucidated.

RET gene expression

The role of *RET* during normal human development is largely unknown. Some clues are provided by expression studies of *RET* mRNA and/or protein product in various tissues and by examination of mice carrying a homozygous disruption of the *RET* gene. In particular, human neuroblastoma cell lines and human tumours originating from neural crest-derived cells, including pheochromocytomas, express the *RET* transcripts at a high level. In addition, the *RET* protein is expressed at low levels in other neural crest-derived cells including human adult adrenal medulla, thyroid and Schwann cells.

In the post-implantation mouse embryo, *RET* transcripts are expressed in a dynamic pattern, mainly in subsets of cells of (i) the peripheral nervous system, including the developing autonomous nervous system, the enteric nervous system and the sensory ganglia of the head and the trunk, (ii) the central nervous system, predominantly the motor neuron lineages of the spinal cord, the hindbrain, and (iii) the urinary system [35].

Mice heterozygous for a site-targetted *ret* mutation (*ret+/−*), seem normal although homozygous mutant mice (*ret−/−*) die within 24 hours of birth [26, 33]. Further examination of the *ret−/−* mice reveal the absence of the myenteric neurons from the small and large intestine (megacolon) and from the oesophagus and stomach, and also absent or rudimentary kidneys showing severe dysplasia with blind ending or absent ureter. The lack of enteric neurons is the main defect in HSCR and emphasizes the role of *RET* in the development of the enteric nervous system [33].

Germline RET mutations in MEN syndromes

MEN 2 is a dominantly inherited cancer syndrome subdivided into 3 types, namely familial medullary thyroid carcinoma (FMTC), MEN of type 2A (MEN 2A) and MEN of type 2B (MEN 2B), differing in the spectrum of tissues involved. Missense mutations of the *RET* gene have been identified in the vast majority of FMTC, and MEN 2A patients [24]. These mutations are clustered in 5 cysteine codons in the cysteine-rich extracellular domain of *RET*. In contrast, a single missense mutation is associated with MEN 2B in almost all patients [18]. This mutation is an ATG → ACG transversion, which results in the replacement of a methionine with a threonine at codon 918 in the catalytic core of the tyrosine kinase domain of *RET*. With regard to tumorigenesis, it is unlikely that the *RET* gene acts as a tumour-suppressor gene. Accordingly, loss of allele for loci on chromosome 10q11.2 is a rare event in MEN 2 tumours. Moreover, *RET* mutations of "MEN 2-type" appear to activate the *RET* product, leading to dominantly inherited cancer syndromes [32]. Germline mutations observed in the MEN 2 syndromes thus appear to be the first example of dominantly acting point mutations leading to human hereditary cancer predisposition.

RET gene mutations in HSCR

Soon after the mapping of a dominant HSCR gene to chromosome 10q11.2, germline mutations of the *RET* proto-oncogene were identified in HSCR families and sporadic cases [13, 31]. Recently, the analysis of 20/21 exons of the *RET* gene by a combination of denaturing gradient gel electrophoresis (DGGE) and single strand conformation polymorphism (SSCP) in a large series of HSCR patients (45 sporadic cases and 35 familial forms), led us to characterize mutations in 50% of familial HSCR [7]. The mean penetrance of the mutant allele in familial HSCR was significantly higher in males (72%) than in females (51%). These penetrances of mutant allele were very similar to those anticipated on the basis of large segregation analyses for a major dominant gene involved in long-segment HSCR (66% and 51% respectively, [8]). Most interestingly, mutations at the *RET* locus accounted for at least ⅓ of sporadic HSCR in that series [7]. These mutations were scattered along the length of the gene (Fig. 1). Finally, among the mutations identified in sporadic cases (16/45), 7 proved to be *de novo* mutations suggesting that new mutations at the *RET* locus significantly contribute to sporadic HSCR [28]. However, the exact prevalence of *RET* mutations in sporadic HSCR is still debatable [3, 4, 7, 21, 36].

As far as genotype-phenotype relationships in HSCR familes are concerned, we found no correlation between the type of *RET* mutation and the length of the aganglionic segment [13]. Further, we found no correlation between *RET* genotype and penetrance among families. Taken together, the low penetrance of the mutant genes, the lack of genotype-phenotype correlation, the sex-dependent effect of *RET* mutations and the variable clinical expression of the disease support the existence of one or more modifier genes in familial HSCR [7].

Only half of our HSCR families (49%) were found to carry mutations in the coding sequence of the *RET* gene, although our 35 pedigrees were consistent with linkage to chromosome 10q11.2. Several explanations could account for this, namely: i) mutations other than those in the *RET* gene coding sequences, including introns and the promoter region; ii) a low rate of mutation detection

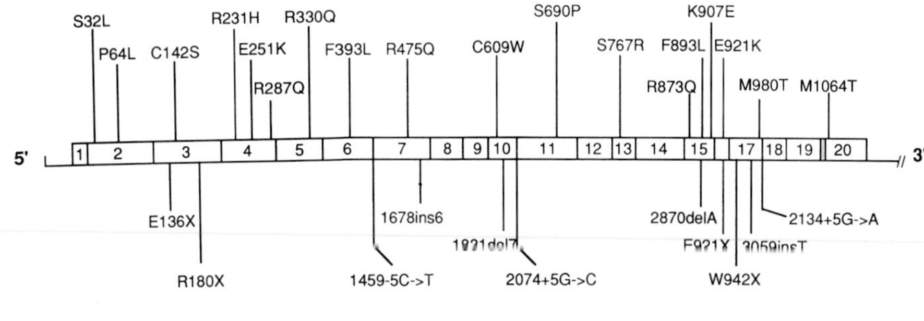

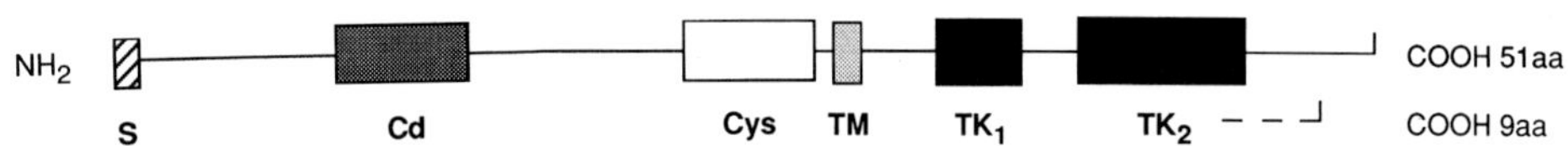

Fig. 1: *Mutations of the RET proto-oncogene in familial and sporadic HSCR. Top = missense mutations, Bottom = mutations resulting in a truncated RET protein. The various domains of the RET receptor tyrosine-kinase are presented: S = signal peptide, Cd = Cadherin, Cys = Cystein-rich, TM = Transmembrane, TK = Tyrosine kinase.*

by using a combination of DGGE and SSCP analyses; and iii) genetic heterogeneity especially as several HSCR families studied were small, and as some substantial evidence for heterogeneity exists in HSCR (see below). Thus, it is still difficult to speculate on the proportion of HSCR families likely to have a *RET* mutation.

Interestingly, one of the patients with long-segment HSCR also had unilateral renal agenesis, a feature that is reminiscent of the phenotype of the *ret−/−* knockout mouse. These data suggest that the *RET* gene may also play a role in renal development, and that mutations at the *RET* locus may result in renal agenesis.

Several lines of evidence suggest that the HSCR phenotype is the result of gene inactivation of haplo-insufficiency at the *RET* locus. First, large deletions of chromosome 10q11 are associated with HSCR. Second, several mutations resulting in premature stop codons are predicted to produce markedly truncated proteins. Finally, Pasini et al. [27] recently reported on a loss of function effect of *RET* mutation *in vitro*. In view of this contrast between the probable inactivating effects of HSCR mutations and activation resulting from MEN 2 mutations, it is of interest that we have recently described *RET* mutations involving the juxtatransmembrane cysteine codons in 4 families in which both HSCR and MEN 2A cosegregated with variable penetrance, both phenotypes apparently resulting from the same mutation [25]. These data underline the allelic heterogeneity and the variable expression of *RET* mutations. Further studies are required to understand how very similar mutations can result in an early developmental defect (HSCR), an inherited syndrome of cancer predisposition (MEN 2A), or both disorders.

Endothelin-signaling pathway mutations in Hirschsprung's disease

EDNRB gene mutations

HSCR has long been regarded as a multigenic condition. Accordingly, several lines of evidence supported the involvement of susceptibility genes different from *RET*, including chromosomal anomalies (trisomy 21, 13q deletions), and *RET* exclusion in some HSCR families [5]. Recently, mutations of the endothelin B receptor (EDNRB) and the endothelin 3 (EDN3) genes were shown to account for megacolon and pigmentary anomalies in the *piebald-lethal and lethal spotting* mouse mutants respectively [16, 17] (Table 1). In addition, we have recently excluded *RET* as the susceptibility locus in HSCR families with pigmentary disorders similar to those observed in the Waardenburg syndrome (WS, [5]), that is also regarded as a neurocristopathy since it results from an abnormal migration of neural crest-derived cells to cephalic mesectoderm, inner ear cells and skin [9]. Accordingly, mutation of the endothelin receptor beta gene have been recently reported in a large HSCR pedigree of mennonite origin with HSCR, deafness and pigmentary abnormalities [29, 30], and in a consanguinous HSCR-WS family (Shah-Waardenburg syndrome, [6]). In the former family, the recessive mutant allele is dosage-sensitive, incompletely penetrant and absent in some patients, suggesting that at least one additional locus controls the disease phenotype [29, 30].

More recently, we have found heterozygous deletions and EDNRB missense mutations in 7 isolated HSCR patients [1]. The EDNRB gene encodes a 442 aminoacid heptahelical receptor that equally binds EDN 1, 2 and 3, and is involved in the intracellular signaling pathway via heterotrimeric G proteins. Large scale 13q21 deletions could be identified in 3 patients harboring chromosome 13q22 deletions. In two of them, the deletion was shown to encompass the EDNRB gene by using flanking polymorphic markers. In addition, in 4/165 of our HSCR patients, heterozygous DNA variations were characterized in exons 1, 5 and 6 predicted missense mutations of the extracellular (G57S), the third intracellular (R319W) and the seventh transmembrane domain (P383L) of the EDNRB protein respectively (Fig. 2). In each of these cases, the mutation was found to be inherited from an asymptomatic carrier. These data support the involvement of EDNRB mutations in isolated HSCR also.

Interestingly, there is also support to the low penetrance of the EDNRB mutant alleles in agreement with the observation that the W276C EDNRB mutation

Table 1: *Genes involved in HSCR in human and megacolon in mice.*

	Humans			Mice			
Genes (disease loci)	Phenotype	Inheritance	Chromosomal assignement	Natural mutants	Knockouts	Inheritance	Chromosomal assignement
RET (HSCR1 [1, 21])	HSCR	AD	10q11.2	–	RET −/− Megacolon Kidney abnormalities [32]	AR	6
EDNRB (HSCR2 [28, 29])	HSCR + WS	AR?	13q22	*Piebald lethal (s')* Megacolon Color spotting	EDNRB −/− Megacolon Color spotting [18]	AR	14
EDN3 (HSCR3 [14])	HSCR + WS	AR?	20q13.2−q.13.3	*Lethal spotting (ls)* Megacolon Color spotting	EDN3 −/− Megacolon Color spotting [15]	AR	2
?	?			*Dominant megacolon (Dom)* Megacolon Color spotting	?	AD	15

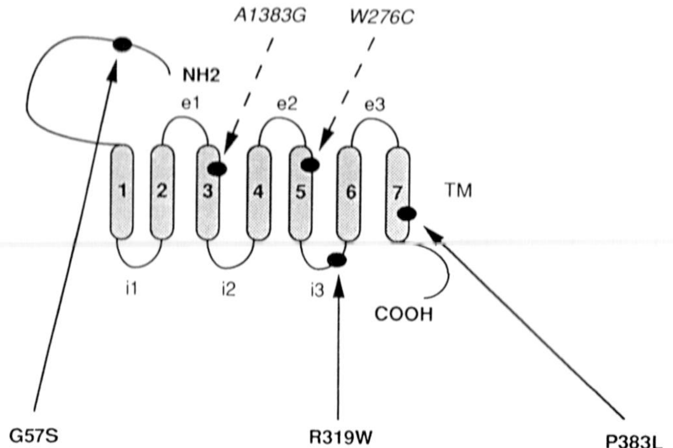

Fig. 2: *Mutations of EDNRB in isolated and syndromic HSCR (see text).*

was neither necessary nor sufficient to produce the HSCR phenotype in the Mennonite kindred. Taken together, these data favour the existence of one or more modifier loci in HSCR individuals carrying heterozygote EDNRB mutations. EDNRB could be regarded therefore as a rare susceptibility locus in non-syndromic HSCR. Finally, these data suggest that EDNRB mutations in human could be dosage sensitive: heterozygosity would predispose to isolated HSCR with incomplete penetrance, while homozygosity would result in more complex neurocristopathies associating HSCR and features of the WS. The question of whether modifying alleles at the EDNRB locus could also account for the low penetrance of *RET* mutations in HSCR families is now open to debate.

EDN3 gene mutations

The EDN3 gene encodes a large inactive preproendothelin-3 precursor which yields a biologically active 21-aminoacid peptide after proteolytic cleavages at furin and endothelin-converting enzyme 1 cleavage sites respectively. EDN3 belongs to a family of oligopeptides, including endothelins 1 (EDN1) and 2 (EDN2), that exert their biological effects through the G protein-coupled heptahelical receptors EDNRA and EDNRB. EDN1 and, to a lesser extent, EDN2 have a high affinity for EDNRA. Since EDN3 (EDNRB ligand) mouse mutants displayed a phenotype similar to EDNRB−/− mutants (megacolon, white coat-spotting), the EDN3 gene was also regarded as an alternative candidate gene in WS-HSCR. Recently, we have reported a homozygous substitution/deletion mutation of the EDN3 gene in a WS-HSCR patient [15]. The mutation located in exon 2 of the EDN3 gene modified the 120 downstream aminoacids and was predicted to result in the complete absence of the active form of the peptide. These data describe EDN3 as a third gene predisposing to HSCR (Table 1).

Finally, while little is known regarding the physiological role of EDN3, the present study demonstrates that EDN3 mutations may account for the pleiotropic features observed in the WS-HSCR association, and suggests that the endothelin-signaling pathways play a major role in the development of neural crest-derived enteric neurons, inner ear cells and melanocytes.

Conclusion

There is thus conclusive evidence for the involvement of various loci in HSCR. In particular, the role of mutations of the *RET* proto-oncogene, the EDNRB and the EDN3 genes in this frequent malformation have been recently demonstrated. The dissection of the genetic etiology of HSCR disease may provide a unique opportunity to distinguish between polygenic diseases and genetically heterogeneous diseases and, thereby, to understand other complex disorders and congenital malformations hitherto considered as multifactorial in origin. The study of the biological basis of HSCR is also a step towards the understanding of developmental genetics of the enteric nervous system in human, and the pathways that govern the embryology of cells derived from the neural crest. Finally, since it has been shown that the *RET* gene is involved in both congenital malformation (HSCR) and inherited syndromes of cancer predisposition (MEN), these studies could shed some light on the relationships between these frequent abnormalities of cell development and proliferation in human.

Summary

Hirschsprung's disease (HSCR, aganglionic megacolon) is a frequent congenital malformation regarded as a multigenic neurocristopathy. Three susceptibility genes have been recently identified in HSCR, namely the *RET* proto-oncogene, the endothelin B receptor (EDNRB) gene, and the endothelin 3 (EDN3) gene. *RET* gene mutations were found in significant proportions of familial and sporadic HSCR, while homozygosity for EDNRB mutations accounted for the HSCR-Waardenburg syndrome (WS) association. More recently, heterozygous EDNRB missense mutations have been reported in isolated HSCR. Finally, mutations of the EDN3 gene were also found in patients with HSCR and WS, uncovering the existence of a third HSCR predisposing gene. Most of these results were obtained after the identification of several mouse genes whose natural or site-directed mutations resulted in megacolon and coat color spotting. These data well illustrate the polygenic inheritance of HSCR, and give support to the role of the *RET* tyrosine kinase and endothelin-signaling pathways in the development of neural crest-derived enteric neurons.

Acknowledgements: We are extremely grateful to the many surgeons, paediatricians and geneticists who have provided us with clinical data and biological samples of their patients and families. This study was supported by the Association pour la Recherche contre le Cancer (ARC), the Association Française contre les Myopathies (AFM), the Ligue Contre le Cancer (Comité de Paris), the Assistance Publique-Hôpitaux de Paris (AP-HP, PHRC 94), the GREG, and the Ministère de la Recherche et de la Technologie.

References

1. Amiel, J., T. Attié, D. Jan et al.: Heterozygous endothelin receptor B (EDNRB) mutations in isolated Hirschsprung disease. Hum. Mol. Genet. 5 (1996) 355−357.
2. Angrist, M., E. Kauffman, S. A. Slaugenhaupt et al.: A gene for Hirschsprung disease (megacolon) in the pericentromeric region of human chromosome 10. Nature Genetics 4 (1993) 351−356.
3. Angrist, M., S. Bolk, B. Thiel et al.: Mutation analysis of the RET receptor tyrosine kinase in Hirschsprung disease. Hum. Mol. Genet. 4 (1995) 821−830.
4. Attié, T., A. Pelet, P. Sarda et al.: A 7 bp deletion of the RET proto-oncogene in familial Hirschsprung's disease. Hum. Molec. Genet. 3 (1994) 1439−1440.
5. Attié, T., M. Till, A. Pelet et al.: Exclusion of the RET and Pax3 loci in Waardenburg-Hirschsprung disease. J. Med. Genet. 32 (1995) 312−313.
6. Attié, A., M. Till, P. Pelet et al.: Mutation of the endothelin-receptor B gene in the Waardenburg-Hirschsprung disease. Hum. Molec. Genet. 4 (1995) 2407−2409.
7. Attié, T., A. Pelet, P. Edery et al.: Diversity of RET mutations in Hirschsprung disease. Hum. Molec. Genet. 4 (1995) 1381−1386.
8. Badner, J. A., W. K. Sieber, K. L. Garver et al.: A genetic study of Hirschsprung disease. Am. J. Hum. Genet. 46 (1990) 568−580.
9. Badner, J. A., A. Chakravarti: Waardenburg syndrome and Hirschsprung Disease: Evidence for pleiotropic effects of a single dominant gene: Am. J. Med. Genet. 35 (1990) 100−104.
10. Bolande, R. P.: The neurocristopathies; A unifying concept of disease arising in neural crest maldevelopment. Hum. Pathol. 5 (1973) 409−429.
11. Bodian, M., C. O. Carter: A family study of Hirschsprung disease. Ann. Hum. Genet. 26 (1963) 261−277.
12. Cass, D. T., A. L. Zhang, J. Morthope: Aganglionosis in rodents. J. Pediatr. Surg. 27 (1992) 351−356.
13. Edery, P., S. Lyonnet, L. M. Mulligan et al.: Mutations of the RET proto-oncogene in Hirschsprung's disease. Nature 367 (1994) 378−380.
14. Edery, P., A. Pelet, L. M. Mulligan et al.: Long segment and short segment familial Hirschsprung's disease: variable clinical expression at the RET locus. J. Med. Genet. 31 (1994) 602−606.
15. Edery, P., T. Attié, J. Amiel et al.: Mutation of the endothelin-3 gene in the Waardenburg-Hirschsprung disease (Shah-Waardenburg syndrome) Nature Genetics 12 (1995) 442−444.
16. Greenstein Baynach, A., K. Hosada et al.: Interaction of endothelin-3 with endothelin-B receptor is essential for development of epidermal melanocytes and enteric neurons. Cell 79 (1994) 1277−1285.

17. Hirschsprung, H.: Stuhlträgheit Neugeborener infolge von Dilatation und Hypertrophie des Colons. Jahrb. Kinderheilkunde 27 (1888) 1−27.

18. Hofstra, R. M. W., R. M. Landsvater, I. Ceccherini et al.: A mutation in the RET proto-oncogene associated with endocrine neoplasia type 2B and sporadic medullary thyroid carcinoma. Nature 367 (1994) 375−376.

19. Hosada, K., R. E. Hammer, Richardson et al.: Targeted and natural (Piebald-Lethal) mutations of endothelin-B receptor gene produce megacolon associated with spotted coat color mice. Cell 79 (1994) 1267−1276.

20. Kapur, R. P.: Contemporary approaches toward understanding the pathogenesis of Hirschsprung disease. Pediatric Pathology 13 (1993) 83−100.

21. Luo, Y., V. Barone, M. Seri et al.: Heterogeneity and low detection rate of RET mutations in Hirschsprung Disease. Eur. J. Hum. Genet. 2 (1994) 272−280.

22. Lyonnet, S., A. Bolino, A. Pelet et al.: A gene for Hirschsprung disease maps to the proximal long arm of chromosome 10. Nature Genetics 4 (1993) 346−350.

23. Martucciello, G., M. P. Bicocchi, P. Dodero et al.: Total colonic aganglionosis associated with interstitial deletion of the long arm of chromosome 10. Pediatr. Surg. Intern. 7 (1992) 308−310.

24. Mulligan, L. M., J. B. J. Kwok, C. S. Healey et al.: Germ line mutations of the RET proto-oncogene in multiple endocrine neoplasia type 2A. Nature 363 (1993) 458−460.

25. Mulligan, L. M., C. Eng, T. Attié et al.: Diverse phenotypes associated with exon 10 mutations of the RET proto-oncogene. Hum. Molec. Genet. 3 (1994) 2163−2167.

26. Pachnis, V., S. B. Mankoo, F. Costantini: Expression of the RET protooncogene during mouse embryogenesis. Development 119 (1994) 1005−1017.

27. Pasini, P., M. G. Borrello, A. Greco et al.: Loss of function effect of RET mutations causing Hirschsprung disease. Nature Genetics 10 (1995) 35−40.

28. Pelet, A., T. Attié, O. Goulet et al.: De novo mutations of the RET proto-oncogene in Hirschsprung disease. Lancet 344 (1994) 1769−1770.

29. Puffenberger, E. G., E. R. Kauffman, S. Bolk et al.: Identity-by-descent and association mapping of a recessive gene for Hirschsprung disease on human chromosome 13q22. Hum Molec. Genet. 3 (1994) 1217−1225.

30. Puffenberger, E. G., K. Hosoda, S. S. Washington et al.: A missense mutation of the endothelin-B receptor gene in multigenic Hirschsprung's disease. Cell 79 (1994) 1257−1266.

31. Romeo, G., P. Ronchetto, Y. Luo et al.: Point mutations affecting the tyrosine kinase domain of the RET proto-oncogene in Hirschsprung's disease. Nature 367 (1994) 377−378.

32. Santoro, M., F. Carlomagno, A. Romano et al.: Activation of RET as a dominant transforming gene by germline mutations of MEN2A and MEN2B. Science 267 (1995) 381−383.

33. Schuchardt, A., V. D'Agati, L. Larsson-Blomberg et al.: Defects in the kidney and enteric nervous system of mice lacking the tyrosine kinase receptor RET. Nature 367 (1994) 380−383.

34. Takahashi, M., Y. Buma, T. Iwamoto et al.: Cloning and expression of the RET proto-oncogene encoding a tyrosine kinase with two potential transmembrane domains. Oncogene 3 (1988) 571−578.

35. Tsuzuki, T., M. Takahashi, N. Asai et al.: Spatial and temporal expression of the RET proto-oncogene product in embryonic, infant and adult rat tissues. Oncogene 10 (1995) 191−198.

36. Yin, L., V. Barone, M. Seri et al.: Heterogeneity and low detection rate of RET mutations in Hirschsprung disease. Eur. J. Hum. Genet. 2 (1994) 272−280.

Diagnosis and management of upper gastrointestinal dysfunctions in children with neurological and neuromuscular diseases

A. Staiano, E. Del Giudice, A. Fanucci

Neuromuscular disorders can affect gastrointestinal motility at level of the: 1) Enteric nervous system, such as in idiopathic, degenerative or inflammatory disorders in the myenteric plexus; 2) Extrinsic nervous system, such as in brain damage and spinal cord injury; 3) Smooth muscle, such as in primary or secondary myopathies [3].

Upper gastrointestinal motor dysfunctions are known to occur frequently in children with different degrees of brain damage, whereas, only recently, several reports are outlining the association of gastrointestinal disorders and congenital myopathies or generalized muscle diseases in pediatric age [15, 17].

In the past, many infants with major respiratory, cardiac, and feeding disorders were not able to survive. The availability of neonatal intensive care units and high-technology diagnostic procedures has led to an increased survival rate of premature and term infants with neurological impairment. The survival of children with severe central nervous system damage has created a major challenge for medical care. The current increase rate of survival has been coupled with an increase in the number of rehabilitation programs to provide therapy and assistance to high-risk infants and children with suspected or identified brain lesion. The prevalence of moderately severe or severe cerebral palsy ranges, in fact, from 1.5 to 2.5 per 1000 live births [8]. Primary diseases of muscle in children are less frequent than neurological diseases and, apart from the rare congenital myopathies, myastenic and myotonic syndromes, the most frequent muscle disorders of childhood are the X-linked progressive muscular dystrophies. Duchenne muscular dystrophy affects 1 : 3.500 male births, and Becker dystrophy affects 1 : 30.000 male births [18].

Differently from children with myopathy in whom GI involvement is often clinically silent, most children with brain damage present a variety of GI symptoms, not always receiving the appropriate attention from the general pediatrician. Swallowing disorders occur in 40% of children with brain damage, recurrent vomiting in 10–15% of mentally retarded children, but if fully investigated up to 75% of these children have gastroesophageal reflux (GER); finally 62% of mentally retarded children present chronic constipation [4, 12, 16].

Swallowing is a very primitive function which is present in most animal species and is vital for the fundamental functions of nutrition and airway protection. Oropharyngeal dysphagia can be caused either by structural or by neuromuscular dysfunction which can be further classified, according to the neuroanatomical level of dysfunction, to include central nervous system, neurogenic and myogenic causes [5]. The most frequent cause of oropharyngeal dysphagia in children is brain damage due to anoxic-ischemic lesions.

It is convenient to classify oro-pharyngeal dysphagia in accordance with the particular motor dysfunction which may affect one or more components of the swallowing sequence. For its complexity, swallowing can be arbitrarly divided in three phases: the oral phase is considered to be largely voluntary, while the pharyngeal and esophageal phases are entirely involuntary. Motor dysfunctions of the oral phase include abnormalities of bolus preparation, salivary lubrication and oral delivery and they are manifest as drooling or escape of food from the mouth and oral stasis. Weakness or incoordination of the tongue impair bolus formation. Most children with cerebral palsy do in fact present poor lip closure with drooling of saliva and, thus, poor lubrication. Lubrication provides an important sensory clue in triggering the pharyngeal swallow response.

Pharyngeal dysfunction can be due to disorders of palatal closure, airway protection, pharyngeal propulsion, whereas disorders of UES opening may induce esophageal dysfunction. It is important to underline that a specific disease may cause dysphagia by affecting several mechanisms involved in the act of swallowing; and, vice versa, dysfunction of a single mechanism is not evidence of a specific disease. Irrespective of etiology, careful evaluation of the precise mechanisms of dysfunction is mandatory for planning management.

Clinical manifestations of altered swallowing in infants are primarily apnea and bradycardia during feeding, although chronic or recurrent respiratory disorders (congestion, cough and wheezing) are also seen.

In the dysphagic child the aims of the diagnostic work-up are to determine the site and the mechanisms of dysfunction as well as to identify the underlying causes. In most instances, the clinical history and the physical examination will differentiate oral and pharyngeal from esophageal dysphagia and provide clues to its etiology. Difficulty in initiating swallowing, nasal regurgitation, cough and apnea during swallowing suggest abnormalities of the oral phase. Additional available investigative techniques include chest radiograph, ultrasonography, videofluoroscopy and manometry. In the last years, dynamic evaluation of the oropharyngeal phases of swallowing by means of fluoroscopic and ultrosonographic videorecording proved to be a reliable method in the evaluation of children with swallowing disorders [10, 6].

Videoultrasonography is the main technique to investigate the oral phase of swallowing, since videofluoroscopy does not allow direct visualization of the tongue musculature and of the floor of the mouth. Radiological techniques provide only an overall view of the dorsum of the tongue in the lateral projection. Videosonography, on the other hand, avoids radiation exposure and provides a direct analysis of any single motor event of swallowing by means of specific multiplanar images [10, 6].

In bottle-fed newborns or infants, longitudinal submental scans of oral cavity show that during sucking the tongue is raised to form a seal with the palatal wall and thus compressing the nipple superiorly. The degree of nipple deformation seems to be related to the strength of suction. The expressed milk initially flows into a median groove and then into a central depression of the posterior part of the tongue where it is subsequently shaped as bolus. The bolus is then pushed posteriorly into the oro-pharynx by a piston-like movement of the tongue. Visualization of the upper larynx and the hyoid bone marks the start of the pharyngeal swallowing.

By videoultrasonography it is possible to evaluate a transverse view of the larynx during quiet breathing, and during swallowing. During quiet breathing vocal cords and arythenoids remain in an abducted position; rima glottidis is clearly visible. During swallowing the vocal cords and the arythenoids adduct while the glottis closes, preventing aspiration of the ingesta into the larynx (Fig. 1 A, B). A suspected aspiration in the respiratory tract should always be confirmed by videofluoroscopy, which, despite its limited capability to visualize the vocal cords, can assess more details of the pharyngo-esophageal phases of swallowing than any other technique (Fig. 2).

The management of oropharyngeal dysphagia includes compensatory strategies which are designed to reduce the symptom with no attempt to modify swallow physiology; indirect therapy designed to improve the neuromuscular control necessary for swallowing without triggering a swallow, or direct therapy designed to modify swallow physiology [9]. Indirect therapy cannot be applied in children, especially in mentally retarded children because this treatment implies the acquisitions of new movements to perform during swallowing. Compensatory strategies include the control of the patient's head and body position, the consistency, the volume and the rate of administration of food. Postural techniques can be extremely effective in preventing aspiration, and can be applied during videosonographic and videofluoroscopic examination so that their effects can be observed and assessed. These non invasive techniques are in fact used to evaluate the efficacy of treatment. For example, neck extension can inhibit muscular movement of swallowing and can align the airway facilitating aspiration.

Throughout any rehabilitation programme for dysphagia the patient's nutrition and hydration should be appropriately controlled and, in the presence of severe swallowing disorders and severe malnutrition it is necessary to feed the patient by parenteral nutrition or tube alimentation [2]. The latter can be achieved

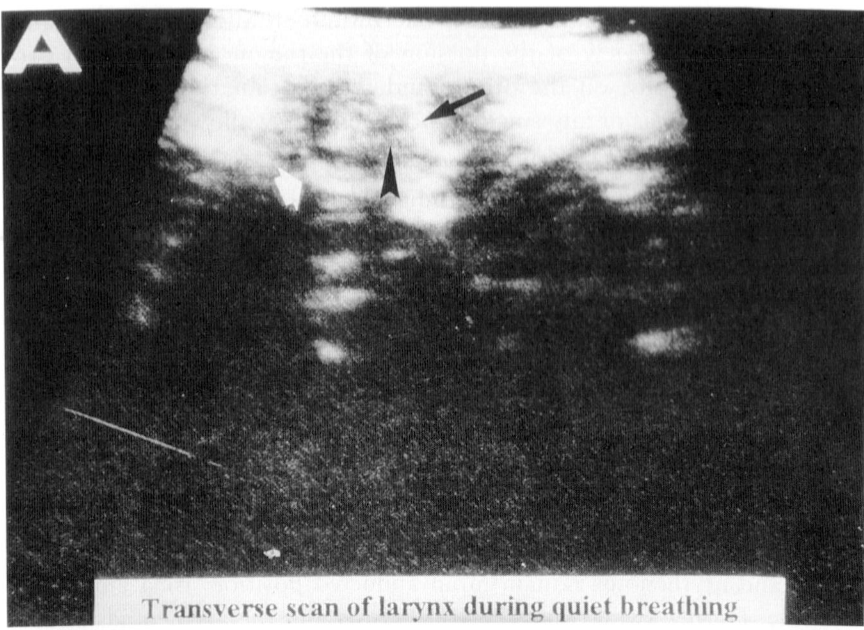

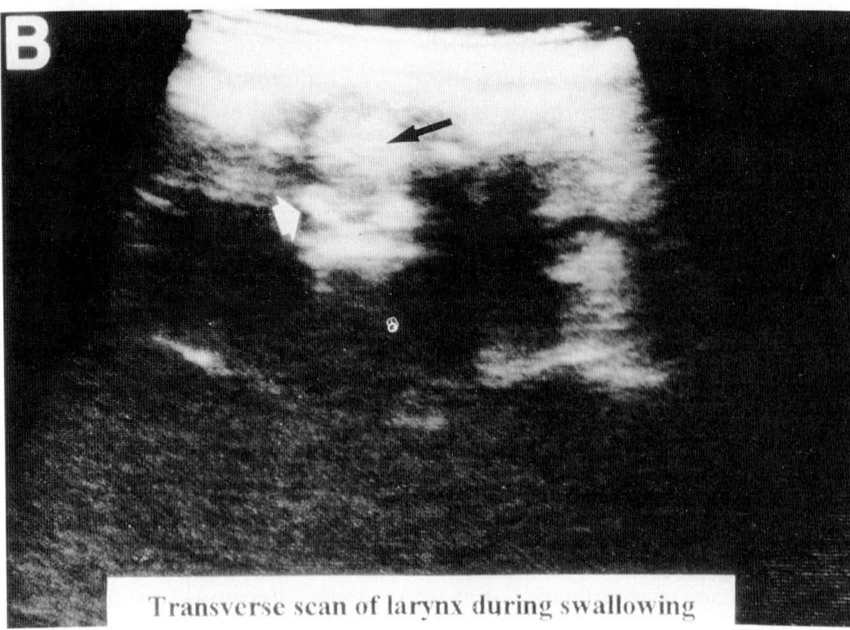

Fig. 1 (A–B): *Transverse scans of the larynx at the level of the vocal cords in a 20-day old infant during quiet breathing (A) and during swallowing (B).*
A: The glottis (black arrowhead) during quiet breathing is easily identified as a median triangular space between the vocal cords (black arrow).
B: During swallowing, vocal cords and arythenoids (white arrow) adduct and glottis disappears.

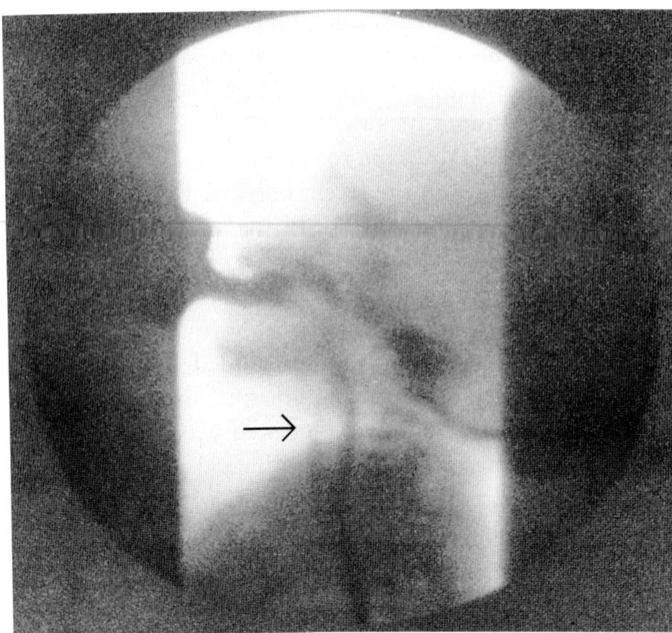

Fig. 2: *Direct laryngeal penetration (arrow) during swallow in a neurologically impaired 3-month-old infant.*

with a nasogastric tube, percutaneous or surgical gastrostomy and jejunostomy. Nasogastric tube is more appropriate for children whose feeding patterns are likely to change rapidly and who may require tube alimentation for no more than 3—6 months. Otherwise, gastrostomy is the procedure of choice. In a child with GER gastrostomy feeding may result in aspiration of regurgitated gastric contents, and a jejunostomy is indicated. Although a preventive antireflux operation at the time of gastrostomy is not indicated, it has been reported that 86% of the children with negative preoperative evaluation for GER would undergo the operation needlessly [19].

Optimal nutrition regimen does not reduce the patient's motivation to resume in due time the oral feeding, but instead keeps the patient physically fit to participate actively in the rehabilitation programme. In order to avoid that patients lose their ability to initiate swallowing, the rehabilitabion programme should be continued, at least in part, during special nutritional support.

Vomiting is another relevant gastrointestinal symptom which frequently affects severely retarded individuals [12]. The majority of them have gastroesophageal reflux (GER); however, recent studies suggest that more widespread dysmotility of the gut may occur. GER is found in 75% of the neurologically impaired children and may be due to different factors. Dysfunction of the autonomous nervous system, with low LES tone, is a likely cause in many children, as no mechanical defect in the cardia has been found. Many of these children have scoliosis, which can dislocate the normal anatomical position of the LES. The supine position and the reduced amounts of swallowed saliva consequent to drooling may alter clearing of the esophagus from reflux material [12]. Independent from scoliosis and the supine position, the later stages of the disease may be the most important factors in determining GER. In the early stages of the disease, most of these children may have abnormal esophageal motility and/or delayed gastric emptying. We reported that children with different degrees of psychomotor retardation may show esophageal motor abnormalities independently from GER. Esophageal motility abnormalities included low amplitude of esophageal contractions, and increased number of abnormal motor responses with presence of simultaneous and double and triple-peaked waves. In children with less severe degrees of mental retardation, mild esophageal motility abnormalities did not persist after proper treatment of esophagitis, whereas in children with severe brain damage esophageal dysmotility did not improve after treatment. These observations suggest that in severely handicapped children, impaired esophageal motor function may aggravate GER and, after treatment, predispose to frequent GER relapses [15].

Delayed gastric emptying is another important factor associated with an increased occurrence of GER in children with cerebral palsy. Fried et al. reported that whey-based formulas reduce the number of episodes of vomiting in children with cerebral palsy by improving the rate of gastric emptying [7]. The percentage of residual gastric radioactivity at 60 e 120 minutes with casein-predominant and whey-based formulas in 8 patients with cerebral palsy was significantly reduced at 60 e 120 minutes in patients fed with whey-based formulas [7]. Recently, Ravelli and Milla reported that children with CNS disorders and vomit have abnormal antral motor activity as often as GER. Following fundoplication more than 80% of the patients with CNS disorders continue to have upper GI symptoms possibly related to antral dysrhythmias, the effect of which may be unmasked by fundoplication. Neurologically impaired children with gastric dysrhythmia have in fact an increased risk of developing severe symptoms of retching following Nissen fundoplication [11].

Electrogastrography may be helpful in detecting antral dysthythmia in such patients for whom alternative therapeutical strategies must be adopted.

In 1989 we diagnosed a primary myopathic condition in two children initially evaluated for hypotonia and recurrent respiratory tract infections and feeding problems due to presumptive disorder of esophageal motility and/or GER. Subsequently we extended GI motility studies to explore more systematically muscle disorders of childhood, and esophageal and gastric motility abnormalities were found in children with progressive muscular dystrophy (MD). These ab-

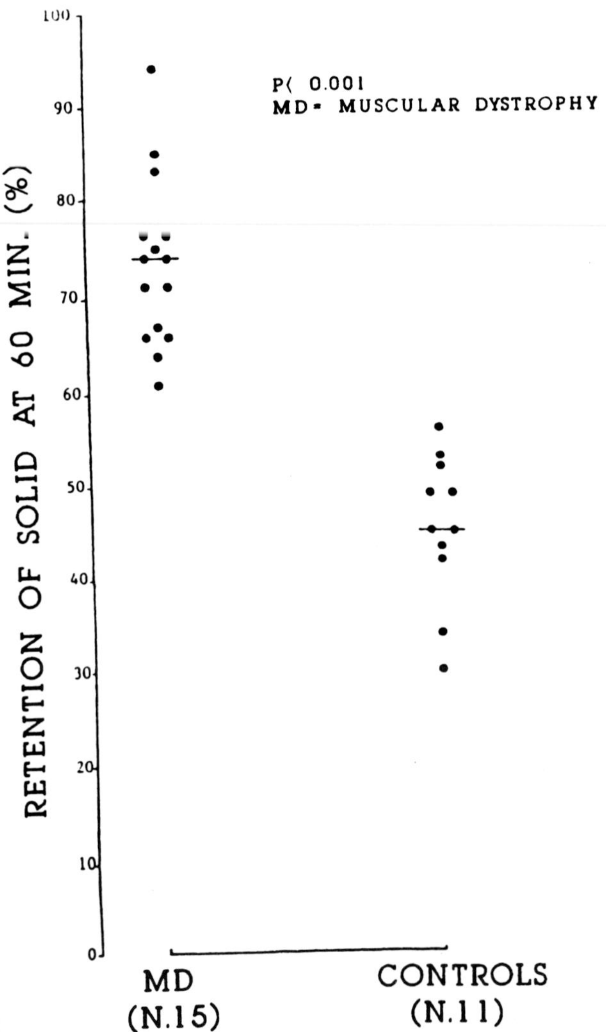

Fig. 3: *Percentage retention of isotope at 60 minutes in children with progressive muscular dystrophy and in 11 age-sex matched control children. The line dividing each group represents the median value.*

normalities were present subclinically early in the course of the disease, even with no evident skeletal muscle involvement. The gastric retention at 60 min of a radiolabelled meal was abnormal in all investigated patients with muscular dystrophy as compared to control subjects (Fig. 3). Furthermore, in 6/15 children with MD the contraction wave amplitudes in the proximal portion of the esophagus were significantly lower than in control subjects.

Fig. 4: Gastroesophageal reflux in brain damaged children: therapy.

H2-blockers + prokinetic drugs

H2-blockers
(1/2 dose for > 6 months)

omeprazole
(1–2 mg/kg/day for 8 weeks)

omeprazole 1 mg/kg/day
H2-blockers
(1/2 dose for 6 months)

fundoplication
± gastrostomy

Children with mental retardation and vomiting respond poorly to conservative treatment [13]. The high failure rate of medical therapy in this special category of patients justifies an aggressive surgical approach, but only after the medical treatment has been given a fair trial. In 1993, Milla's group reported that in spite of the high complication rate and the need for a second operation in 15% of the patients, the quality of life of these children as well as of their parents and caretakers is greatly improved after antireflux surgery. Recently, it has been reported that anterograde percutaneous gastrojejunostomy is a safe alternative method for feeding the neurologically impaired child with GER [1].

Assuming that GER is the most frequent cause of vomiting in children with neurodevelopmental handicap, an algorithm for treatment in children with GER has been proposed (Fig. 4). We usually use prokinetic drug and H2 antagonists. In case of failure we use omeprazole, initially at the dose of 1 mg/kg/die, and then at the dose of 2 mg/kg/die. If symptomatology persists after 2 weeks of treatment or if life-threatening symptoms, such as hematemesis, or severe respiratory symptoms occur, we advise surgery.

In conclusion, GI motor dysfunctions are frequent in children with neuromuscular and other neurological diseases. In children with myopathies, upper GI motor abnormalities do not correlate with symptomatology; it is likely that patients slowly adapt to the disturbance of GI symptoms. Nevertheless, these motility abnormalities may be responsible for significant morbidity. In contrast, in brain damaged children the degree of GI dysmotility correlates with the degree of nervous damage.

Better understanding of the pathophysiology of GI motor disorders in these children may contribute to set treatment strategies which prevent significant secondary causes of morbidity.

References

1. Albanese, C., R. B. Towbin, I. Ulman et al.: Percutaneous gastrojejunostomy versus Nissen fundoplication for enteral feeding of the neurologically impaired child with gastroesophageal reflux. J. Pediatr. 123 (1993) 371–375.
2. Boyle, J. T.: Nutritional management of the developmentally disabled child. Pediatr. Surg. Int. 6 (1991) 76–81.
3. Camilleri, M.: Disorders of gastrointestinal motility in neurologic diseases. Mayo Clinic Proc. 65 (1990) 825–846.
4. Christensen, J. R.: Developmental approach to pediatric neurogenic dysphagia. Dysphagia 3 (1989) 131–134.
5. Cook. I. J. Normal and disordered swallowing: new insights. In: Bailliere's (Ed.): Clinical Gastroenterology, pp. 245–268. Bailliere Tindall, London 1991.
6. Fanucci, A., P. Cerro, E. Fanucci: Sonographic evaluation of physiologic bolus volume in oral swallowing. Am. J. Physiol. Imag. 7 (1992) 73–76.
7. Fried, M. D., V. Khoshoo, D. J. Secker et al.: Decrease in gastric emptying time and episodes of regurgitation in children with spastic quadriplegia fed a whey-based formula. J. Pediatr. 120 (1992) 569–572.
8. Kuban, K. C. K., A. Leviton: Cerebral Palsy. N. E. J. M. 330 (1994) 188–195.
9. Logemann, J. A.: Criteria for studies of treatment for oropharyngeal dysphagia. Dysphagia 1 (1987) 193–199.
10. Newman, L. A., R. H. Cleveland, J. C. Blickman et al.: Videofluoroscopic analysis of the infant swallow. Invest. Radiol. 26 (1991) 870–872.
11. Ravelli, A. M., P. J. Milla: Vomiting and gastroesophageal motility in children with disorders of the central nervous system. Gastroenterology 108 (1995) 675 (A).
12. Sondheimer, J. M., B. A. Morris: Gastroesophageal reflux among severely retarded children. J. Pediatr. 94 (1979) 710–715.
13. Spitz, L., K. Roth, E. M. Kiely et al.: Operation for gastroesophageal reflux associated with severe mental retardation. Arch. Dis. Child 68 (1993) 347–351.
14. Staiano, A., S. Cucchiara, E. Del Giudice et al.: Oesophageal motor involvement in minimal change myopathy. Ital. J. Gastroenterol. 21 (1989) 159–163.
15. Staiano, A., S. Cucchiara, E. Del Giudice et al.: Disorders of esophageal motility in children with psychomotor retardation and gastroesophageal reflux. Eur. J. Ped. 150 (1991) 638–641.
16. Staiano, A., E. Del Giudice: Colonic transit and anorectal manometry in children with severe brain damage. Pediatrics 94 (1994) 169–173.
17. Staiano, A., E. Del Giudice, A. Romano et al.: Upper gastrointestinal tract motility in children with progressive muscular dystrophy. J. Pediatr. 121 (1992) 720–724.
18. Wessel, H. B.: Dystrophin: a clinical perspective. Pediatr. Neurol. 6 (1990) 3–12.
19. Wheatley, M., J. R. Wesley, D. M. Tkach et al.: Long-Term follow-up of brain damaged children requiring feeding gastrostomy: should an antireflux procedure always be performed? J. Ped. Surg. 26 (1991) 301–305.

Diagnosis and management of lower gastrointestinal dysfunctions

C. Di Lorenzo

Introduction

Approximately 25% of children referred to pediatric gastroenterologists have a disorder of defecation. Only a minority of children have organic or anatomic causes for constipation. The incidence of Hirschsprung's disease is only 1 in 6,000 births and Hirschsprung's disease is found in fewer than 1% of children presenting for the first time with constipation [14]. The incidence of anorectal malformations is 1 in 7,000 births. Other common organic causes of childhood constipation include neurologic disease (cerebral palsy, spinal cord disorders, hypotonia), endocrine and metabolic disorders (hypothyroidism, diabetes mellitus, hypercalcemia, renal acidosis, cystic fibrosis) and use of constipating drugs (antacids, iron, codeine-containing medications, imipramine, phenytoin, methylphenidate, atropine, sulcrafate, etc.). Beyond the neonatal period, the most common cause of constipation is functional constipation, which has also been called idiopathic constipation, functional fecal retention or psychogenic megacolon. Childhood functional constipation differs significantly from constipation in adults. It usually begins at the time of toilet training or at school entry and is more prevalent in boys than in girls. Fecal incontinence is more common in childhood constipation than in adults and constipation is associated with withholding behavior in children and straining in adults. Treatment is more successful in children.

Functional constipation

Infants may fail to pass stools because of inadequate water or feeding intake. Sometimes, breast fed babies do not have stools for several days. In these cases, the addition of fruit juices to the diet and an increase in fluid intake is sufficient to make the stool softer and increase the frequency of bowel movements. When the parents overreact to child's struggle to stool, the parental anxiety associated with each defecation is disturbing for the child. The child may respond to the urge to defecate with attempts to withhold, contracting the anal sphincter and the gluteal muscles to avoid defecation and the commotion associated with the act. The rectum accommodates to the fecal mass and the urge to defecate passes. With time, such behavior becomes an automatic response. When suppositories and enemas are used to force the child to have a bowel movement, the child may see this intervention as a punitive measure, reacting with further withholding. Passing a very large stool which painfully stretches the anus, reinforces the conviction that defecation must be avoided at all cost. As the rectum wall stretches and the anal sphincter fatigues, fecal soiling may occur, angering the parents and frightening the child. Attempts to accomplish toilet training at an inappropriately early age (less than 2 years of age), coercive attitudes toward fecal continence and excessive pressure to achieve a perfect daily performance can also trigger a power struggle between the parents and the child and cause the child to withhold. Children are also particularly vulnerable to develop constipation on school entry. Separation anxiety and the poor state of school lavatories may persuade children who are used to defecating at home during the morning to withhold defecation until they are back in the comfort of their own home [5]. At home, watching television, playing with friends and spending time outdoors may represent activities the children enjoy more than stooling, leading to repetitive postponements of defecation.

Children with neurologic diseases

Constipation is an underestimated complaint in children with neurologic diseases. A review of 31 million discharge diagnoses in elderly adults found that the largest group of constipation-associated diseases concerned neurologic and psychiatric diseases [15]. Although similar data are not available in children, pediatric neurologists and gastroenterologists often find constipation in children with neurologic diseases to be a common and formidable challenge. Children with neurologic and developmental delay represent a very heterogeneous population and different pathogenic mechanisms are likely to be important in different groups of children. In tube fed children, the decreased amount of dietary fiber is constipating. The absence of normal skeletal muscle tone and coordination may result in a poor defecatory effort. Immobility and prolonged bed rest may hinder colonic transit, contributing to constipation. The role of such factors is controversial because in other diseases with similar magnitudes of immobility, constipation is rarely a significant clinical problem [15]. Opiates and drugs with anticholinergic properties are often used in neurologically devastated children, with additional impairment of colonic motility. There may be sensory or motor abnormalities due to affected enteric neurons, just as there are abnormalities in the central nervous system. Chronic use of laxatives, especially those containing free anthraquinones, can damage colonic submucosal nerves [28], resulting in abnormal colonic transit. Evidence for an abnormality of colonic motility in children with neurologic diseases comes from a study performed by Staiano and Del Giudice, who found delayed transit in the left colon of constipated children with brain damage [34]. Colonic and rectal motility are modulated by extrinsic nerves consisting both of parasympathetic and sympathetic nervous fibers. The proximal colon receives cholinergic innervation from the vagus and the distal colon receives cholinergic input from the sacral pelvic nerves (S2−S4 roots). The splanchnic nerves, with nerve bodies in the superior mesenteric ganglion, provide adrenergic innervation to the proximal colon and the lumbar nerves, with nerve bodies in the inferior mesenteric ganglia, provide innervation to the distal colon. Lesions to the extrinsic nerves may result in abnormal colonic motility as demonstrated by the association between herpes zoster infection and acute megacolon [4]. In children with spinal cord injury or dysraphism, the rectoanal inhibitory reflex is usually preserved but the external sphincter is often paralytic and the urge for defecation may be lost. As a consequence, children with myelomeningocele may have both constipation and fecal incontinence. Fecal continence is found only in 11% to 30% of children with myelomeningocele [35, 6]. Spinal cord injuries also cause a loss of the gastrocolonic response providing another mechanism for the onset of constipation in children with spinal cord transection.

Treatment of constipation in children with chronic, static CNS disease may include behavioral modification techniques, attempts to increase dietary fiber consumption, routine administration of stool softeners such as mineral oil and lactulose, enemas, oral cathartics, rectal irrigations and biofeedback. Biofeedback training has been helpful in patients who have preservation of some sensorimotor functions in the perianal region and are able to cooperate with biofeedback training [35]. The enema continence catheter has been used to empty the rectum every 48 hours in children with a variety of spinal cord impairments. It consists of a catheter with an inflatable balloon at the end which prevents instant leakage of the enema solution from the incontinent anus and an exterior baffle that locks the balloon in place within the rectum, preventing its displacement. When the total volume of the enema has been admininistered the catheter is removed and the colonic liquid contents are immediately evacuated [18]. Electric stimulation of the sacral nerves using a neuroprosthetic device has also been used in some patients [30].

Colonic neuromuscular diseases

There are "red flags" that should steer the clinician away from a diagnosis of functional constipation, pointing instead towards a neuromuscular colonic disease (Table 1). In children, diseases affecting the submucosal and the myenteric plexus or the colonic smooth muscle are nearly always primary and present during the first year of life. Soiling is often absent and there is no withholding

Table 1: *Comparison of different causes of childhood constipation.*

Signs and symptoms	Functional constipation	Hirschsprung's disease	Other colonic neuromusuclar diseases
symptoms from birth	0	+ + +	+ +
Stool withholding	+ + +	0	+
Obstructive symptoms	+	+ +	+ +
Soiling	+ + +	0	+
Upper GI symptoms	+	+ +	+ + +
Enterocolitis	0	+ +	+ +
Urinary symptoms	Frequent infections in children with encopresis	None	Poor bladder emptying in hollow visceral diseases
Anorectal manometry	Normal sphincter relaxation	No sphincter relaxation	Abnormal sphincter relaxation
Colon manometry	Normal	Normal (?)	Abnormal
Treatment	Medical	Surgical	Varies

behavior. Enterocolitis is a dreaded complication found in Hirschsprung's disease and neuronal intestinal dysplasia (NID). Vomiting, nausea and failure to thrive are found in myopathies or neuropathies extending to the gut proximal to the colon and are not commonly found in functional constipation. Children with colonic neuromuscular diseases may have a hollow visceral neuro- or myopathy causing incomplete bladder emptying while girls with functional constipation and chronic soiling are at risk for developing urinary tract infections from colonic flora.

Pseudo-Hirschsprung's, NID, colonic pseudo-obstruction and visceral neuropathy are some of the labels used to describe neuromuscular diseases of the colon. They represent a heterogeneous and still poorly understood group of disorders which are only now beginning to be recognized. Abnormalities in colonic nervous system range from aganglionosis to hyperganglionosis. *Hirschsprung's disease* is characterized by total absence of ganglion cells in Auerbach's plexus with overgrowth of nerve trunks in the submucosa, muscularis mucosa and lamina propria. In 75% of cases the disease is limited to the rectosigmoid area. It rarely extends beyond the colon. Children with Hirschsprung's disease are treated with a variety of surgical solutions involving the resection of the aganglionic bowel with reanastomosis of the proximal normal bowel to the anal canal. In up to 20% of children, constipation persists after surgery [23, 13]. This may be because of residual disease or an association with NID. There is manometric evidence that a neuropathy is sometimes present in the unresected proximal colon in children who remain symptomatic after surgery [9]. Extracolonic motor dysfunction has been noted in the esophagus [33] and the small intestine (personal observation) of children with Hirschsprung's disease before and after surgery. Both hypo- and hyperganglionosis have been associated with constipation, although a pathologic diagnosis is often difficult due to the lack of age and location control specimens [31].

Neuronal intestinal dysplasia is characterized by hyperplasia of the submucosal plexus and an increase of acetylcholinesterase-positive nerve fibers in the adventitia of submucosal blood vessels. Other common features of NID include increased acetylcholinesterase-positive nerve fibers in the lamina propria and an abnormal distribution of neural elements with neurons found in the lamina propria and within the smooth muscle layers [22]. Caution should be exercised interpreting biopsies obtained from infants because there is a normal hyperplasia of the submucosal ganglia in infants less than four weeks [31, 32]. Inflammation, such as seen in necrotizing enterocolitis, can also cause hyperganglionosis without affecting colon motor function [16]. It has been suggested that the incidence of NID is similar to Hirschsprung's disease and that it can be associated with Hirschsprung's disease in the colon proximal to the aganglionic segment, and with neurofibromatosis and multiple endocrine neoplasia (MEN) type 2b. The association with Hirschsprung's disease raises the possibility that both migration and functional maturation of fibroblasts may be disrupted by the same pathogenic factor [12]. The abnormal segment in NID is almost invariably longer than the aganglionic segment. The classification of NID is likely to undergo changes based on more modern immunocytochemical or histological studies of colonic nervous system.

Hyperplasia of the rectal or colonic myenteric plexus has been reported to account for more than 30% of cases of childhood *chronic intestinal pseudo-obstruction* [25]. A variety of other abnormalities of the myenteric plexus have been described in children with pseudo-obstruction involving the colon [17]. Because colonic histology often does not reflect bowel function it is imperative to perform a careful study of the gut motor function prior to surgical intervention in children with intractable constipation. Fig. 1 summarizes the overlap of colonic neuromuscular diseases with functional constipation and Hirschsprung's disease.

Diagnosis

In most cases, a careful *history* to elicit characteristic behaviors and a thorough *physical examination* are sufficient to diagnose functional constipation. The stool filling the dilated rectum is appreciated as a mobile mass on either side of the rectus sheath. Important findings on physical examination include the presence of fecal seepage, a chronic dermatitis secondary to fecal soiling, an

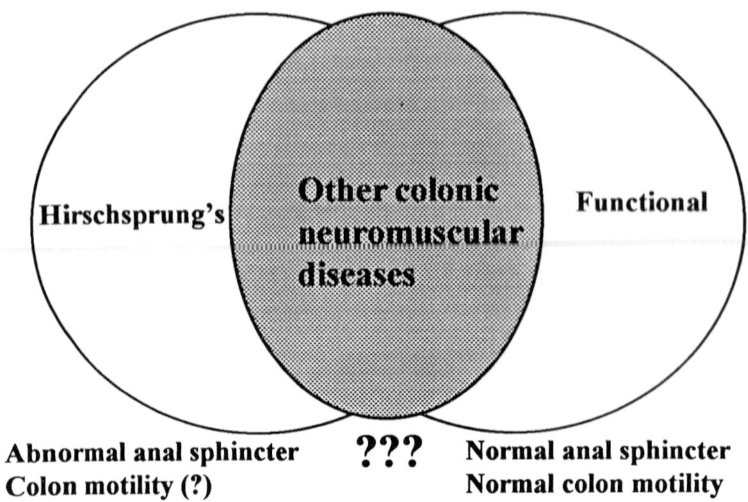

Fig. 1: *Childhood constipation. Colonic neuromuscular diseases may have clinical and manometric features which overlap with functional constipation and Hirschsprung's disease. Little is known on the anorectal and colonic motor function in this group. Colonic motor function in the children who remain symptomatic after Hirschsprung's disease surgery is probably abnormal.*

anteriorly placed anus, and vascular, pigmented or hairy patches over the lumbosacral spine, suggestive of occult spinal dysraphism. The rectal exam shows the presence of a large amount of fecal material occupying a dilated rectal vault in functional constipation and an empty rectal vault in most cases of Hirschsprung's disease. In short segment Hirschsprung's disease and other neuromuscular diseases of the colon stools ranging from hard to soft may be appreciated during a rectal exam. *Anorectal manometry* has been studied extensively in functional constipation, but results are conflicting and often it is unclear if the manometric abnormalities represent a primary disorder or are secondary to the chronic fecal retention and voluntary withholding [20, 19, 36, 21]. The lack of rectoanal inhibitory reflex upon rectal distension has been considered diagnostic of Hirschsprung's disease. There is a sizable subgroup of children with typical or "abortive" NID in which the rectoanal inhibitory reflex is abnormal or even absent (Fig. 2), making the differentiation of NID from Hirschsprung's disease particularly challenging.

Colon manometry may help to clarify pathophysiology of constipation or incontinence in children with neuromuscular colonic disorders. Characteristics of normal colon motility in children of different ages have been defined [8]. Colon manometry has been used to differentiate behavioral from organic causes of constipation [10] and to clarify the pathophysiology of constipation in children with intestinal pseudo-obstruction [11]. In functional constipation, colon motility is normal and shows: 1) presence of high amplitude propagated contractions

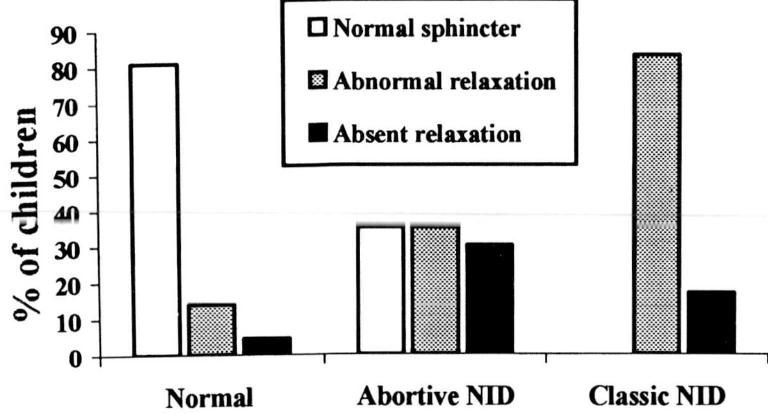

Fig. 2: *Results of anorectal manometry in children with normal histology or abortive or classic neuronal intestinal dysplasia (NID). Children with abortive NID were those with heterotopic ganglion cells without hyperplasia of the submucosal plexus [16].*

(HAPCs) following awakening or a meal, 2) increase in motility index and colonic tone after a meal, and 3) absence of discrete abnormalities. During colonic manometry, HAPCs are easily identified, based upon their characteristically high amplitude (> 80 mmHg), which does not overlap with other contractions, and their duration (> 10 sec.) and propagation over at least 30 cm (Fig. 3) [2]. In adults, HAPCs occur 4–6 times/day in a colon cleansed with cathartics [24] and more infrequently (no more than 2/day) in a normal, unprepared colon [7]. In children, there is an age related decrease in the frequency of HAPCs [8]. A decreased frequency of HAPCs has been reported in adults with colonic inertia [3] and in children with neuropathies involving the colon [11]. Prolonged studies of colon motility coupled with small bowel recordings have been used to predict success of surgery in adults with severe constipation [27, 1]. Thus, colonic manometry, less invasive than a surgical full thickness biopsy, should be considered part of the evaluation for children with intractable constipation prior to considering surgery. Colonic manometry may identify the segment of colon with abnormal motor function (Fig. 4). Colonic manometry can also provide insights in the decision of whether to reconnect a diverted colon. Surgeons commonly divert the colon and place an ileostomy in infants with symptoms suggestive of colonic pseudo-obstruction. Once the child has grown and the symptoms have improved, the decision to reconnect the colon can be based on results of motility studies of the diverted colon, provided that there is no severe diversion colitis [26]. I have also found colon manometry helpful in clarifying pathophysiology of diarrhea or incontinence in children who have received a surgery for Hirschsprung's disease and present with soiling despite good anal sphincter function. Repetitive HAPCs which propagate to the

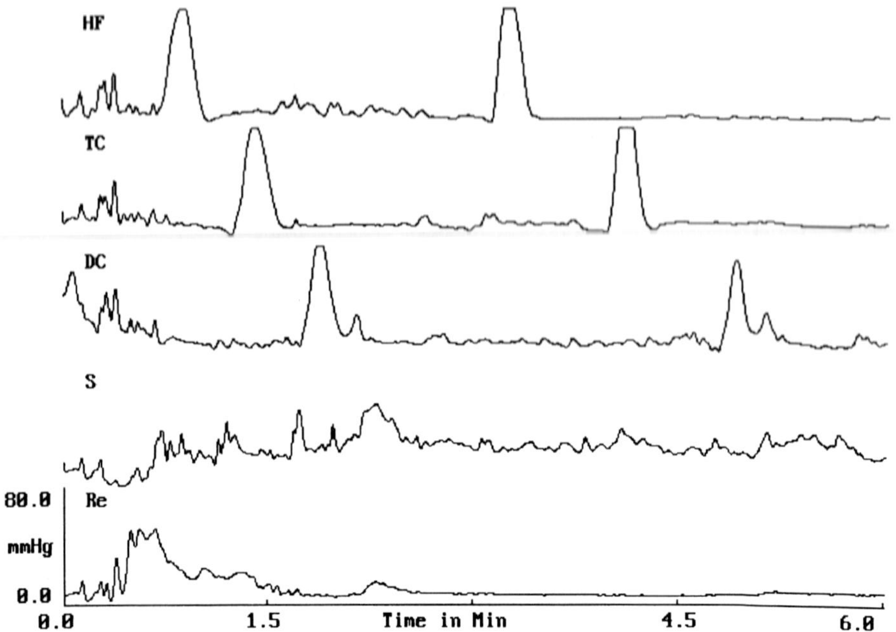

Fig. 3: *Two postprandial HAPCs in a child with functional constipation. The recording sites are 15 cm apart. The first HAPC migrates from the most proximal recording site to the sigmoid colon. The catheter moves distally after the first HAPC and the most distal recording site which is in the rectum is out of the patient's colon at the time of the second HAPC. HF = Hepatic Flexure, TC = Transverse Colon, DC = Descending Colon, S = Sigmoid colon, Re = Rectum.*

neo-rectum just above the anal sphincters (instead of stopping above the pelvic floor) may overcome the resistance produced by the internal and external anal sphincter and produce involuntary passage of stools.

In colonic neuromuscular diseases, *radiopaque markers* may be used to differentiate generalized colonic disease from outlet obstruction. In functional constipation, the markers are found in the rectum within 36 hours. In colonic neuromuscular diseases the markers are scattered throughout the colon for many days. When that happens, full thickness biopsies or colonic manometry studies can differentiate between neuropathy and myopathy. In the absence of generalized colonic dilatation, children whose contractions do not increase following a meal and/or do not produce HAPCs have a colon neuropathy. Children with complete absence of colonic contractions are more likely to have a myopathy. *Anal endosonography* and *defecography* have been only rarely utilized in the evaluation of childhood lower gastrointestinal tract dysfunctions.

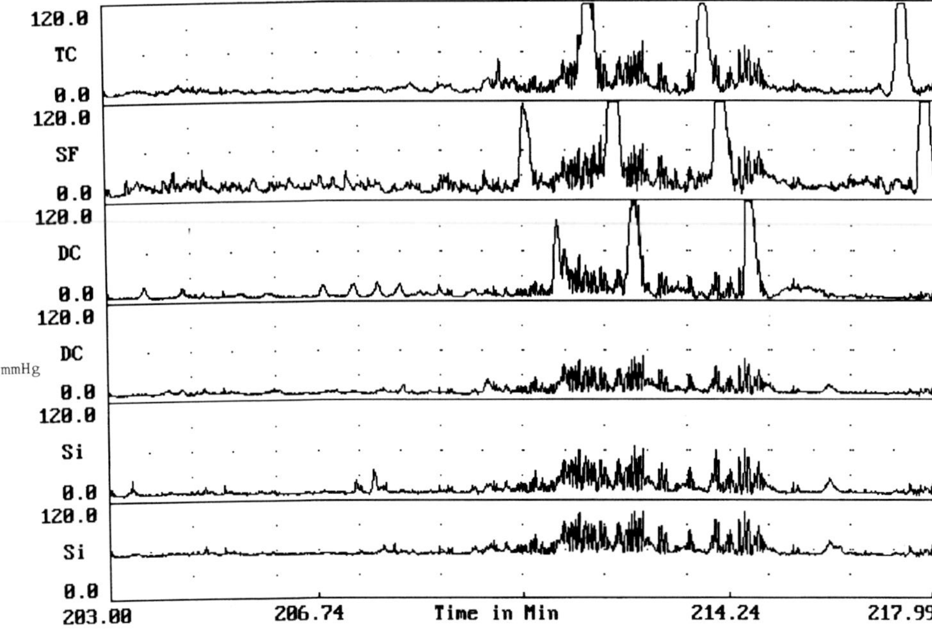

Fig. 4: *Manometric tracing from a child with neuronal intestinal dysplasia. The recording sites are 15 cm apart. There are 4 HAPCs migrating from the transverse colon to the mid-descending colon. There is no propagation of the HAPCs to the distal colon. TC = Transverse Colon, SF = Splenic Flexure, DC = Descending Colon, Si = Sigmoid colon.*

Management

Functional constipation in childhood may be thought of as a maladaptive response to over-control. Educating both the child and parents about the act of defecation and what went wrong in the child's learning process is the cornerstone to an effective treatment. Treatment requires cooperation among the child, the parents and the pediatrician, with the occasional help of a child psychologist and a pediatric gastroenterologist. Drug therapy is directed at making the stools soft and painless to evacuate and behavioral modifications are used to retrain the child to use the toilet. Diets rich in fiber and prokinetic drugs have a limited role in childhood constipation. Biofeedback has been used to teach anal sphincter relaxation to children with abnormal defecation dynamics and to promote continence in encopretic children. Treatment failures occur in a minority of children with functional constipation. When treatment fails, then is time to consider the possibility that an organic disease is causing the symptoms. It has been reported that some children with NID may improve with time [29, 12]. In other patients with NID, surgery may be curative [12]. It should be remembered that there are few conditions as emotionally draining as the daily fight to stool. In children with severe constipation, the emotional toll on the child, the family and the parental-child interaction may be exceptional. When indicated, surgical solutions should not be delayed. The *entire* gastrointestinal motor function should be evaluated to provide the most educated choice of the type of surgery to perform. It has been suggested that a colostomy should be placed at the level of the splenic flexure without resection of the colon showing pathologic evidence of NID until the age of 3 years, because maturational changes in the innervation of the colon may occur up to that age [12]. If the colon continues to show abnormal motility after 3 years of age then a resection of the diseased segment with a take-down of the normal colon should be performed.

References

1. Bassotti, G., C. Betti, M. A. Pelli et al.: Extensive investigation of colonic motility with pharmacological testing is useful for selecting surgical options in patients with inertia colica. Am. J. Gastroenterol. 87 (1992) 143−147.
2. Bassotti, G., M. Gaburri: Manometric investigation of high amplitude propagated contractile activity of the human colon. Am. J. Physiol. 255 (1988) G660−664.
3. Bassotti, G., B. P. Imbimbo, C. Betti et al.: Impaired colonic response to eating in patients with slow transit constipation. Am. J. Gastroenterol. 87 (1992) 504−508.
4. Caccese, W. J., R. L. Bronzo, G. Wadler et al.: Ogilvie's syndrome associated with herpes zoster infection. J. Clin. Gastroenterol. 7 (1985) 309−313.
5. Clayden, G.: Constipation as a behavioural problem in children. In: M. Kamm, J. E. Lennard-Jones (Eds.): Constipation, pp. 117−122. Wringhtson Biomedical Publishing Ltd., Petersfield, UK 1994.
6. Cooper, D. G. W.: Detrusor action in children with myelomeningocele. Arch. Dis. Child 43 (1968) 427−432.
7. Crowell, M. D., G. Bassotti, L. J. Cheskin et al.: Method for prolonged ambulatory monitoring of high amplitude propagated contractions from colon. Am. J. Physiol. 261 (1991) G263−268.
8. Di Lorenzo, C., A. F. Flores, P. E. Hyman: Age-related changes in colon motility. J. Pediatr. 127 (1995) 593−596.
9. Di Lorenzo, C., A. F. Flores, S. N. Reddy et al.: Colon motility in symptomatic children after surgery for Hirschsprung's disease: abnormalities in "healthy" colon. Gastroenterology 100 (1991) A437.
10. Di Lorenzo, C., A. F. Flores, S. N. Reddy et al.: Colonic manometry differentiates causes of intractable constipation in children. J. Pediatr. 112 (1992) 690−695.
11. Di Lorenzo, C., A. F. Flores, S. N. Reddy et al.: Colonic manometry in children with chronic intestinal pseudo-obstruction. Gut 34 (1993) 803−807.
12. Fadda, B., G. Pistor, W. Meier-Ruge et al.: Symptoms, diagnosis, and therapy of neuronal intestinal dysplasia masked by Hirschsprung's disease. Pediatr. Surg. Int. 2 (1987) 76−80.
13. Helij, H. A., X. de Vries, I. Bremer et al.: Long-term anorectal function after Duhamel operation for Hirschsprung's disease. J. Pediatr. Surg. 30 (1995) 430−432.
14. Hyman, P. E., D. Fleisher: Functional fecal retention. Practical Gastroenterology 16 (1992) 29−37.
15. Johanson, J. F., A. Sonnenberg, T. R. Koch et al.: Association of constipation with neurologic diseases. Dig. Dis. Sci. 37 (1992) 179−186.

16. Koletzko, S., A. Ballauff, F. Hadziselimovic et al.: Is histological diagnosis of neuronal dysplasia related to clinical and manometric findings in constipated children? Results of a pilot study. J. Pediatr. Gastroenterol. Nutr. 17 (1993) 59−65.
17. Krishnamurthy, S., Y. Heng, M. D. Shuffler: Chronic intestinal pseudo-obstruction in infants and children caused by diverse abnormalities of the myenteric plexus. Gastroenterology 104 (1993) 1398−1408.
18. Liptak, G. S., G. M. Revell: Management of bowel dysfunction in children with spinal cord disease or injury by means of the enema continence catheter. J. Pediatr. 120 (1992) 190−194.
19. Loening-Baucke, V. A.: Sensitivity of the sigmoid colon and rectum in children treated for chronic constipation. J. Pediatr. Gastroenterol. Nutr. 3 (1984) 454−459.
20. Loening-Baucke, V. A., M. K. Younoszai: Abnormal anal sphincter response in chronically constipated children. J. Pediatr. 100 (1982) 213−218.
21. Meunier, P., J. M. Marechal, M. J. deBeaugeu: Rectoanal pressures and rectal sensitivity studies in chronic childhood constipation. Gastroenterology 77 (1979) 330−336.
22. Milla, P. J., V. V. Smith: Aganglionosis, hypoganglionosis and hyperganglionosis: clinical presentation and histopathy. In: M. Kamm, J. E. Lennard-Jones (Eds.): Constipation, pp. 183−192. Wrightson Biomedical Publishing Ltd., Petersfield, UK 1994.
23. Mishalany, H. G., M. M. Wooley: Postoperative functional and manometric evaluation of patients with Hirschsprung's disease. J. Pediatr. Surg. 22 (1987) 443−446.
24. Narducci, F., G. Bassotti, M. Gaburri et al.: Twenty four hour manometric recording of colonic motor activity in humans. Gut 28 (1987) 17−25.
25. Navarro, J., E. Sonsino, N. Boige et al.: Visceral neuropathies responsible for chronic intestinal pseudo-obstruction syndrome in pediatric practice. J. Pediatr. Gastroenterol. Nutr. 11 (1990) 179−195.
26. Ordein, J. J., C. Di Lorenzo, A. F. Flores et al.: Diversion colitis in children with severe gastrointestinal motility disorders. Am. J. Gastroenterol. 87 (1992) 88−90.
27. Redmond, J. M., G. W. Smith, I. Barofsky et al.: Physiological tests to predict long term outcome of total abdominal colectomy for intractable constipation. Am. J. Gastroenterol. 90 (1995) 748−753.
28. Reimann, J. F., H. Schmidt, W. Zimmerman: The fine structure of colonic submucosal nerves in patients with chronic laxative abuse. Scand. J. Gastroenterol. 15 (1980) 761−768.
29. Scharli, A. F.: Neuronal intestinal dysplasia. Pediatr. Surg. Int. 7 (1992) 2−7.
30. Schmidt, R. A., B. A. Kogan, E. A. Tanagho: Neuroprosthesis in the management of incontinence in myelomeningocele patients. J. Urol. 143 (1990) 779−782.
31. Schofield, D. E., E. J. Yunis: Intestinal neuronal dysplasia. J. Pediatr. Gastroenterol. Nutr. 12 (1991) 182−189.
32. Smith, V. V.: Intestinal neuronal density in childhood: a baseline for the objective assessment of hypo- and hyperganglionosis. Pediatr. Pathol. 13 (1993) 225−237.
33. Staiano, A. M., E. Corazziari, M. R. Andreotti et al.: Esophageal motility in children with Hirschsprung's disease. A. J. D. C. 145 (1991) 310−313.
34. Staiano, A. M., E. Del Giudice: Colonic transit and anorectal manometry in children with severe brain damage. Pediatrics 94 (1994) 169−173.
35. Wald, A.: Use of biofeedback in fecal incontinence in patients with meningomyelocele. Pediatrics 68 (1981) 45−49.
36. Wald, A., R. Chandra, D. Chiponis et al.: Anorectal function and continence mechanisms in childhood encopresis. J. Pediatr. Gastroenterol. Nutr. 5 (1986) 346−351.

Bladder replacement: experience with an ileocecal segment with multiple transverse teniamyotomies

E. Alcini, A. D'Addessi, M. Racioppi, A. Alcini

Introduction

In 1980 we started the experience in orthotopic bladder replacement working at first with the integral ileocecal segment [1] and then, since 1983, with detubularized ileal reservoir [2]. This fact has allowed us to evaluate the advantages and disadvantages of each [3].

In 1987 we developed a technique using an ileocecal segment which was not detubularized but was made more distensible by multiple transverse teniamyotomies [4]. The goal of the procedure is to reduce the intestinal wall tension and so the internal pressures lowering the incidence of incontinence during the first year and avoiding meanwhile an excessive dilatation of the new bladder over time.

Patients and methods

Since 1987, 60 patients with invasive bladder cancer have undergone cystoprostatectomy and bladder replacement using an ileocecal segment with multiple transverse teniamyotomies.

After the cystoprostatectomy is performed using the traditional technique, the last 5–6 cm of the terminal ileum and about 10 cm of the cecum are isolated based on the ileocolic artery. The anterior tenia coli and the tenia omentalis are located on the cecum segment. Transverse incisions are then performed about 3–4 cm apart extended down to the submucosal layer. Performing such incisions on the tenia coli results in an almost spherical cecal neobladder without significantly weakening wall resistance. In the first 12 operated patients manometric pressures within the cecum were measured intraoperatively, which allowed us to standardize the number of incisions from 5 to 7. The incisions reduced the internal pressure at capacity of 15 and 20 mmHg compared to the pressure of the intact intestine and increased the capacity almost twofold (Table 1). The segment is then positioned in the pelvis and the ureters anastomosed directly end-to-side to the ileal segment with no attempt to construct an anti-reflux mechanism. The antimesenteric wall of the cecum is then anastomosed to the membranous urethra. An appendectomy was performed in all the

Table 1: *Capacity and intraluminal pressure at 120 ml of filling recorded in 12 patients before and after performing teniamyotomies.*

Patients	Capacity (ml)		Pressure (mmHg)	
	before	after	before	after
1	130	255	50	32
2	145	300	42	25
3	150	275	40	25
4	155	285	40	23
5	160	310	35	20
6	130	285	45	24
7	160	285	35	17
8	135	255	48	32
9	130	260	44	24
10	135	270	46	30
11	160	300	35	22
12	130	250	48	30

patients. The ileocecal sphincter acts as a natural anti-reflux mechanism; we did not use any technique to reinforce it to avoid possible obstacles to the urinary flow from the kidney.

The average follow-up of patients is 33.6 months (range 3−95).

Results

Of the 60 operated patients 19 died: one of them during the post-operative period of mesenteric artery embolism in a patient with mitral valve prosthesis, 15 of them of neoplastic progression with an average survival of 19.4 months (3−59) and 3 of different causes.

Complications: The early complication rate was limited. Overall there were 2 wound dehiscences, one of which needed abdominal wall plastic, 2 reoperation for intestinal obstruction for adhesions, 1 reoperation for dehiscence of the ileocolostomy and finally 1 patient with prolonged lymphorrhoea. Among the late complications of the 59 investigated patients, we found during control void-ing cystograms the presence of monolateral ureteral reflux in 6 patients (10.2%), but it did not cause any clinical or functional disturbances. During an average follow-up of 18.9 months (range 2−47), stenosis at the uretero-ileal anastomosis level was found in 7 patients (11.9%); one case needed a reopera-tion for ureteral reimplantation, 4 cases needed a percutaneous dilatation of the stenosis, whereas 2 of them did not need any manoeuvre and were routinely observed at follow-up. In no subject did the renal function change in comparison to the preoperative status. Even in the patients with refluxes or stenosis no change in the blood nitrogen and creatinine values was found at follow-up.

Functionality: Continence was assessed in 56 patients, who were followed-up for at least 6 months. Patients with usual or significant urinary escapes which needed the use of absorbants were considered incontinent. In order to compare the time evolution we reevaluated the patients dividing them in two groups, the first one consisting of patients with less than 3 years of follow-up, and the second one with more than 3 years of follow-up.

Group 1 (28 patients, average follow-up of 16.7 months, range 6−33). The diurnal continence is reached at once: 50% of the patients have intervals of 2−3 hours, whereas the second half have intervals of 3−5 hours. In the night 71.4% of the patients are continent with intervals of 2−3 hours, 7.2% with intervals of 3−4 hours, whereas 21.4% of them suffer from enuresis.

Group 2 (28 patients, average follow-up of 54 months, range 36−95). During the diurnal period 32.1% of the patients are continent with intervals of 2−3 hours, whereas the remaining 67.9% with intervals of 3−5 hours. During the night 57.1% of the patients are continent with intervals of 2−3 hours, 28.6% with intervals of 3−4 hours, whereas the percentage of enuretic patients is reduced to 14.3%. Among all the enuretic patients of both groups (10 cases), some of them (4 cases) chose freely to be incontinent at night because they refused to train themselves with programmed awakening between the micturitions and then progressively prolonging these intervals.

An urodynamic evaluation was made in 12 patients with a follow-up of 12 months and in 14 patients with a follow-up of 5 years; data are summarized in Tables 2 and 3.

Up until now, as we have already said, we never found any renal failures after the operation. The average values of blood nitrogen and creatinine in the pa-

Table 2: *Urodynamics of 12 patients after 1 year.*

Patients	12
Max. capacity (ml)	$285.8 \pm 34.6\ (227-464)$
Pressure at max. capacity (cmH$_2$O)	$31.3 \pm 13.2\ (13-\ 63)$
Max. intravesical pressure (cmH$_2$O)	$47.4 \pm 21.4\ (15-\ 80)$
Q max. (ml/sec)	$18.7 \pm\ 7.3\ \ (9-\ 38)$
Post-micturition residual (ml)	$22\ \ \pm 12.7\ \ (0-\ 48)$

Table 3: *Urodynamics of 14 patients after 5 years.*

Patients	14
Max. capacity (ml)	469 $\pm$ 75.8 (359−578)
Pressure at max. capacity (cmH$_2$O)	30.4 $\pm$ 14.3 (13− 70)
Max. intravesical pressure (cmH$_2$O)	47.6 $\pm$ 16.7 (25− 72)
Q max. (ml/sec)	20.8 $\pm$ 7.8 (11− 42)
Post-micturition residual (ml)	28 $\pm$ 16.3 (0− 65)

tients investigated were 22.7 mg/dl (normal values 10−23 mg/dl) and 1.16 mg/dl (n. v. 0.7−1.4 mg/dl) respectively. Also serum electrolytes did not vary significantly.

The average metabolic values in arterial blood samples were 7.399 $\pm$ 0.027 (n. v. 7.340−7.440) of pH, 39.9 $\pm$ 4.1 mmHg (n. v. 32−45) of pCO$_2$, 88.1 $\pm$ 12.4 mmHg (n. v. 74−108) of pO$_2$, 21.9 $\pm$ 2.8 mmol/l (n. v. 21−29) of HCO$_3$ and −1.7 $\pm$ 2.6 mmol/l (n. v. from − to 2) of bases excess. The average serum values of vitamin B$_{12}$ were 264.6 $\pm$ 96.2 pg/ml (n. v. 160−1138) and of folic acid were 5.75 $\pm$ 2.06 ng/ml (n. v. 1.5−17.3).

Discussion

Following the correct oncological indications, the possibility to reconstruct a new bladder after its exeresis has been a major progress in urology, as it is also evident considering the continuing interest in this issue and the vast contribution of technical approaches proposed over these last years.

The evaluation of our experience drawn over 15 years [5] and the analysis of anatomophysiological considerations have led us to advocate the ileocecal tract with transverse teniamyotomies as the most suitable intestinal segment for the replacement of the bladder. It is thought that intestinal motility is an important determining factor in relation to urinary continence. Electrophysiological studies have demonstrated that the most important control over intestinal motility is myogenic [7], depending upon the frequency of the intrinsic electrical activity of the smooth muscle cells of the intestine: theoretically there could be less motor activity in the ileocecal tract [8]. Also, as indicated by the oscillators theory [11], such activity consisting of uncoordinated oscillations would be essentially aimed at regulating the storage function in the cecum.

In addition to the theoretically scarce contractility, the cecal tract has another important motor characteristic, receptive relaxation, which implements the storage function [10]. This term indicates the ability of the viscera to adapt to the increasing volume of the internal contents with little or no increase of the endoluminal pressure. It is likely that this functional characteristic, when comparing several intestinal segments, makes the cecum capable of resembling bladder functions. Moreover, this functional characteristic is regulated by a dedicated anatomical structure, since the cecum has a large lumen and a muscular structure which, relatively to other segments, is not as much developed. The particular muscular structure of the cecum with an internal circular layer present over the entire segment and an external longitudinal layer gathered in three teaniae coli, suggested the authors to perform transverse teniamyotomy. With this technique it is possible to obtain a consistent relaxation of the wall and a reduction in wall tension of the new bladder, which acquires a near spherical configuration [9]. An initial capacity of 250–300 ml is reached at the operation and it eventually stabilizes between 400 and 500 ml.

Overall, the analysis of our series seems to confirm that the teniamyotomies are much easier and more rapid to be made than the detubularization. The bisection of the teniae is performed over its whole width without extending the incision beyond the submucosal layer. Thus, by performing a limited number of sutures, the potential risk of dehiscences and complications is reduced. The volume of the new bladder does not tend to increase out of proportion but, rather, its capacity remains within a paraphysiological range after many years after surgery. In addition, differently from detubularized neobladder, the cecal neobladder with teniamyotomies maintains basal tone similar to the normal bladder. Similar observations were reported by other authors. Planche et al., in their experience [12] with different cecal neobladders, recorded and compared the endoluminal pressure secondary to contraction waves: it is 100–120 cm H_2O in the intact cecal neobladder and 30–60 cm H_2O in those where our technique of teniamyotomies has been performed. This basal tone of 10–20 cm H_2O is maintained during filling with 100–120 ml, a functional condition which may offer some advantages in comparison to the intact and detubularized newbladders. In this way a late atony, often present after the detubularization, is prevented, post micturition residual results negligible and no patient needs self-catheterizations. The diurnal continence is ensured at once for all patients, even if with variable intervals between micturitions. The nocturnal continence is reached by a significant number of patients within the first months and by many more in the subsequent periods.

The average reservoir capacity is 285 ml, after one year from the surgical procedure, and then it increases progressively to reach an average value of less than 500 ml after 5 years from the operation, a value which appears to be relatively stable since it is not different from that recorded after 3 years from the operation (9 patients evaluated, average capacity 407 ml). The average internal pressure of the reservoir, recorded at end filling, is 31.3 cm H_2O after one year and 30.4 cm H_2O after 5 years from the operation. The neovesical wall tone is preserved without any leakage signs. The average maximum pressure peak is almost identical after one and 5 years (47.4 cm H_2O and 47.6 cm H_2O, respectively). The simplicity of the operation is obtained even for the use of the ileocecal junction, which possibly acts as an antireflux mechanism. The more recent anatomophysiologic data seem to indicate that the ileo-cecal junction may react as a sphincter to oppose reflux and facilitate transit of its contents to be stored into the cecum. The reduced occurrence of ureteral refluxes, and overall the absence of clinical complications such as dilatations or recurrent infections, shows that it adequately performs its peculiar task with no need of additional reinforcement. This anatomofunctional characteristic is further reinforced by the teniamyotomy, which reduces the internal pressures [6].

Based on our experience, it would seem logical to conclude that the use of the ileocecal tract with teniamyotomies is a worthwhile surgical approach for its simplicity and for its functional results.

References

1. Alcini, E., M. Vincenzoni, A. Destito et al.: Ileocaeco-urethroplasty after total cystectomy for bladder cancer. Brit. J. Urol. 57 (1985) 160.
2. Alcini, E., M. Pescatori, A. D'Addessi et al.: Bladder reconstruction after cystectomy for cancer: use of the ileal reservoir. Brit. J. Urol. 57 (1985) 245.
3. Alcini, E., F. Grassetti, A. D'Addessi et al.: Bladder replacement by ileocaeco-urethrostomy or ileo-urethrostomy with a reservoir after cystoprostato-vesiculectomy. A functional evaluation. Br. J. Urol. 63 (1989) 36.
4. Alcini, E., M. Pescatori, A.D'Addessi et al.: Multiple taeniamyotomy of the replaced caecum after restorative cystoprostatovesiculectomy for bladder cancer. Br. J. Urol. 66 (1990) 441.
5. Alcini, E., A. D'Addessi, M. Racioppi et al.: Four years' experience with bladder replacement using an ileocecal segment with multiple transverse teniamyotomies. J. Urol. 149 (1993) 735.
6. Alcini, E., M. Racioppi, A. D'Addessi et al.: Refluxes in orthotopic neobladders: can the ileocecal sphincter be considered an adequate antireflux mechanism? Urology 44 (1994) 38.
7. Bortoff, A.: Myogenic control of intestinal motility. Physiol. Rev. 56 (1976) 418.
8. Christensen, J.: The controls of gastrointestinal movements: some old and new views. New Engl. J. Med. 285 (1971) 85.
9. Hinman, F., Jr.: Selection of intestinal segments for bladder substitution: physical and physiological characteristics. J. Urol. 139 (1988) 519.
10. Netter, F. H.: Digestive System. Lower digestive tract, p. 86. E. Oppenheimer, New York: CIBA 1975.
11. Sarna, S. K., E. E. Daniel: Electrical stimulation of gastric electrical control activity. Am. J. Physiol. 225 (1971) 125.
12. Truong, T. T.: Etude de 101 cystectomies suivies de coecystoplastie. Mémoire pour le Diplôme Inter-Universitaire de Spécialité de Chirurgie Urologique. Université D'Aix−Marseille, Marseille, France 1994.

Orthotopic ileal bladder by "Vescica Ileale Padovana"

W. Artibani, F. Pagano, G. Maio, A. Ruffato, G. Mulonia,
R. Piazza, E. Pescatori

Introduction

The goal in constructing an intestinal urinary reservoir is to obtain an adequate-capacity low-pressure non-refluxing reservoir, employing the shortest possible length of bowel in order to minimize bowel and metabolic disturbances. This goal is achievable by detubularization and reconfiguration [6].

The double-folding Kock principle [9, 10] is the gold-standard in constructing a spheric reservoir from a cylindric bowel segment. Other detubularized and reconfigurated intestinal urinary reservoirs obtained similar results, namely the Mainz pouch [14, 15], the Hautmann's ileal bladder [5], and the Vescica Ileale Padovana [11, 12].

The fact that, having the same initial length of the bowel segment, the capacity and the intraluminal pressure of reservoir depend upon the geometric configuration is well established and easily demonstrable [6]. Due to geometrical considerations, the larger the radius the larger the volume is, i.e. the best "performance" is obtained by a sphere. This explains geometrically why the double-folding technique obtains the largest possible volume from the same initial length. The grossly spheric configuration offers other advantages due to the laws of Laplace and Pascal: at the same pressure, the larger diameter will accommodate a larger volume.

Beside these geometrical considerations, viscoelastic properties are important. The true capacity of a reconfigured intestinal urinary reservoir is obtained after a "maturation" of about six months. The long-term behaviour of intestinal detubularized and reconfigured urinary reservoirs is a fascinating, incompletely explored field.

Having established the Kock pouch as the gold-standard, many of the proposed detubularized and reconfigured intestinal reservoirs achieved good results in terms of adequate capacity and low pressure (Mainz, Hautmann, Studer [13], Camey II, Vescica Ileale Padovana). The possible pros and cons regard the type (ileal, colic, ileo-colic, gastric) and the length of the bowel segment, and the simplicity/reliability of the surgical technique. At present, it is difficult to indicate objectively the best techniques. In the absence of data relating to ten years follow-up on large series, it is a matter of opinion.

Development of the "Vescica Ileale Padovana" (VIP)

The "Vescica Ileale Padovana" (VIP) was first performed on September 9th, 1987. The VIP was developed as a practical application of the concepts of vesical physiopathology [1] expressed by Camey [3, 8], Kock [4, 9, 10] and Hinman [6], to the construction of an intestinal urinary reservoir. Detubularization, reconfiguration, search for sphericity and good capacity using the shortest possible bowel segment are the main principles of the VIP procedure. VIP comprises features from Camey I ileal reservoir [8], Bramble's clam enterocystoplasty [2], and double folding Kock principle [9].

The original points of VIP are the construction of a lower funnel and the type of geometric reconfiguration.

The advantages offered by VIP are the following: use of ileum, very short bowel segment preserving ileocecal valve, simple and quick procedure, final anatomy closely resembling the original (the lower funnel resembles an empty prostatic fossa, ureters lying in their place without crossing or dislocating), and the reservoir fitting naturally into the pelvis.

Surgical technique

The membranous urethra is managed as in radical prostatectomy [16] and is incised as close as possible to the prostatic apex in order to preserve the distal urethral sphincter. In selected cases nerve-sparing cystoprostatectomy may be performed.

A 40 cm ileal segment is isolated starting at a convenient point 15—20 cm from the ileo-cecal valve. The distal (ab-oral) mesenteric incision is very deep at the level of the ileo-colic artery in order to provide good mobility. On the other hand, the proximal (oral) mesenteric incision can be very short because it does not contribute to the mobility of the lower loop and because the medial folding of the upper loop requires minimal mobility. Intestinal continuity is restored by end-to-end anastomosis.

The ileal segment is split open all along the antimesenteric border. A lower funnel is created by means of a running suture about 5 cm in length. The proximal loop is medially folded on itself in a reversed 'U' shape and the inner opposite borders are then sutured side-to-side so as to form an upper ileal cup. This will be tied to the edges of the lower ileal cup, in order to obtain an oval re-fashioned reservoir. The ileal anastomotic hole is created at the lowest end of the anterior suture of the funnel. A Le-Duc's uretero-ileal anastomosis [7] is carried out bilaterally. The urethro-ileal anastomosis is performed with six 3/0 chromic catgut stitches.

Since its first applications, there have been minor changes to the surgical technique, in order to simplify and shorten the procedure.

Initially the sequence of manoeuvres was that described in Eur. Urol. [11]: ileo-urethral anastomosis, detubularization, lower funnel, bilateral Le Duc, posterior reconfiguration, anterior reconfiguration.

In April 1990, the sequence of manoeuvres was definitely established as follows: detubularization, construction of the lower funnel, mucosal eversion in the anastomotic hole, posterior reconfiguration, bilateral Le Duc, subcomplete anterior reconfiguration, ileo-urethral anastomosis, complete reconfiguration. With this sequence of manoeuvres the main part of the procedure is performed on surface, thus reducing the surgical time (at present around two hours).

The ureters are drained by means of 6−8 F stents, which are removed after 8−9 days. The reservoir is drained by a transurethral 22 F catheter. A radiologic control is performed after 14 days. Special attention is paid to train the patient to completely void the reservoir by abdominal straining plus simultaneous perineal relaxation and to develop surrogates to the normal voiding desire.

Patient series

From September 1987 through November 1994, 188 VIPs were performed following radical cystectomy for invasive bladder cancer. The age of patients varied from 38 to 76 years with a mean age of 59.5 years.

4 patients were lost at follow-up or their documentation was incomplete. This series thus includes 184 evaluable patients.

Beside the usual oncological contraindications − urethral involvement and pelvic lymphadenopathy −, VIP was not indicated in case of urethral stricture, significant ureteral dilation, lowering of functional renal reserve. However, as in any other series, some exceptions from the contraindications were sometimes made according to specific cases. 33 out of 184 patients were submitted to neoadjuvant chemotherapy (MVAC). The pathological staging was the following: 37 pTO, 13 pTis, 31 pT1b, 28 pT2, 34 pT3a, 27 pT3b, 14 pT4. 24 patients had positive lymphnodes. In 17 cases incidental prostatic cancer was detected.

12 patients were submitted to adjuvant systemic chemotherapy, without complications related to the ileal reservoir (an indwelling catheter was not needed to avoid resorption). In 5 patients pelvic recurrence was observed. 2 patients were submitted to nephroureterectomy due to secondary upper tract transitional cancer. To date no urethral recurrence has been observed. 1 patient presents posi-

tive urinary citology without visible lesions (occult urothelial disease) at 6 years follow-up.

Pelvic recurrences occurred at 4, 6, 10, 34, and 65 months after surgery. Three patients were partial responders to MVAC neoadjuvant chemotherapy.

The first patient was submitted to mass removal, nephroureterectomy due to ureteral involvement and partial demolition of the reservoir. Radiotherapy followed. The patient died after 7 months.

The second patient died 3 months after mass removal (pre-rectal lymphangitis) and radiotherapy.

The third patient was submitted to adjuvant chemotherapy and died after 3 months.

The fourth patient had a pelvic mass plus aorto-iliac lymphadenopathy; he died after 5 months without oncological treatment.

The fifth patient died after 5 months without oncological treatment.

All patients continued to void spontaneously until the pre-terminal phases.

Results

Oncological status

The oncological status was evaluated in 159 patients, 132 of them with a follow-up longer than 6 months.

128 are now alive and disease-free, 5 patients are alive with metastases, 22 died due to disease progression − among these the 5 patients with local recurrence −, 2 died due to non-oncological causes, 1 due to massive pulmonary embolus, and 1 due to miocardial infarction. 1 patient is alive after more than 5 years with occult urothelial disease.

Early and late complications

The early complications of VIP, evaluated on 176 patients are reported in Table 1.

The overall rate of early complications was 6.25%.

Late complications of VIP evaluated in 132 patients with a follow-up longer than 6 months are reported in Table 2.

The overall rate of late complications was 43.9%.

In regard to the urethral strictures, two were very short at bulbar level and were treated by endoscopic incision; the remaining involved almost all the penile and bulbar urethra and required open urethrotomy.

Table 1: *Early complications of VIP.*

5 prolonged paralitic ileus
3 mechanical bowel obstruction
1 fistula between stapler ileal anastomosis and reservoir
1 fatal pulmonary embolus
1 deep venous thrombosis
1 acute unilateral pyelonephritis
1 casual ablation of ureteral catheters on the second post-operative day with subsequent paralitic
  ileus and evisceratio
3 pelvic hematoma (1 required surgery)

Table 2: *Late complications of VIP.*

18 stenoses in the ileo-urethral anastomosis (13.6%)
21 stenoses in the uretero-ileal anastomosis (15.9%)
 3 urethral strictures (2.4%)
11 laparoceles (8.3%)
 2 posterior "ileocele"
 2 reservoir stones
 1 renoureteral litiasis

As to the 18 stenoses in the ileo-urethral anastomosis, the diagnosis was made 3−31 months after surgery, with a mean latency of 12 months. All were treated by endoscopic incision: 16 with very good results. In 1 case the incision was repeated twice and the patient later died of pelvic recurrence. In 1 case the stenosis was treated successfully by endoscopic resection. This kind of complication was progressively reduced, probably due to the introduction of the mucosal eversion in the anastomotic hole.

The 21 uretero-ileal stenoses occurred after a mean interval of 15 months (with a minimum of 2 and a maximum of 42 months). 17 stenoses were unilateral (7 right, 10 left, 1 single right kidney), 4 were bilateral.

Treatment required conversion to a Bricker in 1 patient, with a right single kidney, in whom the situation had not been revealed until a severe renal failure. Taking down the reservoir and tapering it to form a ileal conduit with redoing of the uretero-ileal anastomosis was easily achieved.

In 7 patients the anastomosis was surgically redone, in one of them with a simultaneous nephroureterectomy for secondary upper tract transitional cancer. 2 patients with atrophic kidneys were submitted to nephroureterectomy.

Eleven patients were submitted to endourological treatment by means of nephrostomy, antegrade catheterization and dilation or incision, followed by stenting for 30—40 days. Short-term results were good. In our experience reflux was rare: 8 patients showed 2nd degree unilateral persistent reflux.

Complications at uretero-ileal anastomosis were frequent in patients with pre-operative dilated ureters: out of 12 patients with dilated ureters, 3 patients developed stenosis and 2 reflux.

The absence of episodes of acute pyelonephritis following orthotopic ileal reservoir must be outlined.

Clinically relevant metabolic or intestinal disturbances have not occurred. No patient needed bicarbonate or B12 supplementation.

Day-time and night-time continence

Complete day-time continence (no protection) was achieved in more than 90% of our patients (Table 3).

Night-time continence (dry sleep for 6—7 hours or 1 spontaneous awakening due to voiding desire) was observed in around 75% of our patients after a 4-year follow-up (Table 4).

Table 3: *Complete day-time continence.*

84% at 6 months	(89 evaluable patients)
91% at 1 year	(77 evaluable patients)
91% at 2 years	(61 evaluable patients)
98% at 3 years	(42 evaluable patients)
98% at 4 years	(30 evaluable patients)
100% at 5 years	(19 evaluable patients)

Table 4: *Complete night-time continence.*

65% at 6 months	(89 evaluable patients)
77% at 1 year	(77 evaluable patients)
79% at 2 years	(61 evaluable patients)
74% at 3 years	(42 evaluable patients)
79% at 4 years	(30 evaluable patients)
88% at 5 years	(19 evaluable patients)

Nocturnal continence/incontinence is a complex phenomenon, due to the balance of several variables: residual urethral resistances during sleep, reservoir capacity, nocturnal diuresis, contractile activity of the reservoir, capacity of feeling and recognizing the voiding desire, complete reservoir emptying.

Urodynamic features

Mean VIP-manometric capacity was constantly around 400 ml during actuarial follow-up, with a maximal capacity of 650 ml. VIP pressures at capacity showed similarly constant behaviour during follow-up, averaging 17 cm H_2O with peaks of 35–40 cm H_2O. In our series, 32.7% (52/159) of the patients showed pressure waves at manometry during reservoir filling, with a mean width of 39 cm H_2O (min/max: 15–70) and a mean threshold volume of 226 ml (min/max: 42/400); 37 patients out of 159 (23%) showed voiding problems with a mean post-micturition residual of 151 ml (min/max: 20–600). These situations were difficult to categorize and varied from patient to patient. Altered abdominal straining or perineal relaxation were often present. Some patients showed a dramatic improvement by means of reeducation of abdominal contraction and voluntary perineal relaxation. In these patients with chronic urinary retention, reservoir overdistension or rupture has not been observed so far. Two patients eventually required clean intermittent self-catheterization.

Sexual activity

Sexual activity was evaluated in 95 patients interested for age and psychology to the issue. 23 patients referred spontaneous erections which were sufficient for penetration, but only in 3 of them were the erections normal. 34 patients had a PGE_1 test, which resulted to be positive in 27. Only 9 patients adopted a regimen of self-administration: 7 were satisfied, 2 later opted for hydraulic penile prosthesis.

Conclusions

VIP offers a simple and easy to perform surgical technique, which does not require a long learning curve for the urologist who is used to performing radical prostatectomy, ileal conduit and antireflux surgery. The morbility is low. VIP obtains a good capacity, low-pressure, non-refluxing reservoir employing a 40 cm ileal segment. Clinical and urodynamic results are comparable to those of the best reservoirs available at present. The main advantage offered by VIP seems to be its simplicity and straightforwardness.

References

1. Artibani, W., V. Pegoraro, S. Guazzieri et al.: Presupposti di fisiopatologia all'ampliamento e alla sostituzione vesicale con intestinto. Atti 59° Congresso della Società Italiana di Urologia, pp. 95 ff. Milano 1966.

2. Bramble, F. G.: The treatment of adult enuresis and urge incontinence by enterocystoplasty. Br. J. Urol. 54 (1982) 693–696.

3. Camey, M., F. Richard, H. Botto: Bladder replacement by ileocystoplasty. In: L. R. King, A. R. Stone, G. D. Webster: Bladder reconstruction and continent urinary diversion, pp. 336–359. Year Book Medical Publishers, Chicago 1987.

4. Ekman, H., B. Jacobsson, N. Kock et al.: The functional behaviour of different types of intestinal urinary bladder substitutes. In: Proceedings of the XIII Congrès de la Société Internationale d'Urologie, Vol II, Discussions and free communications, p. 213. E & S Livingstone, London 1965.

5. Hautmann, R. E., G. Egghart, D. Frohneberg et al.: The ileal neobladder. J. Urol. 139 (1988) 39–42.

6. Hinman, F., Jr.: Selection of intestinal segments for bladder substitution: physical and physiological characteristics. J. Urol. 139 (1988) 519–523.

7. Le Duc, A., M. Camey: Un procédé d'implantation urétéro-ileale anti-reflux dans l'enterocystoplatie. J. d'Urol. 85 (1979) 449.

8. Lilien, O. M., M. Camey: A 25-year experience with replacement of the human bladder (Camey procedure). J. Urol. 132 (1984) 886–891.

9. Kock, N. G., A. E. Nilson, L. O. Nilsson et al.: Urinary diversion in a continent ileal reservoir: clinical results in 12 patients. J. Urol. 128 (1982) 469–475.

10. Kock, N. G.: The development of the continent ileal reservoir (Kock pouch) and application in patients requiring urinary diversion. In: R. L. King, A. R. Stone, G. D. Webster: Bladder reconstruction and continent urinary diversion, pp. 269–289. Year Book Medical Publishers, Chicago 1987.

11. Pagano, F., W. Artibani, P. Ligato et al.: Vescica Ileale Padovana: A technique for complete bladder replacement. Eur. Urol. 17 (1990) 149–154.

12. Pagano, F., W. Artibani: Kontinente ileumblase: Vesica Ileale Padovana (V.I.P.). Aktuelle Urologie 22 (1991) I–VI.

13. Studer, U. E., D. Ackermann, G. A. Casanova et al.: Three years experience with an ileal low pressure bladder substitute. Br. J. Urol. 63 (1989) 43–52.

14. Thuroff, J. W., P. Alken, H. Riedmiller et al.: The MAINZ pouch (Mixed Augmentation Ileum and Zecum) for bladder augmentation and continent diversion. J. Urol. 136 (1986) 17–26.

15. Thuroff, J. W., P. Alken, H. Riedmiller et al.: 100 cases of Mainz pouch: continuing experience and evolution. J. Urol. 140 (1988) 283.

16. Walsh, P. C.: Radical retropubic prostatectomy. In: P. C. Walsh, R. F. Gittes, A. D. Perlmutter et al.: Campbell's Urology, 5th ed., vol. 3, pp. 2769–1772. Saunders, Philadelphia 1986.

Metabolic and colonic mucosal abnormalities following urinary-intestinal diversion

R. Caprilli, G. Latella, G. Frieri, A. Marcheggiano

Introduction

Bowel is commonly used in urological surgery for creation of continent urinary diversions. A variety of operative procedures have been developed including the ureterosigmoidostomy, the ileal or colonic conduit and the neo-bladder that empties via the anus (neorectal bladder) or via the urethra (ileal or colonic orthotopic bladder) or that acts as a continent reservoir that drains through a catheterizable stoma (continent ileal or colonic pouches) [2, 4, 16, 33, 36, 41, 42, 47, 48, 55]. With improvement of the new reconstructive techniques the use of the intestinal orthotopic bladder has increased in children with bladder extrophy as well as in older patients submitted to cystectomy for cancer [16, 55].

The goals in bladder reconstruction are to reduce the length of the segments of bowel employed, to protect the upper urinary tract from urinary reflux, to reinstate continence with expulsion of urine under voluntary control, and to avoid both the metabolic complications and the increased risk of local cancer observed following the traditional urinary diversions [31, 39].

Metabolic abnormalities

The intestine does not act as an inert conduit or storage vehicle for urine, but it is actively involved in the pathogenesis of the metabolic complications which may occur in the short and long term. These complications include systemic electrolytes and acid-base disorders, hepatic metabolism alterations, drug metabolism abnormalities, nutritional disturbances, calculus formation, bone mineralization defects (osteomalacia), growth retardation etc. Many of these metabolic complications are influenced by the type of bowel segment employed (stomach, small bowel, colorectum) and by the degree to which absorption of urinary solutes occurs across the bowel segment [24, 25, 26, 31, 39]. The factors that influence solute absorption include the segment and the surface area of the bowel used, time of urine retention, concentration of solutes in the urine, pH and osmolality of urine, renal function and the duration the intestinal segment has been in the urinary tract. It has been suggested that the activity of mucosal transport processes decreases with time.

When the stomach is used either to augment the bladder or to construct an orthotopic bladder hypokalemia, hypochloremic metabolic alkalosis and dysuria occur [1, 24, 31, 32]. Hypochloremic metabolic alkalosis develops only in patients with impaired renal function. In this condition the secretion of hydrogen ion by the stomach segment occurs in parallel with bicarbonate release into the circulation which the kidney is not able to remove. The severe acidity of urine (aciduria) which may induce a marked dysuria becomes a limiting factor in the use of pure gastric reservoirs. Hypochloremic metabolic alkalosis and dysuria may improve with the administration of H2 receptor antagonists (ranitidine) or proton pump inhibitors (omeprazole) by reducing hydrogen ion secretion by the stomach segment. In composite gastroileal storage systems there is a tendency for electrolytic neutrality; the stomach and ileum compensate their absorptive and secretory properties, and clinically significant changes in serum or urinary pH do not occur [31, 32].

The electrolyte disorders that occur when jejunum is used include hyponatremia, hypochloremia, hyperkalemia, and acidosis. These alterations have been observed in about one third of patients [23]. They develop as a consequence of an increased secretion of sodium and chloride and an enhanced reabsorption of potassium and hydrogen by the jejunal segment. The loss of large amounts of sodium and chloride determine a loss of a large volume of water which may induce severe dehydration and increase of serum nitrogen. The treatment of such disorders is the intravenous infusion of solution containing sodium chloride and sodium bicarbonate. As long-term therapy oral supplement with sodium chloride is recommended.

The electrolyte abnormalities more commonly observed after ileum or colon urinary diversion are hyperchloremia and metabolic acidosis [3, 8, 13, 25, 39]. The incidence of such alterations is very high in patients with ureterosigmoidostomy (up to 80%), whereas in the other types of urinary diversion using either ileum or colon segment the incidence ranges from 10% to 70%. It is assumed that the occurrence and the degree of acidosis are related directly to the surface area of bowel exposed to the urine and the duration of the contact exposition. This may account for the high incidence of metabolic abnormalities in patients with ureterosigmoidostomy in which the entire colon is exposed to urine and the urine is retained for prolonged periods. For the same length of bowel segment employed, both incidence and severity of acidosis are higher in ileal than colonic urinary diversion [25]. This may be explained by a recent experimental study showing that colonic segments absorb less acid and secrete less alkali than ileal segments when electrolyte transport is examined as a function of bowel surface area by urine [27].

Numerous studies have been conducted to elucidate the pathophysiology of hyperchloremic metabolic acidosis and most have demonstrated that it is mainly

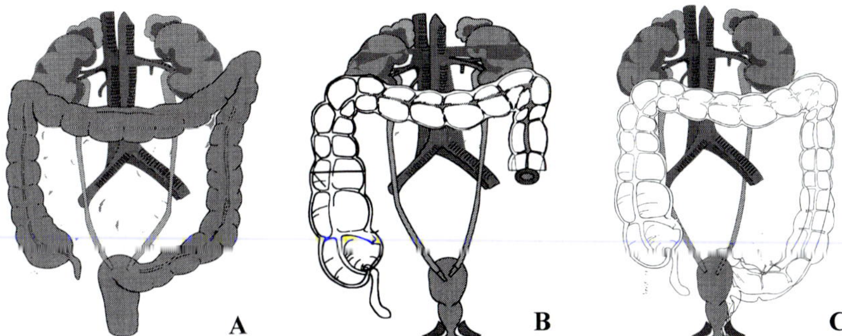

Fig. 1: *Representation of the 3 different types of colonic urinary diversion studied: A = USS; B = RSB according to Mauclaire tecnique, C = RSB according to Boyer-Movelacque tecnique.*

Table 1: *Systemic metabolic alterations in urinary diversion.*

Systemic alterations	RSB	p	USS
Metabolic acidosis	86%		80%
blood pH	7.34 ($\pm$ 0.04)	0.01	7.29 ($\pm$ 0.07)
HCO3 (mEq/l)	18.91 ($\pm$ 1.50)	0.005	15.77 ($\pm$ 3.93)
Hyperchloremia	27%		20%
Cl (mEq/l)	111.7 ($\pm$ 2.3)	ns	113.3 ($\pm$ 3.2)
Increased anion gap	50%		70%
anion gap (mEq/l)	21.2 ($\pm$ 3.2)	ns	23.9 ($\pm$ 5.6)

due to the reabsorption of chloride, ammonia and hydrogen ions and to the secretion of bicarbonate by the intestinal mucosal segment [5, 24, 25, 26, 39].

In previous studies conducted in patients with colonic urinary diversion we found a high incidence of normochloremic metabolic acidosis with increased anion gap [5, 34]. The systemic metabolic consequences were investigated in patients with ureterosigmoidostomy (USS) and rectosigmoid bladder (RSB) performed either according to Mauclaire or Heitz–Boyer–Movelacque [4] (Fig. 1). Two series of patients have been studied prospectively: 45 adult patients submitted to cystectomy for cancer (25 USS, 22 RSB) and 10 children affected by bladder extrophy (2 USS, 8 RSB).

Acid-base balance, serum electrolytes, renal function, analysis of urine from RSB and urine-feces mixture (UFM) from USS were evaluated.

In the group of *adult patients* metabolic acidosis occurred in 86% of RSB and in 80% of USS, but it was significantly (p < 0.01) less severe in patients with RSB (pH 7.34 $\pm$ 0.04) than in those with USS (pH 7.29 $\pm$ 0.07) (Table 1). This finding corresponded to a significantly lower intestinal loss of HCO_3- in the

RSB than in the USS. The frequency of hyperchloremia was very low both in RSB and USS (27% and 20% respectively), whereas the incidence of an increased anion gap was surprisingly high (50% and 68% respectively).

In the group of *young patients* metabolic acidosis was observed in 60%, while an increase in the anion gap was present in only 30%. The less frequent increase in the anion gap encountered in this group may be due to the relatively preserved renal function of the young patients.

The pathogenesis of metabolic acidosis of colonic urinary diversion is not yet completely clear. One of the proposed mechanisms is considered to be the increased intestinal loss of bicarbonate. In normal subjects the overall daily loss of bicarbonate in the feces and urine is about 6 mEq, while in patients with USS and RSB it increases eight and three folds respectively [5, 6, 34]. These results may account for the high incidence of metabolic acidosis observed in both groups of patients studied, and at the same time explain why in patients with RSB the metabolic change is less severe and often clinically silent. Considering that the time interval the urine or the urine-feces mixture stayed in the colon was comparable, the lower intestinal loss of bicarbonate observed in the RSB group is probably due to the smaller area of intestinal mucosa exposed to hydroelectrolytic exchanges. This may also account for the increased concentration of sodium and chloride found in urine of RSB (Table 2).

Table 2: *Composition of urine (RSB) and urine/faeces mixture (USS).*

	RSB	p	USS
pH	6.87 ($\pm$ 0.4)	0.001	7.85 ($\pm$ 0.7)
HCO3 (mEq/l)	11.2 ($\pm$ 8.0)	0.001	24.4 ($\pm$ 15.2)
Na (mEq/l)	88.6 ($\pm$ 32.1)	0.001	47.5 ($\pm$ 25.2)
Cl (mEq/l)	93.6 ($\pm$ 33.0)	0.001	61.6 ($\pm$ 26.2)
K (mEq/l)	29.5 ($\pm$ 12.6)	ns	23.8 ($\pm$ 8.0)

It would appear, therefore, that even 30 cm of large bowel used in the surgical construction of the new reservoir result in such a high ion exchange that systemic metabolic changes occur.

Metabolic acidosis in USS is generally considered to be of the hyperchloremic type and to have a normal anion gap [3, 13]. In our series of patients, however, hyperchloremia was present in less than a third of cases, whereas the anion gap was increased in more than 50% of cases. It has been suggested that hyperchloremia may be due to enhanced colonic reabsorption of chloride, which is related in part to anionic exchange with the secretion of bicarbonate, in part to active sodium absorption [12, 37]. The enhanced anionic Cl/HCO_3 exchange may explain the metabolic acidosis but does not explain the hyperchloremia and especially why this finding is present only in some patients. If the pathogenesis of hyperchloremia would result from this mechanism, hyperchloremia and the base deficit should always be associated. This was not the case in our series of patients. On the other hand, it is known that only 25% of intestinal absorption of chloride occurs through Cl/HCO_3 exchange, with the remainder diffusing passively via intercellular pathways down the electrochemical gradient generated by electrogenetic Na absorption [12]. Despite the continuous reabsorption of chloride, chloremia was normal in most of our patients with internal urinary diversion (IUD), thus indicating that the enhanced intestinal absorption of chloride was balanced by the increased renal excretion of this ion. It is possible that hyperchloremia, when present, is produced on the basis of the law of electroneutrality in order to balance the reduction in plasma bicarbonate. When chloremia was normal, the balance was maintained through the increase of the anion gap [45]. The increased anion gap found in our patients may result from the increase in unmeasured anions, i. e. inorganic acids such as phosphates and sulphates, probably due to defective renal excretion of these ions [5, 34]. These inorganic acids are in part buffered by the bicarbonate system, in part metabolized and excreted by the kidney. In urinary diversion both these mechanisms are deficient and contribute to the increase of the anion gap. In fact a low serum bicarbonate was present in more than 80% and an impaired renal function in about 50% of patients [5, 34]. In the series of our young patients with IUD the increase in the anion gap was encountered less frequently, compared with what was found in adult IUD patients [34]. This may be due to the preserved renal function shown by these young patients. Thus the commonly accepted theory that USS leads to hyperchloremic acidosis and a normal anion gap should be reconsidered. The metabolic disturbance in USS and RSB is more frequently normochloremic with an increased anion gap. These studies demonstrate that metabolic acidosis develops even after RSB surgery, thus indicating that the reduction in the area of the colonic mucosa in contact with urine is not itself sufficient to prevent the metabolic changes. In addition, no correlation between the severity of metabolic changes and the time interval elapsing from surgery has been observed.

Beside hyperchloremia other electrolyte disorders may occur when ileum or colon are used including hypokalemia, hypocalcemia, hypomagnesemia and hyperammonemia.

Hypokalemia and total body depletion of potassium are more frequent in ureterocolonic diversion (about 30%) than ileal conduit (about 15%) [14, 59]. This difference may be due to the fact that ileal segment when exposed to the high potassium concentrations of urine reabsorb part of the potassium, whereas the colon is less able to do so [27]. In our series of patients with ureterocolic diversions hypokalemia was found in only a few cases (11% of USS and 6% of RSB)

[5]. It is of clinical relevance to remember that if hypokalemia is associated with severe acidosis, the treatment of the latter must be associated always with potassium replacement. Correction of acidosis without replacement of potassium may further aggravate hypokalemia with the consequence of flaccid paralysis.

Hypocalcemia and hypomagnesemia are infrequent, but when they occur they may be responsible for severe neuromuscular dysfunction. Hypocalcemia may occur as a consequence of excessive renal loss and its depletion of body storage. The systemic acidosis increases calcium depletion probably by decreasing renal tubule calcium reabsorption [30]. Metabolic acidosis may alter calcium balance by impairing vitamin D metabolism [29]. Altered sulphate and phosphate metabolism present in urinary diversion also results in renal loss of calcium. An increased and prolonged calciuria may lead to bone demineralization (osteomalacia in adults, rickets in children) [18, 40, 51]. In addition, the increased urinary excretion of calcium increases also the incidence of urinary tract calculi, especially in patients with ileal urinary diversion.

Hypomagnesemia is almost always associated with hypocalcemia because magnesium shares many of the calcium transport processes at the level of renal tubules. Acidosis and altered metabolism of calcium and sulphate impair renal magnesium reabsorption.

Hyperammonemia or even a hyperammonemic encephalopathy condition have frequently been reported in patients with intestinal urinary diversion, and particularly in those with ureterosigmoidostomy [21, 22, 38]. In the urinary diversion there is an increased absorption of ammonia by intestinal segment due mainly to the increased load of ammonia from the urine. Ammonia is generated in large amount by renal tubules and then excreted with the urine. In addition, ammonia may also be produced from urea by urease of intestinal bacteria, especially in presence of an intraluminal alkaline pH. Therefore in urinary diversion the liver is exposed to an increased load of ammonia which is cleared by the activation of the high functional reserve of liver ornithine cycle, producing urea. In normal conditions, one observes only a slight elevation of ammonia serum levels, whereas if liver dysfunction or chronic disease coexist, severe hyperammonemia, encephalopathy or coma occur. The risk of hyperammonemic encephalopathy is increased by ureasic bacteria infections which are frequent when obstruction of urinary tract develops.

In conclusion, the metabolic alterations of intestinal urinary diversion involve a complex omeostatic mechanism in which the intestine, the kidney, the liver and the lung interact (Fig. 2).

Large amounts of ammonia and chloride arrive into the intestinal segment with the urine. Chloride is avidly reabsorbed by intestinal mucosa, in part in ex-

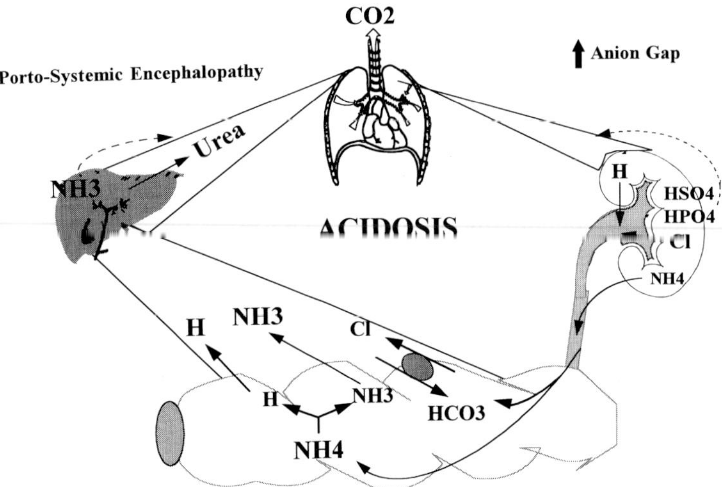

Fig. 2: *Schematic representation of omeostatic mechanism involved in metabolic alterations following intestinal urinary diversion. For details see the text.*

change for bicarbonate, leading to iperchloremia and alkali defect, that is to say metabolic acidosis. Ammonia is reabsorbed too, contributing to metabolic acidosis and accumulating into the blood. In conditions of liver failure it may induce hyperammonemic encephalopathy. The renal function is of great importance in the homeostatic response. If the renal function is normal, the kidney is able to increase the excretion of hydrogen ions, chloride and ammonia and then compensate the excess of acid. When these mechanisms are impaired acidosis develops and anion gap is increased for the accumulation of sulphate and phosphate produced by catabolism of proteins. In our series of patients renal function was impaired in about 50% of the cases. A normal lung function in part compensates metabolic acidosis eliminating CO_2, otherwise contributing to aggravate it.

Since systemic metabolic changes are also present in asymptomatic patients, it is obvious that they require a regular follow-up. Continuous clinical surveillance, periodic assessment of renal function, serum electrolytes, acid-base balance and anion gap, and continuous treatment with oral bicarbonate or citrate are necessary.

Risk of local cancer

Urinary diversion is associated with an increased risk of local carcinoma. The risk has been assessed with particular reference to ureterosigmoidostomy, but there is growing evidence that other types of intestinal urinary diversion (colon conduit, ileal conduit, bladder augmentation cistoplasty, rectal bladder) should also be regarded as pre-neoplastic conditions [19, 35, 39, 43, 49, 52, 53, 54, 60]. In patients who have undergone USS the risk is increased by as much as 500 fold, compared with the general population, and it is even higher in young adults. The latency period is 3 to 50 years, with a mean of 20 to 25 years for young patients, but the period is shorter for older patients in whom the diversion has been performed for malignant conditions. The most frequent type of tumor is adenocarcinoma (85% of all cases). Transitional cell carcinoma account for 10% and other histological types for the remaining 5%.

A cause and effect relationship undoubtedly exists between urinary diversion and the subsequent development of neoplasia of the ureterocolic junction. Many theories have been put forward to explain this phenomenon but none seems to be satisfactory. It is unlikely to be attributable to a single factor but it may represent the sum of several factors, the relative importance of each being difficult to assess. Factors claimed to be significant in the induction of neoplasia include the irritative effect of urine, the high concentration of electrolytes, the glandular metaplasia of the ureteric stump, the chronic inflammation and atrophy of colonic mucosa adjacent to the ureteric implant sites, an increased activity of ornithine decarboxylase in colonic mucosa, the production of N-nitrosamine [9, 10, 15, 20, 34, 44, 52, 58]. In experimental conditions it has been reported that the highest incidence of carcinoma occurs when urethelium is juxtaposed to the colonic epithelium and both are bathed by the mixture of urine and feces [11, 50]. It has been therefore hypothesized that in USS the local activation of fecal carcinogens by the diverted urine, or of urine carcinogens by fecal bacteria may be the cause of cancer. However, the development of tumors has also been reported in patients who have undergone diversion surgery that does not result in the mixture of urine with feces, suggesting that in these cases other risk factors are involved [35, 43, 53, 54].

In previous studies we found abnormal patterns of epithelial mucin secretion in both USS and RSB [20, 34]. Morphological, histochemical and lectin binding characteristics of colorectal mucosa were prospectively investigated on endoscopy biopsy specimens obtained from both adult patients submitted to cistectomy for cancer (12 USS, 14 RSB) and young patients effected by bladder extrophy (2 USS, 8 RSB). Twenty biopsies taken from uninvolved transitional mucosa adjacent to colorectal carcinomas in 10 patients and 20 normal rectal biopsies from 10 patients with hemorrhoids, were used as controls. Serial biopsy sections were stained with hematoxyline eosin for routine histologic examination. For histochemical studies the high iron diamine-alcian blue method at a pH of 2.5 was used. FITC-conjugated Dolichos biflorus agglutinin (DBA) and Arachis hypogaea agglutinin (PNA) were used for the study of lectin binding characteristics. Mild chronic inflammation and changes in the mucosal architecture with

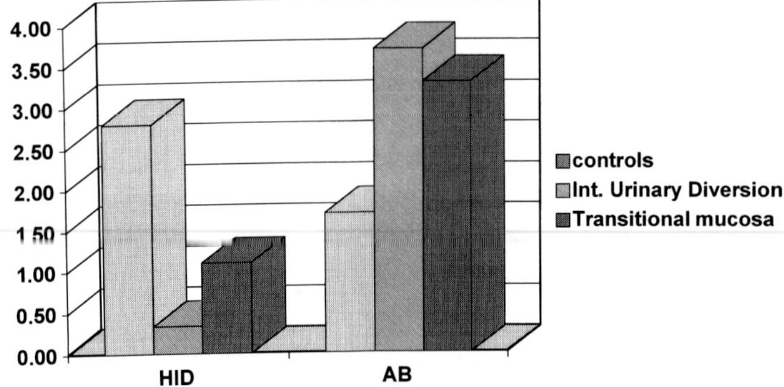

Fig. 3: *Scores for high iron diamine (HID) and alcian blu (AB) positive epithelial cells in colonic crypts assigned according to the following semiquantitative evaluation: 0 = no positive cells; 1 = one third of cells positive; 2 = one half of cells positive; 3 = two thirds of cells positive; and 4 = all cells positive.*

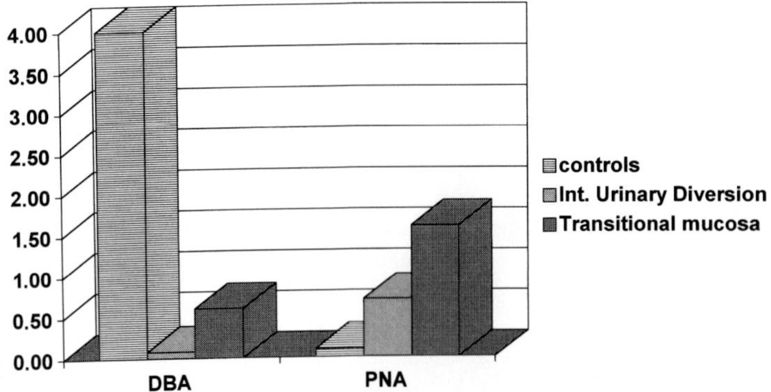

Fig. 4: *Scores for FITC-DBA and FITC-PNA positive epithelial cells in the colonic crypts assigned according to the following semiquantitative evaluation: 0 = no positive cells; 1 = one third of cells positive; 2 = one half of cells positive; 3 = two thirds of cells positive; and 4 = all cells positive.*

crypt distortion were observed in the majority of biopsy specimens taken from patients with RSB. Histochemical and/or lectin binding changes were found in the majority of patients of both groups (USS and RSB) and were identical to those observed in premalignant and malignant condition of the colon. The changes were characterized by an increase in the number of sialomucin-containing goblet cells, the dramatic decrease in DBA labeling and the appearance of substantial number of PNA labeled goblet cells (Fig. 3, 4, 5). An interesting finding is the persistence of the changes in the rectal mucosa of young patients with urinary diversion after 3 years.

Factors responsible for morphological and mucin secretion abnormalities of colorectal mucosa found in our series of patients with IUD are unknown. Some

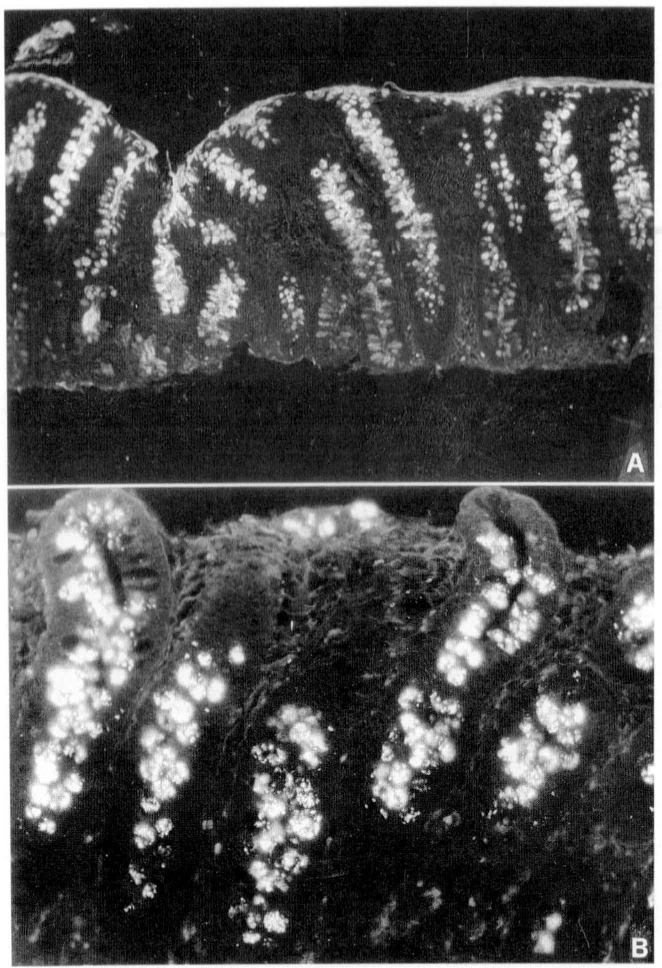

Fig. 5: *Rectal mucosa from a normal subject showing intense labelling of goblet cells in the upper two thirds of the crypts. (Fluorescein-conjugated Dolichos biflorus agglutinin; × 100) (A). Biopsy specimen from a patient who underwent rectal bladder surgery showing PNA labelling of several goblet cells in each crypt. (Fluorescein-conjugated Arachis hypogaea agglutinin; × 250) (B).*

roles may be played by intraluminal short chain fatty acids (SCFA) and pH. SCFA, end products of intestinal bacteria fermentation, represent the main energetic fuel of colorectal epithelium. The colonocyte functions dependent on SCFA metabolism include cell respiration, cell turnover, ionic exchanges and enzymatic activities. SCFA act also as substrates for gluconeogenesis, lipogenesis, protein synthesis and mucin production. It is worthwhile to note that among SCFA, butyrate is responsible for regulatory mechanisms of gene expression, cell proliferation and differentiation [7, 28]. Butyrate experimentally shows an antitumorigenic effect being able to reverse the transformed characteristics of cells to normal morphological and biochemical pattern, reducing proliferation and increasing cellular differentiation. In urine of RSB we found the absence of SCFA. The mucosal chronic inflammation observed in RSB may be due to the lack of intraluminal SCFA as it occurs in diversion colitis. In this condition the mucosal lesions represent the expression of an extreme form of nutritional deficit of the colonic mucosa since restoration of fecal transit or irrigation with SCFA of the excluded colon will bring on a complete histological regression of the mucosal lesions [17]. In RSB the longstanding SCFA deficit could not only reduce the colonocyte metabolism therefore altering the epithelial barrier, but could also intervene to increase the risk of local cancer by eliminating the protective antineoplastic action of butyrate on the mucosa.

In patients with USS we did not find any mucosal inflammation, probably because, although the SCFA were present in the urine-feces mixture, their levels were significantly lower in comparison to the normal values. The reduction of SCFA concentration in urine-feces mixture may result from urine dilution or from the reduced production by bacteria. The latter condition may be induced by the intraluminal alkaline pH. The intraluminal alkaline environment present in USS may play an important role for the increased risk of cancer of these patients [56]. This hypothesis seems to be supported by several observations. Patients with colorectal neoplasia present an alkaline fecal pH [46, 57]. Among SCFA the high pH mainly reduce butyrate, which has antineoplastic properties. The intraluminal pH between 7 and 8, as found in MUF of USS, is the optimum for degradation by 7-alpha-dehydroxylase of primary into secondary bile acids, which have been involved in the genesis of colorectal cancer. An alkaline pH shifts the reaction $NH_3 \leftrightarrow NH_4$ to the left, resulting in an excess of NH_3, a potentially cocarcinogen metabolite. Finally, the high pH promotes the production of carcinogenetic nitrose compounds.

In conclusion, our data confirm that endoscopic and histologic follow-up may be of great value in assessing the neoplastic risk in urinary diversions, especially in young patients with long life expectancy. It is also important to stress that all the patients candidate for urinary diversion operation, particularly those operated for malignant conditions, should be submitted to a preliminary colonoscopy to rule out the presence or colorectal mucosa abnormalities.

References

1. Adams, M. C., M. E. Mitchell, R. C. Rink: Gastrocystoplasty: an alternative solution to the problem of urological reconstruction in the severely compromised patient. J. Urology 140 (1988) 1152.

2. Bennet, A. H.: Extrophy of bladder treated by ureterosigmoidostomies: long term evaluation. Urology 2 (1973) 165−168.
3. Boyd, S. D., W. M. Schiff, D. G. Skinner et al.: Prospective study of metabolic abnormalities in patients with continent Kock pouch urinary diversion. Urology 33 (1989) 85.
4. Bracci, U.: Rectal bladder. In: G. Mayor, E. Zingg (Eds.): Urologic surgery, diagnosis, techniques and postoperative treatment, pp. 556−585. George Thieme, Stuttgart 1976.
5. Caprilli, R., G. Frieri, G. Latella et al.: Electrolyte and acid base imbalance in patients with rectosigmoid bladder. J. Urology 135 (1986) 148−150.
6. Caprilli, R., G. Frieri, G. Latella et al.: Faecal excretion of bicarbonate in ulcerative colitis. Digestion 35 (1986) 136−142.
7. Caprilli, R., G. Latella: Colonocyte metabolism and colorectal cancer. In: F. P. Rossini, S. J. Lynch, S. J. Winawer (Eds.): Recent Progress in Colorectal Cancer: Biology and Management of high risk groups, pp. 115−118. Excerpta Medica, Amsterdam−London−New York−Tokyo 1991.
8. Castro, J. E., M. D. Ram: Electrolyte imbalance following ileal urinary diversion. Br. J. Urol. 42 (1970) 29.
9. Chiarelli, S. M., F. Sandei: Polyps at the site of ureterosigmoidostomy. Tumori 70 (1984) 209−215.
10. Cohen, M. S., M. E. Hilz, C. P. Davis et al.: Urinary carcinogen (nitrosamine) production in a rat animal model for ureterosigmoidostomy. J. Urol. 138 (1987) 449.
11. Daher, N., R. Gautier, H. Abourachidet et al.: Rat colonic carcinogenesis after ureterosigmoidostomy. Pathogenesis and immunohistological study. J. Urology 139 (1988) 1331−1336.
12. Davis, G. R., S. G. Morawski, C. A. Santa Ana et al.: Evaluation of chloride bicarbonate exchange in the human colon in vivo. J. Clin. Invest. 71 (1983) 201−207.
13. Ferris, D. O., H. M. Odel: Electrolyte pattern of the blood after bilateral ureterosigmoidostomy. JAMA 142 (1950) 634.
14. Geist, R. W., J. S. Ansell: Total body potassium after ureteroileostomy. Surg. Gynec. Obstet. 113 (1961) 585.
15. Gilchrist, K. W., D. T. Vehling, J. R. Starling: Cancer surveillance after ureterosigmoidostomy: colonic microscopic changes. J. Surg. Res. 36 (1984) 251.
16. Goldwasser, B.: The colonic orthotopic bladder. Urology 45 (1995) 190−192.
17. Harig, J. M., K. H. Soergel, R. A. Komorowsi et al.: Treatment of diversion colitis with short chain fatty acid irrigation. N. Engl. J. Med. 320 (1989) 23−28.
18. Hossain, M.: The osteomolacia syndrome after colocystoplasty: a cure with sodium bicarbonate alone. Brit. J. Urol. 42 (1970) 243.
19. Husmann, D. A., H. M. Spence: Current status of tumor of the bowel following ureterosigmoidostomy: a review. J. Urol. 144 (1990) 607.
20. Iannoni, C., A. Marcheggiano, F. Pallone et al.: Abnormal patterns of colorectal mucin secretion after urinary diversion of different types: histochemical and lectin binding studies. Hum. Pathol. 17 (1986) 834−840.
21. Kaufman, J. J.: Ammoniagenic coma following ureterosigmoidostomy. J. Urology 131 (1984) 743.
22. Kaveggia, F. F., J. S. Thompson, E. C. Schafer et al.: Hyperammonemic encephalopathy in urinary diversion with urea-splitting urinary tract infection. Arch. Inter. Med. 150 (1990) 2389.
23. Klein, E. A., J. E. Montie, D. K. Montague et al.: Jejunal conduit urinary diversion. J. Urology 135 (1986) 244.
24. Koch, M. O., W. S. McDougal: The pathophysiology of hyperchloremic metabolic acidosis after urinary diversion through intestinal segments. Surgery 98 (1985) 561−570.
25. Koch, M. O., W. S. McDougal, P. K. Reddy et al.: Metabolic alterations following continent urinary diversion through colonic segments. J. Urology 145 (1991) 270−273.

26. Koch, M. O., W. S. McDougal, C. O. Thompson: Mechanisms of solute transport following urinary diversion through intestinal segments: an experimental study with rats. J. Urology 146 (1991) 1390—1394.
27. Koch, M. O., E. Gurevitch, D. E. Hill et al.: Urinary solute transport by intestinal segments: a comparative study of ileum and colon in rats. J. Urol. 143 (1990) 1275.
28. Latella, G., R. Caprilli: Metabolism of large bowel mucosa in health and disease. J. Colorectal Dis. 6 (1991) 127—132.
29. Lee, S. W., J. Russell, L. V. Avioli: 25-Hydroxycholecalciferol to 1,25-dihydroxycholecalciferol: conversion impaired by systemic metabolic acidosis. Science 195 (1977) 994.
30. Lemann, J., J. R. Litzow, E. J. Lennon: Studies of the mechanism by which chronic metabolic acidosis augment urinary calcium excretion in man. J. Clin. Invest. 46 (1987) 1318.
31. Lockhart, J. L., R. Davies, L. Persky et al.: Acid-base changes following urinary tract reconstruction for continent diversion and orthotopic bladder replacement. J. Urol. 152 (1994) 338—342.
32. Lockart, S. L., R. Davies, C. Cox et al.: The gastroileal pouch: an alternative continent urinary reservoir for patients with short bowel, acidosis and/or extensive pelvic radiation. J. Urology 150 (1993) 46.
33. Mahran, M. R., A. M. Ghaly, K. Z. Sheir et al.: The modified rectal bladder (the augmented and valved rectum) for urine diversion in children. Urology 44 (1994) 737—741.
34. Marcheggiano, A., C. Iannoni, G. Latella et al.: Abnormalities of colonic mucin secretion and metabolic changes after internal urinary diversion for bladder extrophy: a prospective study. Br. J. Urol. 67 (1991) 477—482.
35. Marchetti, D. L., M. S. Piver, Y. Tsukada: Adenocarcinoma in an isolated sigmoid urinary conduit. Obstet. Gynecol. 63 (1984) 54S—56S.
36. Marks, S. D., G. D. Webster: Simplified urinary drainage following orthotopic or continent bladder replacement. J. Urology 153 (1995) 334—335.
37. McConnel, J. B., J. Murison, W. K. Stewart: The role of the colon in the pathogenesis of hyperchloremia acidosis in ureterosigmoid anastomosis. Clin. Sci. 57 (1979) 305—312.
38. McDermott, W. V.: Diversion of urine to the intestine as a factor in ammoniagenic coma. N. Engl. J. Med. 250 (1957) 460.
39. McDougal, W. S. et al.: Metabolic complications of urinary intestinal diversion. J. Urol. 147 (1992) 1199—1208.
40. McDougal, W. S., M. O. Koch, C. Shands et al.: Bone demineralization following urinary intestinal diversion. J. Urol. 140 (1988) 853.
41. Mogg, R. A.: Urinary diversion using the colonic conduit. Br. J. Urol. 39 (1967) 687—689.
42. Montie, J. E., J. E. Pontes, B. G. Parulkar et al.: W-stapled ileal neo-bladder formed entirely with absorbable staples. J. Urol. 151 (1994) 1188—1192.
43. Moorcraft, J., C. E. Duboulay, P. Isaacson et al.: Changes in the mucosa of colon conduits with particular reference to the risk of malignant changes. Br. J. Urol. 55 (1983) 185—188.
44. Mostofi, K. K., R. V. Thompson et al.: Mucous adenocarcinoma of the urinary bladder. Cancer 8 (1955) 741—745.
45. Oh, M. S., H. J. Carrol: The anion gap. N. Engl. J. Med. 297 (1977) 814—817.
46. Pietroiusti, A., R. Caprilli, M. Giuliano et al.: Faecal pH in colorectal cancer. It. J. Gastroenterol. 17 (1985) 88—91.
47. Pitts, W. R. Jr., E. C. Muecke: A 20 year experience with ileal conduit: the fate of the kidneys. J. Urol. 122 (1979) 154—157.
48. Rogers, E., P. T. Scardino: A simple ileal substitute bladder after radical cystectomy: experience with a modification of the Studer pouch. J. Urol. 153 (1995) 1432—1438.
49. Schwab, A., P. Merkle, H. Bader: Das Dickdarmcarcinom — eine Spätfolge der Ureterosigmoidastomie. Chirurg. 57 (1986) 394—396.

50. Shands, C., W. S. McDougal, E. P. Wright: Prevention of cancer at the urothelial enteric anastomotic site. J. Urol. 141 (1989) 178.
51. Specht, E. E.: Rickets following ureterosigmoidostomy and chronic hyperchloremia. J. Bone Joint Surg. 49 (1969) 1422.
52. Stewart, M., F. A. Macrae, C. B. Williams: Neoplasia and ureterosigmoidostomy: colonoscopy survey. Br. J. Surg. 69 (1982) 414—416.
53. Stone, A. R., T. P. Stephenson: Tumors associated with lower urinary tract reconstruction using isolated bowel segments. In: L. R. King, A. R. Stone, G. D. Webster (Eds.): Bladder reconstruction and continent urinary diversion, pp. 93—112. Yearbook Medical Publishers, Chicago 1987.
54. Strand, W. R., H. J. Albert: Nefrogenic adenoma occurring in an ileal conduit. J. Urol. 137 (1987) 491—492.
55. Studer, U. E., W. H. Turner: The ileal orthotopic bladder. Urology 45 (1995) 185—189.
56. Thornton, J. R.: High colonic pH promotes colorectal cancer. Lancet I (1981) 1081—1083.
57. Vernia, P., P. Ciarniello, M. Cittadini et al.: Stool pH and SCFA in colorectal cancer and polyps. Gastroenterology 96 (1989) A528.
58. Weber, T. R., S. H. Westfall, G. F. Steinhardt et al.: Malignancy associated with ureterosigmoidostomy: detection by mucosa ornithine decarboxylase. J. Ped. Surg. 23 (1988) 1091.
59. Williams, R. E., T. J. Davenport, L. Burkinshaw et al.: Changes in whole body potassium associated with uretero-intestinal anastomosis. Br. J. Urol. 39 (1967) 676.
60. Zabo, A., R. Kay: Ureterosigmoidostomy and bladder extrophy: a long-term follow-up. J. Urol. 136 (1986) 396.

Digital fluoroangiographic video-urodynamics in the follow-up of the urinary diverted patients

A. Carbone, H. Gezeroglu

Introduction

The ileal conduit has been regarded as the best method for supravesical urinary diversion in cystectomized patients [5]. More recently, however, long term follow-up studies have revealed that impairment of renal function is not infrequent following this procedure [3]. The continent ileostomy was introduced by Kock in 1969 as an alternative to conventional ileostomy [2, 8].

Nowadays bladder replacement is a valuable alternative for continent urinary reconstruction in selected patients after radical cystectomy. Reservoirs for urine are created mostly from ileum, colon or a combination of these two intestinal segments.

The anatomo-physiological characteristics of the normal vesico-sphincteric complex enable to assure some fundamental functions: a reservoir function, an absolute continence during the filling phase without vesico-ureteral reflux and complete and voluntary emptying of the bladder during the voiding phase.

It is evident that when a urinary diversion is planned after cystectomy to guarantee a satisfactory quality of life for the patients, the surgeon should remember the importance of reconstructing a neobladder that satisfies such functions. This goal should be pursued irrespective of the indications for cystectomy, whether oncological or not, unless objective conditions exclude the possibility to carry out a continent diversion.

Moreover, in reconstructing an intestinal diversion the surgeon should make every effort to obtain what is considered the most important anatomical outcome: the spherical shape of the reservoir [1].

In the patients diverted by means of an orthotopic bladder or a continent reservoir, continence will be easily achieved after surgery, but only the orthotopic diverted patient will be able to pass urine spontaneously.

It is not always so easy to reconfigurate the bowel in a spherical shape during the tailoring of the neobladder. Nevertheless, during the neobladder reconstruction every effort has to be made to obtain the essential goal of reservoirs with excellent biomechanical characteristics. The spherical shape of the reservoirs is in fact a basic feature to prevent neovesico-ureteral reflux and to avoid overflow incontinence. This shape, according to Laplace's law, is necessary to assure neobladders characterized by low pressures, low wall tension, high volume and high compliance.

The continent diversions, whether orthotopic or not, represent a valuable reconstructive technique in the patients candidate to radical cystectomy, assuring them an excellent quality of life.

Aim of the study

It is thus necessary to submit the patients to an adequate follow-up in the postoperative period to ascertain that the scheduled goals are reached and that these goals are able to guarantee normal renal and vesical functions and also to assure that the obtained results will be maintained over time. For this reason it is necessary to include, in the follow-up, both morphological and functional evaluations to exclude postoperative complications, such as hydronephrosis and vesico-ureteral reflux, and to control that the biomechanical characteristics of neobladder walls are able to assure an adequate compliance of the neoreservoir.

The authors report their experience in assessing urinary diverted patients by means of digital fluoroangiographic video-urodynamics (DRFVU).

Patients and methods

27 patients diverted by means of continent urinary reservoirs (16 Vescica Ileale Padovena (VIP), 5 Studer ileal bladder, 6 Indiana pouch) underwent video-urodynamic evaluation six months postoperatively. This method fits perfectly the requirements of an accurate follow-up as it enables simultaneous morphological and functional assessment of the reconstructed lower urinary tract. It has, in fact, the advantage of carrying out two different examinations (cystography and cystometry with pressure/volume and pressure/flow studies) at the same time. The video-urodynamic tests were performed by means of a digital fluoroangiographic method (DRFVU) using SIEM urodynamics equipment combined with a General Electric Prestilix DRS digital fluoroangiograph. This instrument is particularly apt for the high definition monitors, the digitalized control in acquiring and storing the radiological images and the opportunity to process the previously stored images.

After flowmetry, the cystometry and the pressure/flow study study were performed with patients in a standing position simultaneously recording bladder, abdominal and detrusorial pressures and perineal EMG, the latter carried out with surface electrodes.

Pressure/volume characteristics of the reservoirs

All the 16 VIP pouches evaluated in our series showed well shaped neobladders (Fig. 1 a−b−c) with a maximum capacity ranging from 410 ml to 560 ml with internal pressures ranging from 16 cm H_2O to 25 cm H_2O at the maximum filling. In 3 patients a vesico-ureteral reflux was observed (2 pts passive complete monolateral and 1 pt passive complete bilateral) (Fig. 2 a−b). The residual urine always ranged from 10 to 70 ml, exceeding 100 ml only in 1 pt.

The 5 Studer neobladders showed a satisfying shape of the reconstructed lower urinary tract with a maximum capacity ranging from 440 ml to 620 ml with internal pressures ranging from 15 cm H_2O to 29 cm H_2O at the maximum filling. All the cases showed ureteral reflux in absence of uninhibited contraction of the neobladder wall and with an optimal neobladder compliance (Fig. 3 a−b).

The Indiana pouches had maximum capacities from 250 to 800 ml with a mean volume of 580 ml. The intraluminal pressures at maximum filling ranged from 15 to 90 cm H_2O with some peristaltic contractile activity. Reflux to the ureters was present in 3 cases.

The ureters reimplantation, in all Indiana pouch and VIP cases, was performed according to Le Duc's technique.

Discussion

A low reservoir pressure is relevant to prevent high resistance to urinary flow, facilitating the inflow of the urine into the reservoir and thus avoiding the possible consequent impairment of the renal function, since long-lasting obstruction to urinary flow leads to renal deterioration. Pyelorenal backflow occurs as a result of an obstruction, sometimes even at a pelvic pressure of approximately 20 cm H_2O. With increasing pressure there is a substantial increase of the backflow [14]. Net glomerular filtration pressure is calculated to 25−30 cm of H_2O and the amplitude of the peristaltic waves in the ureters is normally less than 10 cm H_2O [13].

Considering these figures, long-lasting periods with pressure exceeding 25 cm H_2O in the urinary reservoirs will probably obstruct urine flow and impair the renal function [4].

Moreover a low reservoir pressure is essential also for the preservation of continence both when the reservoir is connected to the urethra and when the reservoir is used for supravesical urinary diversion and is provided with a valve mechanism for incontinence [7].

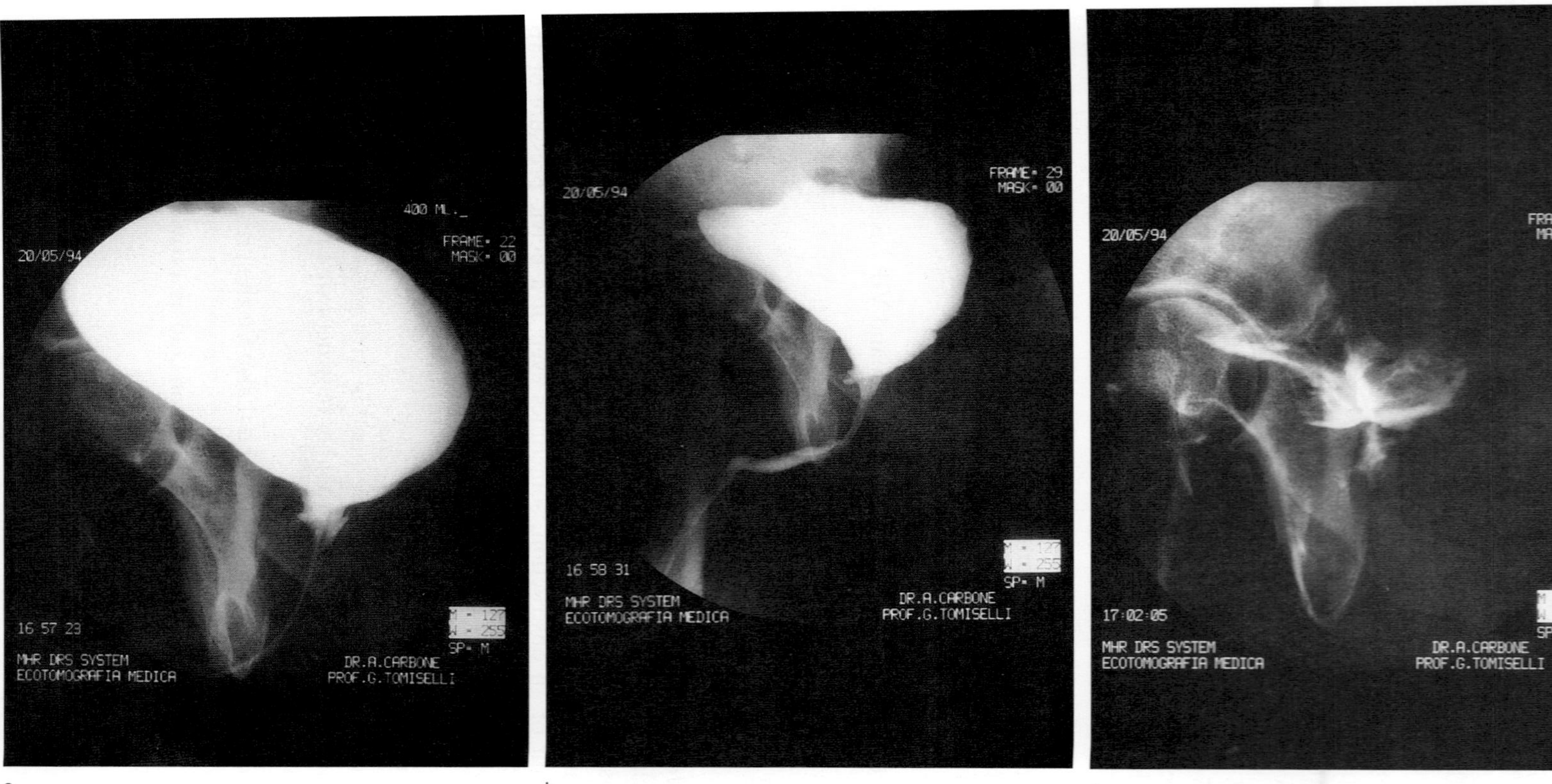

Fig. 1a: *Orthotopic Padovana ileal bladder (VIP) has an excellent spherical shape.*
Fig. 1b: *Micturition phase in a VIP.*
Fig. 1c: *Complete emptying of the neobladder occurs with abdominal strain in VIP.*

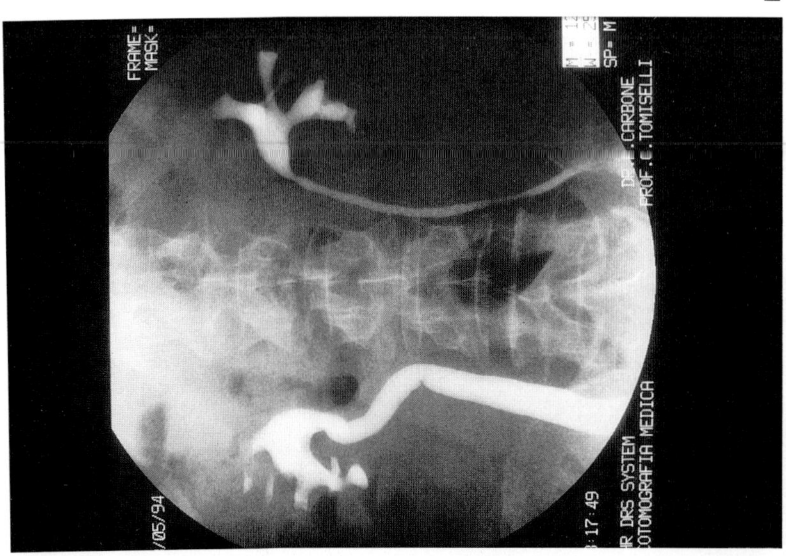

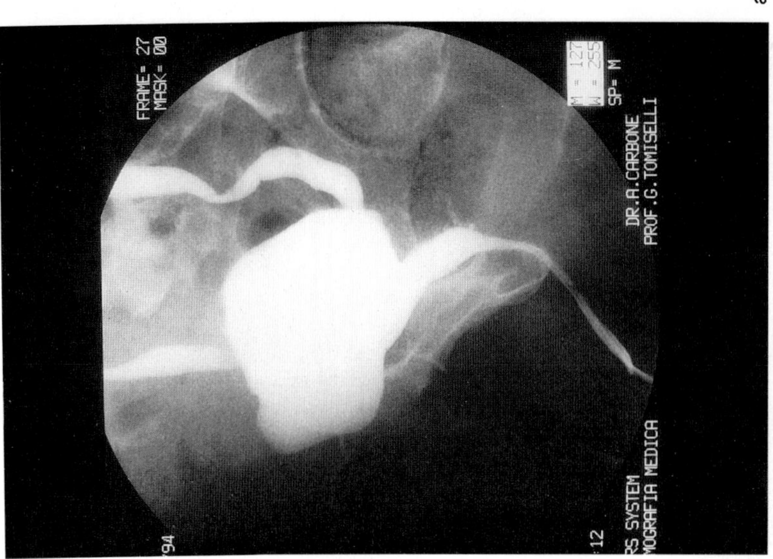

Fig. 2a: *Bilateral active reflux in a VIP.*
Fig. 2b: *The reflux involves all the pyelocaliceal system bilaterally.*

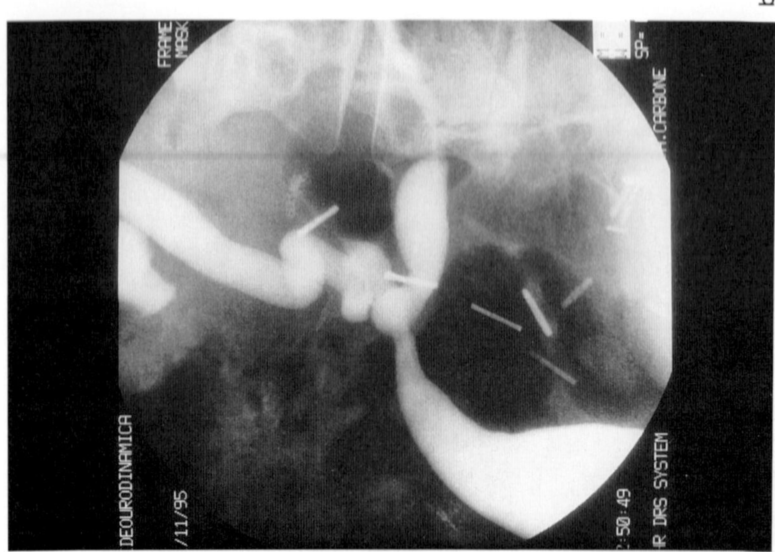

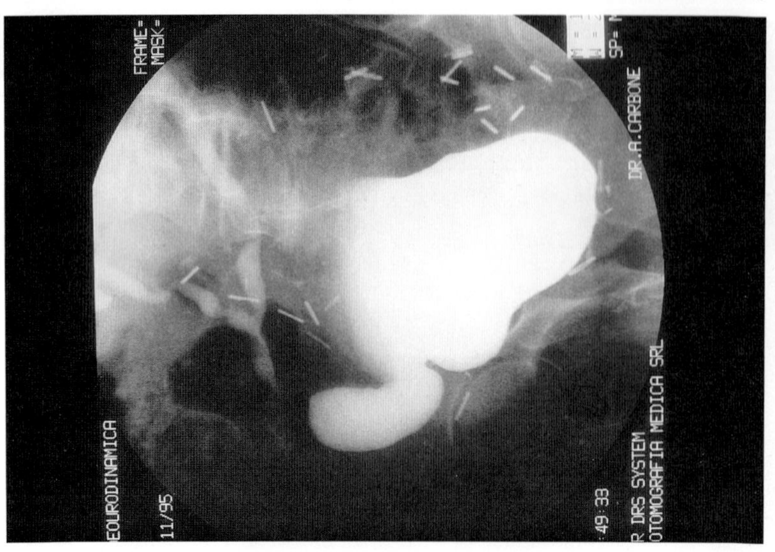

Fig. 3a: *Studer type orthotopic bladder with reflux.*
Fig. 3b: *The massive reflux involving pyelocaliceal system bilaterally in the Studer orthotopic bladder.*

Reflux from the reservoir to the upper urinary system is a relatively frequent event. In most patients the magnitude of the reflux was parallel to the maximal reservoir pressure, while in some patients the reflux was moderate despite high pressure and substantial at low pressure. However, discussing the variability in the quantity of the reflux is beyond the aim of this study.

When in continuity to the urethra, the reservoir pressure should not exceed 50 cm H_2O, which is the approximate resistance of the relaxed membraneous sphincter in the supine position [10].

Conclusions

The reported data indicate how important the use of pressure/flow studies and radiographic techniques is in the follow-up of the urinary diverted patient for monitoring the morpho-functional aspects of the reservoir, which prevents the deterioration of the upper urinary systems.

The DRFVU is a highly sophisticated technique which allows to carry out simultaneously a morphological (cystography) and a functional (cystometry and pressure/flow study) assessment of these patients. The use of a digital fluoroangiograph allows to obtain images of high qualitative value submitting the patient to a low X-ray exposure. Moreover the digital storage of the images enables their re-elaboration at the end of the examination (zoom, substraction of the images) for a more detailed and accurate morphological evaluation. The high imaging quality, executive efficiency and possibility of simultaneous morphological and functional evaluation are further advantages of the use of this method in the follow-up of the urinary diverted patients.

Costs of the equipment represent the major disadvantage, limiting the use of DRFVU to few centres.

References

1. Benson, M. C., C. A. Olsson: Urinary diversion. In: Campbell's Urology, 6th ed., pp. 2654–2716. W. B. Saunders Company, Philadelphia 1992.
2. Berglund, B., N. G. Kock: Volume capacity and pressure characteristics of various types of intestinal reservoivs. World J. Surg. 11 (1987) 798–803.
3. Berglund, B., N. G. Kock, H. E. Myrvold: Volume capacity and pressure characteristics of the continent ileostomy reservoir. Scand. J. Gastroenterol. 19 (1984) 683–690.
4. Berglund, B., N. G. Kock, L. Norlen et al.: Volume and capacity and pressure characteristics of the continent ileal reservoir used for urinary diversion. J. Urol. 137 (1987) 29–34.
5. Bricker, E. M.: Bladder substitution after pelvic evisceration. Surg. Clin. N. Amer. 30 (1950) 1511.

6. Goldwasser, B., W. Mansson, T. Davidson et al.: Cystourethrometric findings in patients with detubularized right colonic segment for bladder replacement. J. Urol. 145 (1991) 538—541.
7. Hedlund, H., K. Lindstorm, W. Mansson: Dynamics of a continent caecal reservoir for urinary diversion. Brit. J. Urol. 56 (1984) 366—372.
8. Kock, N. G.: Intraabdominal reservoir in patients with permanent ileostomy. Arch. Surg. 99 (1969) 223.
9. Koraitim, M., M. Atta, M. Foda: Early and late cystometry of detubularized and non detubular-ized intestinal neobladders: New observations and physiological correlates. J. Urol. 154 (1995) 1700—1703.
10. Lapides, J., E. P. Ajemian, P. E. Stewart et al.: Further observations on the kinetics of the ureter-ovesical sphincters. J. Urol. 84 (1960) 86.
11. Mansson, W., A. Matiasson, T. White: Acute effects of full urinary bladder and full caecal urinary reservoir on regional renal function. Scand. J. Urol. Nephrol. 18 (1984) 299—306.
12. Pagano, F., W. Artibani, P. Ligato et al.: Vescica Ileale Padovana: a technique for total bladder replacement. Eur. Urol. 17 (1990) 149—154.
13. Rattner, W. H., S. Fink, J. J. Murphy: Pressure studies in the human ureter and renal pelvis. J. Urol. 78 (1957) 359.
14. Risholm, L., K. J. Obrink: Pyelorenal backflow in man. Acta Chir. Scand. 115 (1958) 144.
15. Rowland, R. G., M. E. Mitchell, R. Bihrle et al.: Indiana continent urinary reservoir. J. Urol. 137 (1987) 1136—1139.
16. Studer, U. E., D. Ackermann, G. A. Kazanova et al.: Three years of experience with an ileal low pressure bladder substitute. Brit. J. Urol. 63 (1989) 43.

Index